How To

Cure

Diabetes!

Sherry A. Rogers, M.D.

Sand Key Company, Inc.
PO Box 19252
Sarasota FL 34276
2013

How To Cure Diabetes

Sherry A Rogers, M.D.

Sand Key Company, Inc.
PO Box 19252
Sarasota, FL 34276

1-800-846-6687
www.prestigepublishing.com

Library of Congress Control Number: 2012948994

ISBN: 978-1-887202-08-4
Printed in the United States of America

Table of contents

How To Cure Diabetes

Introduction
Is Your Diabetes Doctor a Dinosaur or a Dynamo?

Chapter 1
Dinosaur Diabetes Docs Depend on Drugs

Chapter II
Dinosaur Diabetes Docs Deny Disparity

Chapter III
Dinosaur Diabetes Docs Don't Diagnose Deficiencies

Chapter IV
Dinosaur Diabetes Docs Deny Dysbiosis

Chapter V
Dinosaur Diabetes Docs Don't Deliver Doses for Cure

Chapter VI
Dinosaur Diabetes Docs Don't Detoxify

Chapter VII
Dinosaur Diabetes Docs Dismiss Deity

Dedication

To God's greatest earthly gift to me, Luscious,
who has continued to grow more luscious over 44 blessed years.
He is infinitely more than the unseen, the powerful yet lovingly
gentle
"Wind Beneath My Wings".
He is much more than my hero, my idol, my Superman, ….. my
life.

And after a particularly creative day, when we are both contentedly
tired,
Luscious helps me prepare our libations, for he knows I'm no
longer "wired".
Then with a twinkle in my eye, I tell him "Luscious, you don't
look so fine …..
Even your lips look tired ……. so why not rest yours on mine?"

About the Author

Sherry A. Rogers, M.D., board certified by the American
Board of Family Practice, is board certified by the American
Board of Environmental Medicine, a Fellow of the American
College of Allergy, Asthma and Immunology, and a Fellow
of the American College of Nutrition. She has been in solo
private practice in environmental medicine for over 40 years
in Syracuse, NY where she saw patients from all over the
world. She has lectured at Oxford and in 6 countries where
she has taught well over 100 physician courses, has
published over 16 books including the landmark books
*Detoxify Or Die, The Cholesterol Hoax, The High Blood Pressure
Hoax* and *Is Your Cardiologist Killing You?*
(prestigepublishing.com), over 20 scientific papers, textbook
chapters, was environmental medicine editor for *Internal
Medicine World Report*, received the American Academy of
Environmental Medicine's Dr. Herbert Rinkle, M,D. Award

i

for Teaching Excellence, has a referenced monthly newsletter for over 24 years, a non–patient consulting service, a lay and professional lecture service, is the guest on over 100 radio shows a year, and much more. Her goal is to empower folks with sufficient referenced knowledge to enable them to heal themselves, against all odds.

Introduction

Is Your Diabetes Doc a Dinosaur or a Dynamo?

You've been told there's no cure for diabetes? Wrong! That's because the medical education for us physicians is strongly influenced by the drug industry. We do not learn in medical school how to cure diseases, but rather how to *manage* them with expensive drugs. Have you noticed how every symptom seems to be the deficiency of some drug? And have you noticed that you're told most diseases have "no known cause and no known cure"? Could it have anything to do with the fact that as the *Journal of the American Medical Association* reports **over 87% of the medical "experts" who make the rules for the practice of medicine** (called practice guidelines) **are financially linked to the pharmaceutical industry** (Choudhry)? Further evidence from the *Journal of the American Medical Association* proves the ugly fact that **less than 11% of recommendations made by cardiologists,** as another blatant example, **are based on scientific evidence** (Winslow). And for the remainder? **The rest of the practice of medicine dealing with the top cause of death, serious heart disease, 89% is wrapped around a pharmaceutical focus.**

As Dr. Marcia Angell, a member of Harvard Medical School's Department of Social Medicine and former editor of the *New England Journal of Medicine* for 25 years has written, "Drug companies have enormous influence over what doctors are taught about drugs and what they prescribe." And she details how **drug marketing masquerades as education, since the pharmaceutical industry funds not only medical research and physician continuing education courses, but also hires prestigious medical school department heads as spokespersons and designated "experts".** But just because the largest for-profit industry, pharmaceutical, owns medicine does not mean that every symptom and disease is a drug deficiency. In fact **I'll prove to**

you how drugs not only fail to cure, but make the sick get sicker, quicker.

Best of all, I will show you here a glimpse of some of the thousands of references proving, as we and others have experienced in clinical practice, that **diabetes is curable**. Once you have seen the incontrovertible evidence you will realize how misguided the field of medicine is, but more importantly that **you have the ultimate control over your health**. You find this all too hard to believe? How do you think I felt as a trained medical physician for over 4 decades?

I have been asked by many of our readers to make this shorter and more user-friendly for their friends, for whom this concept of cure is new. Hence, I'll resort to the old **80/20 rule**: 80% of the people will get better using only 20% of what we have to offer. Most folks won't need everything here to cure their diabetes. For infinitely much more detail and the scientific backup for every statement that is not referenced here, you are referred to the books on the back pages and our over 2 decades of referenced newsletter, *Total Wellness* (*TW*). Meanwhile, I have provided you here with enough evidence for any doctor and the discerning person intent on healing.

Meanwhile, folks who know me know that I never leave anyone out when I write a book, regardless of its title. For new readers who have never encountered my works before, you're going to feel *overwhelmed* at times and think that this is all beyond you. But it's not. Health is a process and the more you stick with this and read, and **re-read**, the more it will become a part of you. Besides I owe it to my faithful readers to take them to newer levels of wellness by quantum leaps with each new book. So for whatever level you are entering this journey with, just dig in and enjoy. And realize that my goal is to make you too smart to fail in your health goals. Regardless of how overwhelmed you may feel at certain points, and even if your eyes glaze over, I offer this: If you persevere to the end, your understanding of how to attain the health you want will have taken a quantum leap (and I promise some easy tips).

References:

• Winslow R, Search for better **diabetes therapy falls short. Current treatments,** while effective, **fail to also help prevent heart attacks and stroke,** in blow to researchers, patients, *Wall Street Journal*, A5, Mar. 15, 2010

• Winslow R, **Study questions evidence behind heart therapies**, *Wall Street Journal*, D1, Feb. 25, 2009

• Winstein, KJ, **A simple health-care fix fizzles out**, *WSJ*, 2/11/10, A1, A18

• Choudhry NK, et al, **Relationships between authors of clinical practice guidelines and the pharmaceutical industry**, *Journal of the American Medical Association* 287; 5:612-17, Feb. 6, 2002

• Angell M, *The Truth About The Drug Companies. How They Deceive Us and What To Do About It*, Random House, New York 2004

• Tricoci P, et al, Scientific evidence underlying the ACC/AHA clinical practice guidelines, *Journal of the American Medical Association,* 301:831-41, 2009

• Shaneyfelt TM, et al, Reassessment of clinical practice guidelines. Go softly in that good night, *J Am Med Assoc*, 301:868-9, 2009

• Kjaergard LL, et al, Association between competing interests and author' conclusions: Epidemiological study of randomized clinical trials published in the BMJ, *Brit Med J,* 325-249, 2002

• Als-Nielsen B, et al, Association of funding and conclusions in randomized drug trials, *J Amer Med Assoc*, 290:921-8, 2003

• Burton TM, **Study sites cardiology conflicts**, *Wall Street Journal* A4, March 29, 2011

Who Needs This Book?

Diabetes is merely an example of accelerated aging. For that reason, **this book is essential for anyone who wants to retard aging**. And folks who know me through the other dozen and a half books and couple of decades of newsletters, know that **regardless of the title, I never leave anyone out.** Even though a title focuses on one disease entity, the information contained in it is crucial for the health of all of us, even those who do not have the disease in the title, or any disease, for that matter.

Diabetes is also a perfect example of why one third of the population that doesn't even have diabetes is obese. Once you understand how we get diabetes and then how we cure it, you also will understand **how to get rid of that immovable weight gain**. So anyone who wants to lose weight should read this. In addition to immoveable weight gain, anyone with **Syndrome X (also called Metabolic Syndrome or insulin resistance), with either accompanying high blood pressure, high cholesterol, high triglycerides, or hypoglycemia (low blood sugar that leads to mood swings, headaches, weakness, dizziness), or NASH (non-alcoholic steatohepatitis or fatty liver disease) is potentially pre-diabetic** and needs to read this to prevent and/or cure themselves. And unfortunately, obesity, insulin resistance, and diabetes, formerly seen mainly in adults, are increasing at epidemic rates in children (over one in eight kids in some areas).

Furthermore, **much of what heals the diabetic also reverses other diseases**, from "incurable" Alzheimer's and arthritis to many other "incurables", like macular degeneration to mysterious nerve conditions like motor neuron diseases. For **medicine merely labels diseases "incurable" if there is no drug or surgery for them**. Furthermore, **conventional medicine finds most diseases incurable because it fails to look for the underlying correctable causes that you will learn about** in these pages. The bottom line? **<u>There isn't anyone who could not benefit from this book.</u>**

And I promise you that even though there are times when your eyes may glaze over and you may feel overwhelmed with chemistry, if you persevere through the whole book, you will be rewarded with life-altering tips that you'll never fine elsewhere.

References:

- Rosenbloom AL, et al, Emerging epidemic of type II diabetes in youth, *Diabetes Care* 22:345-54, 1999

- SEARCH for Diabetes in Use Study Group, Liese AD, et al, The burden of diabetes mellitus among U.S. youth: prevalence estimates from SEARCH for Diabetes In Use Study, *Pediatrics* 118:1510-18, 2006

- Hurley D, Child's Plague, *Discover* magazine, 51-5, May 2010

How Can I Claim to Cure Diabetes When I Am Not a Diabetologist?

I'm no smarter than any other doctor, I was just sicker. Having been challenged early with over two dozen "incurable" maladies, I realized all that I learned in medical school (and the decades of training beyond) was useless. It was focused merely on drugs and surgery. But when I was forced to study in more depth about the biochemistry and physiology of the human body, it became obvious that the molecular biochemical design of the human body is nothing short of miraculous.

If we get over a flu bug, heal a laceration or mend a broken ankle, then we also ought to be able to heal colitis, asthma, osteoporosis, rheumatoid arthritis, multiple chemical sensitivities with toxic encephalopathy, super-ventricular tachycardia, amnesia, an egg-sized uterine fibroid, 12 rocky-hard painful breast fibroadenomas, a trapped nerve with a paralyzed leg for six weeks, six back fractures, sciatica, unwarranted depression, ruptured discs, hundreds of allergies, pesticide and mercury poisonings, etc., etc., all of which I personally did, without surgery or drugs. And now at nearly 70 I am healthier than ever in my life, with no major surgery, no implants and no drugs. I play 2 hours of tennis often 5 days a week, and don't even have grey hair yet. But this pales in comparison to what others have done, once they were shown that the body is designed to heal. They have cured such "incurables" as macular degeneration, high blood pressure, Alzheimer's, end-stage cancers with just days to live, and yes...... diabetes.

And that's exactly what I've seen in **over 40 years of practice as a medical physician.** Clearly **the body was designed to heal**. And **I will give you the irrefutable evidence for it here.** I believe it was merely another of God's plans. **As a drug-trained medical doctor, I had to be brought to my knees with over 2 dozen "incurable" maladies in order to become interested enough to ferret out the causes and the cures.** Otherwise, I would probably still be a licensed "pill-pusher". Perhaps this has a bearing on the fact that at my medical school 40th re-union over 15% of my class was already dead. This doesn't speak well for the "experts" in health who were only in their mid-60's. Yet the more encouraging fact is that thanks to the efforts of thousands of researchers across the globe, the answers have been here all along, many of them for decades. But there is a powerful force with obscene financial incentives that has worked hard to keep this information secret.

For those readers whose first reaction to sections on blood pressure, cholesterol, arrhythmias, and heart failure is that they have already been covered in the other books or newsletters, consider these 3 facts. (1) All folks with any of these diseases are at heightened risk of getting diabetes and in fact are called pre-diabetic. (2) Most all diabetics eventually get one or more of these diseases. And (3) by refreshing your knowledge about these, you increase your chances of avoiding both. So don't let repetition annoy you, but rather relish in the fact that it's one more area you have mastered or conquered.

Dinosaurs: As beautifully fascinating as the pre-historic dinosaur era was, these magnificent beasts are no longer with us. They have become extinct for many reasons. In no way do I intend to malign these awesome creatures, but only to playfully make an analogy in the hope that the dinosaur doctors of the present will also become extinct, leaving medicine focused, as it should be, on cure. For the current dinosaur doctors wallow in the past decades of relentless pharmaceutical influence over the practice of medicine.

Consequently, dinosaur doctors see every symptom as a deficiency of the latest drug. And it's very quick, easy and profitable to prescribe a drug and get out the door to the next patient. On the flipside are the doctors who have seen through this ruse and realize the body was designed to heal. They are eager to *teach* you how to heal, and are eager to become *partners* with you in curing whatever disease you have. They are the dynamos of medicine. So now, I humbly invite you to join me while I let the secrets for healing diabetes and its litany of complications be revealed.

Chapter I

Dinosaur Diabetes Docs Depend on Drugs

In my "semi-retirement" I promised to indulge myself in my long time desire to learn how to play "cocktail piano", primarily the incomparably romantic tunes of the 1920-40 jazz eras. I recently flipped open one of my jazz theory books and stumbled onto a paragraph that I must have read at least three times in the past, but frankly in the past I wasn't ready for it. This day I was. And it provided a quantum leap in my understanding of how to arrange a piece from "fake book" chords and begin to play by ear.

My point? Regardless of what you are learning, some parts will be over your head in the beginning. Then suddenly one day you will make quantum leaps as well. So don't give up with just one "read". In over 44 years of being a medical doctor, I've seen that <u>a key to learning is to read and re-read</u>, especially when it concerns something as complex as control over your own health. So just plow through the first time and get what you can. For I guarantee you the second time around you'll learn many new things that you could swear you had never read before. But now the difference will be you have made a quantum leap and are infinitely more knowledgeable and empowered, and ultimately *in control of your health.*

My goal? Only one thing: to make you too smart to fail!

Proof That Diabetes Drugs Don't Work, In Fact They Shorten Your Life

You might stop me right here and say, "Wait a minute! My doctor prescribes drugs for my diabetes and we watch my sugar and hemoglobin A1C (hgb A1C). He says everything is fine." But this is not true, as you will learn. A report in the *Wall Street Journal* came from studies that were unveiled at the American College of Cardiology meeting and published in *the New England Journal of*

1

Medicine (Winslow). What did this expensive research show? The sad fact is that **our great medical system doesn't work for diabetics.**

And surprise, surprise! It shouldn't. **None of the diabetes drugs has anything to do with the cause and cure of diabetes. Drugs merely poison enzyme systems to make the laboratory blood sugar levels look more normal, while they double your risk of dying.** If you find this as difficult to believe as I did, let me quote directly for you from the *PDR (Physician's Desk Reference 2001*, the book in any library that describes prescription drugs). Let's look at Diabinese (tolbutamide), an old diabetes drug used on millions of Americans. It states "patients treated for 5 to 8 years with diet plus a fixed dose of tolbutamide (1.5 g per day) had **a rate of cardiovascular mortality 2 1/2 times that of patients treated with diet alone**." Did you get that? **The leading diabetes drug for decades more than doubled your chance of dying of a heart attack,** while mere diet was twice as good as the drug! Yet millions of diabetics were duped for years with this category of drugs, as just one tiny example. And the deception continues, as you will learn.

As a more modern example, **Metformin, the current most commonly prescribed diabetes drug lowers B12** (over 18 % lower!)**, folic acid, and CoQ10. But these hidden deficiencies in turn lead to insidious memory and vitality loss that are both blamed on aging** (Pelton). And these drug-created deficiencies trigger heart disease, Alzheimer's, cancers and more. Again this is not new as researchers have warned for decades that the depletion of folic acid and B12 raise a blood protein called homocysteine, which in turn promotes many of the serious side effects that diabetes is known for, such as early death (Sahin, Pongchaidecha).

And yet **diabetologists rarely supplement the nutrients that their prescribed medications destroy.** As Harvard researchers showed over 2 decades ago, just a silent insidious B12 deficiency (as from a leading diabetes drug, Metformin) can lead to

2

psychiatric diseases like depression, schizophrenia, memory loss and dementia (Lindenbaum). And what was even worse is that this B12 deficiency may not cause the standard changes in blood tests to make doctors think of checking for it. So brain deterioration, memory loss and even eventual institutionalization are chalked up to "normal" aging.

Consequently, the leading drug for diabetes can bring on the very same symptoms that diabetes does, in spades. Plus these hidden deficiencies raise your homocysteine, a blood factor that increases your likelihood of having accelerated arteriosclerosis; the very thing diabetes does (deJager). But this is why you take the drug, to slow down aging and early death. And in addition to poisoning the liver's ability to make sugar, the drug also has a chemotherapy-like action (meaning it can also foster cancer). In addition it can act like fertilizer for cancers (Giovannucci). No wonder many **cancers occur twice as commonly in diabetics**, while many newer diabetes medications warn of side effects like body swelling, low white blood cell counts, thyroid tumors, fatal pancreatitis, interference with other drugs, and increased cancers (*PDR, MPR,* Giovannucci).

And many drug studies have been way too short to delineate more serious effects that occur with extended years of use. Even insulin use can increase cancers, since nobody has fixed what was broken (Bowker, Barone). As another example of **diabetes drugs' hidden side effects, they cause bone loss, osteoporosis, the need for joint replacements**, and increased falls and fractures (Yaturu). And I haven't even begun to tell you about the price you pay for stifling symptoms through poisoning body pathways instead of repairing them.

And it gets even worse with other drugs. In fact **adding one additional drug to a drug you are currently taking raises your side effects not twice, but twenty-fold** (*TW*). That's right. One plus one does not equal two in terms of potential side effects, but twenty. As another example, as you will learn later, a common

3

drug given to diabetics for high triglycerides increases your risk of pancreatic cancer 33%, while a commonly prescribed cholesterol drug increases your cancer risk a walloping 70%!

When even **the *New England Journal of Medicine* publishes a study proving that 5 years of the standard drugs for diabetics does not change the death rate or even lower the rate of heart attack one iota,** we are in deep trouble. And yet these studies are not all new. Researchers for years have shown that **neither of the top two** categories of **diabetes drugs** appreciably **alters the** rate of **progression of complications** in patients with type 2 diabetes (Kohlstadt, Krentz). Even the Mayo Clinic has reported the most prescribed classification of diabetes drugs like Metformin (the class is called thiazolidinediones) can create heart failure as well as fluid retention in the lungs (Kermani).

One in four Americans over the age of 60 now has diabetes and three quarters of them have high blood pressure and die from cardiovascular diseases. As **26 million Americans have diabetes, they are on a path of accelerated aging that propels them faster toward heart attacks, strokes, amputations, blindness, Alzheimer's, dialysis,** and much more. And *thrice* that staggering number is pre-diabetic. Truly **abnormal sugar metabolism is our planet's largest epidemic**. Yet it doesn't stop with diagnosed diabetes. Twice as many folks are pre-diabetic with metabolic syndrome (also called Syndrome X or insulin resistance) and the most common liver disease NASH (non-alcoholic steatohepatitis), which are related (Marchesini). In fact, **having NASH predicts that the person will develop diabetes** (Musso, Shibata). We are truly a nation of "sickos" and it's just beginning to snowball. The good news is these are all curable.

But un-cured diabetes also brings on painful neuropathy with loss of nerve function or numbness, erectile dysfunction, cataracts and glaucoma. As well it destroys the kidneys leading to renal dialysis, which in turn loads the body with toxic aluminum and plasticizers which then further accelerate all diseases..... a veritable avalanche

4

of diseases.   By attacking blood vessels, un-cured diabetes also leads to gangrene and amputation of toes and legs as well as tooth loss and even cancers. Furthermore, un-cured diabetes leads to cataracts, retinal damage and blindness. The good news is it is all preventable, regardless of how severe your diabetes it.   Why? Because you have not had the care that this book proves you need. Tough it out through this chapter and it will get easier as you go along, plus you will have taken the first step in providing your health with a quantum leap. **Clearly you are going to <u>need to read this book more than once</u>, for your mind is taking a quantum leap into the land of cure that medicine ignores.**

(For your information, here are some Metformin trade names: Fortamet, Glucophage, Glumetza, Riomet.   Plus Avandamet contains Avandia with metformin for double jeopardy, while Janumet contains Metformin plus a newer drug category. There are many more continually being introduced.)

References (evidence from medical journals):

- DeJager J, et al, Long term **treatment with metformin** in patients with type 2 diabetes and **risk of vitamin B12 deficiency**: randomized placebo-controlled trial, *Brit Med J* 340:2181, 2010

- Giovannucci E, et al, **Diabetes and cancer**: a consensus report, *CA Cancer J Clin* 60:207-21, 2010

- Barone BB, et al, Long-term all-cause **mortality in cancer patients with pre-existing diabetes** mellitus: a systemic review and meta-analysis, *J Am Med Assoc*, 300:2754-64, 2008

- Stafylas PC, et al, The controversy of effects of thiazolidinediones on cardiovascular morbidity and mortality, *Int J Cardiol* 131; 3:298-304, 2009

- Bowker SL, et al, **Increased cancer-related mortality in patients with type 2 diabetes** who use sulfonylureas or insulin, *Diabetes Care* 29:254-8, 2006

- *PDR, Physician Desk Reference 2010*, www.pdr.net

- *MPR, Monthly Prescribing Reference*, July 2010, www.eMPR.com

- Pelton R, et al, *Drug-Induced Nutrient Depletion Handbook*, 2nd Ed, 1-877-837-LEXI (5394), 2001

- Sahin M, et al, Effects of **metformin or rosigliatazone** on serum concentrations of **homocysteine, folate, and vitamin B12** in patients with type 2 diabetes mellitus. *J Diabetes Complic* 21; 2:118-23, Mar-Apr 2007

- Pongchaidecha M, et al, Effect of **metformin on plasma homocysteine, vitamin B12 and folic acid**: a cross-sectional study in patients with type 2 diabetes mellitus, *J Med Assoc Thai*, 87; 7:780-87, Jul 2004

- Carlsen SM,et al, **Metformin increases total serum homocysteine** levels in non-diabetic male patients with coronary heart disease, *Scand J Clin Lab Invest* 57; 6:521-7, 1997

- Kohlstadt I, Ed., *Food and Nutrients in Disease Management*, CRC Press, Boca Raton, 2009

- Krentz AJ, et al, Oral antidiabetic agents: current role in type 2 diabetes mellitus, *Drugs* 65; 3:385-411, 2005

- Lindenbaum J., et al., **Neuropsychiatric disorders caused by cobolamin deficiency in the absence of anemia** or macrocytosis, *New Engl J Med* 318:1720-28, 1988

- Marchesini G, et al, **Association of nonalcoholic fatty liver disease with insulin resistance,** *Am J Med*, 107:450-5, 1999

- Musso G, et al, Lipoprotein metabolism mediates the association of MTP polymorphism with beta cell dysfunction in healthy subjects and in nondiabetic normolipidemic patients with nonalcoholic steatohepatitis, *J Nutr Biochem* 21:834-40, 2010

- Shibata M. et al, **Nonalcoholic fatty liver disease is a risk factor for type II diabetes** in middle-aged Japanese men, *Diabetes Care* 30:2940-4, 2007

- Anonymous, **CDC raised the estimate of Americans with diabetes to nearly 26 million**, *Wall Street Journal*, Jan. 27, 2011, A1

- Gerstein HC, et al, Action to control cardiovascular risk in diabetes study group. Effects of intensive glucose lowering in type II diabetes, *New Engl J Med* 358; 24:2545-59, 2008 (ACCORD study, more later on this)

- Kermani A, et al, Thiazolidinedione-associated congestive heart failure and pulmonary edema, *Mayo Clinic Proceedings* 78:1088-91, 2003

What About the Newer Diabetes Drugs?

As an example, the **two leading diabetes drugs, Avandia (rosiglitazone) and Actos (pioglitazone) are associated with an increased risk of heart problems, including heart failure (which is usually fatal in five years**). If that weren't enough, these **two leading diabetes drugs increase the risk of bone fractures by 43%** (their category of diabetes drugs is called thiazolidinediones in the references). And the loss of bone strength occurred very quickly, within six months. And this has been known for over six years without the FDA doing anything about it, except periodic reports in the *Wall Street Journal* that they are looking into it. History shows the FDA procrastinates until a drug patent nears expiration while the company reaps literally billions a year. In 2010 they merely restricted the use of Avandia®

to new patients only if they are unable to take any other medications including Actos®, which is in the same chemical category (Anonymous *MPR).*

Furthermore, the *Wall Street Journal* was full of articles in 2010 on how this one popular diabetes medication, **Avandia®, doubles the heart attack rate and raises the bad cholesterol LDL, increases the chance of heart failure and made folks anemic** (Nissen). In fact even these authors who write about nothing to cure diabetes pointed out that **it is wrong to treat laboratory numbers as opposed to looking at the actual resulting deaths and heart attacks**. And it should come as no surprise that Avandia (rosiglitazone) doesn't cure diabetes since it poisons over a dozen genes. And this is a survey of 42 studies not just one, plus analysis of data by the study's author shows that this study even underestimates the damage done by drugs.

In fact, the author states in the *Journal of the American Medical Association* that even the manufacturer of Avandia knew the heart attack rate was 30-43% higher using their drug (Nissen). Meanwhile, even top FDA drug safety scientists' warnings have been ignored for years, in spite of studies showing **a minimum 13-17% increase in death and an even higher percentage of heart failure from the two leading diabetes drugs on the market** (Whalen). Also, this medication category can trigger heart failure, pulmonary edema (fluid retention in lungs), and more (Thomas, Hirsch, Tang). And this is the best medicine has to offer!(?)!

If that were not enough, this class of **diabetes drugs increases the chance of cancer** (Rubenstrunk), as can other categories of diabetes medications like sulfonylurea's (like Diabinese), insulin and newer long-acting insulin analogues (Bowker, Currie, Hemkens). In fact it looks like the further you get away from real insulin and into more fabricated drug forms, the more they can increase cancer risk (Giovannucci).

References:

- Winstein KJ, Diabetes study questions expensive treatments. **NIH finds patients** with heart disease **fared equally well without** stents and **drugs such as Avandia, Actos**, *Wall Street J*, B1, June 8, 2009

- Nissen SE, Setting the RECORD straight, *J Am Med Assoc,* 1194-5 Mar 24, 2010

- Nissen SE, et al, **Effect of rosiglitazone on the risk of myocardial infarction and death** from cardiovascular causes, *New Engl J Med* 356; 24:2457-71, June 14, 2007

- Sahin M, et al, Effects of **metformin or rosigliatazone** on serum concentrations of **homocysteine, folate, and vitamin B12** in patients with type 2 diabetes mellitus. *J Diabetes Complic* 21; 2:118-23, Mar-Apr 2007

- Yaturu S, et al, **Thiazolidinedione treatment decreases bone mineral density** in type 2 diabetic men, *Diabetes Care* 30:1574-76, 2007

- Mundy A, Favole JA, **Study ties drugs to fractures**, *Wall Street J*, B2, June 8, 2009

- Ali AA, et al, **Rosiglitazone causes bone loss** in mice by suppressing osteoblast differentiation and bone formation, *Endocrinol* 146:1226-35, 2005

- Stafylas PC, et al, The controversy of effects of thiazolidinediones on cardiovascular morbidity and mortality, *Int J Cardiol* 131; 3:298-304, 2009

- Chaggar PS, et al, Review article: Thiazolinediones and heart failure, *Diab Vasc Dis Res* 6; 3:146-52, 2009

- Whalen J, et al, **FDA scientist attacks Avandia safety**, *Wall Street Journal,* B4, June 11, 2010

- Anonymous, Avandia access restricted, *MPR, Monthly Prescribing Reference* (www.eMPR.com) page A10, Nov. 2010

- Giovannucci E., et al., **Diabetes and cancer**: a consensus report, *CA Cancer J Clin* 60: 207-21, 2010

- Hemkens LG, et al, **Risk of malignancies in patients with diabetes treated with human insulin** or insulin analogues: a cohort study, *Diabetologia* 52:1 732-44, 2009

- Currie CJ, et al, The **influence of glucose lowering therapies and cancer risk in type II diabetes**, *Diabetologia*, 52:1766-77, 2009

- Bowker SL, et al., **Increased cancer-related mortality for patients with type II diabetes who use sulfonylurea's or insulin,** *Diabetes Care* 29:254-8, 2006

- Rubenstrunk A, et al, Safety issues and prospects for future generations of PPAR modulators, *Biochim Biophys Acta* 1771:1065-81, 2007

- The Associated Press, Study of **diabetes drug draws criticism**, *The Portland Press Herald*, A4, July 10, 2010

- Rockoff JD, Regulators scould drug for diabetes, *Wall Street Journal*, A1, September 24, 2010

- Anonymous, FDA reviews safety data on diabetes drug Actos, *Wall St J*, B8, Sept. 20, 2010

- Thomas ML, et al, Pulmonary edema associated with rosiglitazone and troglitazone, *Ann Pharmacother,* 35:1 to 3-4, 2001

- Hirsch IB, et al, Pulmonary edema associated with troglitazone therapy, *Arch Intern Med* 159:1118, 1999

- Tang WH, et al, Fluid retention after initiation of troglitazone therapy in diabetic patients with established chronic heart failure, *J Am Coll Cardiol* 41:1394-8, 2003

"My Doctor Says I Need Drugs to Lower My Hgb A1C"

An elevated hemoglobin A1C also called glycated hemoglobin (or also glycosylated hemoglobin A1C or hgb A1C) is a serious indicator of accelerated deterioration of body cells due to persistently high sugars. It is a blood test that shows if your sugar level has been out of control over the last 120 days. It is so sensitive an indicator that **a 1% rise in hemoglobin A1C increases the chance of going blind from diabetic retinopathy 37%,** and **increases your chance of a heart attack 18%** (Action to Control Cardiovascular Risk in Diabetes Study Group). But this **study showed that intensive <u>lowering of the hemoglobin A1C</u> to less than 6** (the top limit of normal for most labs) **with all medications available actually <u>increased the relative death rate 22%</u>.** Why? *Because the drugs don't repair your body chemistry, they just lower a laboratory number.* You look great on paper while you silently and mysteriously deteriorate.

Furthermore, in this study after taking common diabetes drugs to improve the hemoglobin A1C, researchers found that **after 3 1/2 years on diabetes drugs, the death rate was higher for folks who took the drugs than for folks who did not take them,** and the drug-takers gained about 10 pounds, while those not taking them did not. And why don't drugs work? Because they don't find and fix the underlying cause. They do not fix what's broken.

So how does nature lower or repair the elevated Hgb A1C? In many ways, depending on what the individual person is deficient in. For example, **a marked reduction in hemoglobin A1C occurs with** many nutrients (which you will learn about in much more detail), alone or in combination, depending on the damage the individual has. Not only **ALC (Acetyl L-Carnitine), but R-Lipoic Acid, P5P (Pyridoxal-5-Phosphate), Magnesium** and much more can protect proteins from being "fried" (glycosylated or destroyed). And most of these nutrients (and you will learn more about them plus their doses and sources) are low in most diabetics (Bonnefont, Sales).

No wonder drugs don't work! If for example, the person was deficient in magnesium and that caused the elevated hgb A1C along with loss of diabetic control, then no wonder adding a drug that does not add magnesium (but in fact depletes it faster) leads to a higher death rate in folks taking the drug compared with folks not taking it. Now you are beginning to understand why **the death rate is higher if you take a drug than not. With drugs the sick get sicker, quicker.** They use up nutrients that are needed to heal.

Yet when you use nutrients to actually correct what was needed, you fix what's broken and may also cure the person. And with nutrients you get an additional bargain, secondary beneficial side effects. For example, **when you correct a hidden magnesium deficiency it may not only improve the glycosylated hemoglobin**, it may also lower blood pressure, cholesterol, raise HDL (the good cholesterol) (Song), **protect against sudden cardiac arrest**, control depression, migraines, angina, arrhythmias, bowel spasm, back spasm, muscle pain, and much more. And an even more important fact for you to memorize is that *the average person gets only about a third of the magnesium he needs in a day.* So most folks are low already. So the poor **diabetic whose specialist is not checking his RBC magnesium is doomed for earlier sudden cardiac death....while his blood hgb A1C test looks deceivingly good.** Herein lies *one of the best kept secrets and dangerous facts about "modern" medicine; the treatment is considered a success (by self-imposed laboratory standards) even though the patient dies prematurely (of preventable and curable causes!).*

On the flip side, consider that when you **use acetyl L-carnitine (ALC) to lower sugars and reduce damaged proteins (hgb A1C),** once again as with all nutrients, you get many additional good side effects. **ALC** benefits include **lowering the dangerous lipoprotein(a)** (Derosa), reducing the **bad oxidized LDL cholesterol** (Malaguarnera), **improves walking distance** and **reduces pain from clogged leg arteries (claudication)** (Santo), makes new brain, etc. And combined with other nutrients **ALC improves erectile dysfunction and even regenerates nerves** (Gentile, Sima). Wow! Who could ask for anything more? Are you beginning to appreciate the power of fixing what's broken? So why is cure not standard in "modern" medicine? Just refer back to the facts in the introduction. Now you are starting to understand a wee bit about why I was so compelled to take years out of my life to give you this information. And these are only 2 nutrients.

References:

- Action to Control Cardiovascular Risk in Diabetes Study Group, Effects of intensive glucose lowering in type 2 diabetes, *New Engl J Med* 358; 24:2545-59, 2008

- Higuchi O, et al, Amino phospholipid **glycation** and its inhibitor screening system: a new role of **pyridoxal 5'-phosphate as the inhibitor**, *J Lipid Res*, 47:964-74, 2006

- Rhabar AR, et al, Effect of L-**carnitine on plasma glycemic** and lipidemia profile in patients with type II diabetes mellitus, *Eur J Clin Nutr* 59; 4:592-6, 2005

- Derosa G, et al, The affect of L-carnitine on plasma lipoprotein (a) levels in hypercholesterolemic patients with type II diabetes mellitus, *Clin Ther* 25; 5:1429-39, May 2003

- Malaguarnera M, et al, L-**carnitine supplementation reduces oxidized LDL** cholesterol in patients with diabetes, *Am J Clin Nutr* 89; 1:71-6, 2009

- Santo SS, et al, Effect the PLC on functional parameters and oxidative profile in type II diabetes-associated PAD, *Diab Res Clin Pract* 72; 3:231-7, 2006

- Gentile V, et al, Effect of propionyl-L-carnitine, L-arginine, and nicotinic acid on the efficacy of vardenafil in the treatment of **erectile dysfunction in diabetes**, *Curr Med Res Opin* 25; 9:2223-8, 2009

- Sima AA, et al, **Acetyl-L-carnitine improves pain, nerve regeneration** and vibratory perception in patients with chronic **diabetic neuropathy**: an analysis of two randomized placebo-controlled trials, *Diabetes Care* 28; 1:89-94, 2005

- Sales CH, et al, Magnesium and diabetes mellitus: their relation, *Clin Nutr* 25; 4:554-62, 2006

- Bonnefont-Rousselot D, et al, The role of **antioxidant micronutrients in the prevention of diabetic complications**, *Treat Endocrin*, 3; 1:41-52, 2004

- Rodriguez-Moran M, et al, **Oral magnesium supplementation improves insulin sensitivity and metabolic control in type 2 diabetes** subjects: a randomized double-blind controlled trial, *Diabetes Care* 26; 4:1147-52, April 2003

- Song Y, et al, Effects of oral **magnesium supplementation on glycemic control** in type 2 diabetes: a meta-analysis of randomized double-blind controlled trials, *Diab Med* 23; 10:1050-56, Oct 2006

- Bierhaus A, et al, Advanced glycation-induced activation of NF-kappa B is suppressed by a-lipoic acid in cultured endothelial cells, *Diabetes* 46; 9:1481-90, Sept 1997

- Ruggenenti P, et al, Ameliorating hypertension and insulin resistance in subjects at increased cardiovascular risk: effects of acetyl-L-carnitine therapy, *Hypertension* 54; 3:567-74, 2009

"My Doctor Says I Need Drugs to Lower My Triglycerides"

Wrong and doubly dangerous! Would you lower your triglycerides with a drug that gives you a chance of getting cancer of the pancreas? Let's, as an example, take a look at one of the newer drugs for triglycerides, Trilipix®. What doctor would think that lowering your triglycerides is a rational trade-off for not **only increasing your risk of cancer, but your chances of lung clots (pulmonary embolus), pancreatitis, or the need for gallbladder surgery**? More importantly it has a **heart attack rate of 11%**, the same as placebo (taking nothing). So how does it protect you? To quote from page 550 of the *2010 PDR*, "There was a.... 19% increase in ... coronary heart disease mortality.... with fenfibrate (Trilipix) as compared to placebo".

The *PDR* also says Trilipix is **a cousin to the first drug of this category** (fibrates), **clofibrate (Atromid S), known for decades for its strong cancer-inducing qualities.** I again quote from page 550 of the *2010 PDR* "In a study conducted by the World Health Organization, 5000 subjects without coronary artery disease were treated with placebo or clofibrate for five years and followed for an additional one year. There was a statistically significant higher age-adjusted all course of mortality in the clofibrate group compared with the placebo group. **Excess mortality was due to a 33% increase in non-cardiovascular causes including malignancy,** post cholecystectomy complications and pancreatitis. **This confirmed the higher risk of gallbladder disease seen in clofibrate-treated patients** studied in the Coronary Drug Project."

12

This is right out of the book which describes prescription drugs for all doctors!

I say "Nix on Trilipix". On the flipside many nutrients, as you are beginning to learn, work in harmony in the body to lower triglycerides naturally. For example, eicosapentaenoic acid or EPA (the main fatty acid in **Cod Liver Oil**) lowers triglycerides (Minami), while l-carnitine as in ALC (**Acetyl L-Carnitine) lowered triglycerides 25-39% in just 10 days** (Abdel-Aziz). Meanwhile, multiple other studies show that **lowering triglycerides with drugs does not lower the death rate** (Winslow, Winstein, *PDR*, page 550).

References:

- Winslow R, Search for better **diabetes therapy falls short. Current treatments,** while effective, **fail to also help prevent heart attacks and stroke,** in blow to researchers, patients, *Wall Street Journal*, A5, March 15, 2010

- Winslow R, **Study questions evidence behind heart therapies**, *Wall Street Journal*, D1, Feb. 25, 2009

- Winstein, KJ, **A simple health-care fix fizzles out**, *WSJ*, 2/11/10, A1, A18

- *PDR or Physicians Desk Reference, 64th edition, 2010*, www.PDR.net

- Minsami A, et al, Effect of eicosapentaenoic acid ethyl ester v. oleic acid-rich safflower oil on insulin resistance and type II diabetic model rats with hyper triglyceridemia, *Brit J Nutr* 82; 2:157-62, 2002

- Abdel-Aziz MT, et al, Effective carnitine on blood lipid pattern in diabetic patients, *Nutr Rep Int* 29:1070-79, 1984

"I Need Medication for My High Blood Pressure"

If you take HCT or hydrochlorthiazide, a common diuretic (fluid pill) then you lower magnesium. This makes not only diabetes worse but the blood pressure (recall the references you just read that prove magnesium is crucial for diabetic control). And recall **most folks get less than a third of the magnesium they need in a day**. If your doc doesn't check the right magnesium (erythrocyte or RBC or intracellular versus **the wrong one, serum magnesium**) then he won't even know your undiagnosed magnesium deficiency is setting you up for a sudden cardiac arrest and instant death (yes, even if you don't have diabetes). You must see your lab result. If it just says "magnesium", he ordered the dangerously wrong one as you will learn.

The next drug for the treatment of high blood pressure is often the category of **calcium channel blockers** which includes such names like Norvasc, Amlodipine, Lotrel, Adalat, Procardia, Calan, Cardizem, Dilacor, Cardene, Verapamil, and many other disguises. These actually **are used to create diabetes in experimental animals!!** (Vilches-Flores). These are not just prescribed for high blood pressure but also prescribed for angina, heart failure, and after a heart attack or stents. I'll be telling you more later.

Meanwhile, calcium channel blockers make diabetes worse by inhibiting insulin secretion and turning down the action of genes that properly regulate sugar metabolism. And if you think that is all the harm they do, guess again. **They also literally shrink the brain.** Within less than five years of use of calcium channel blockers, MRI x-rays show that the brain has shrunk away from the skull. Furthermore, testing of the I.Q. shows that the intellect has also taken a dramatic nosedive. But not to worry, all this brain loss is chalked up to "normal aging". Of course as you will learn, many nutrients totally repair the calcium channels such as the correction of nutrient deficiencies of fatty acids, zinc, selenium, vitamin D, phosphatidyl choline, and many others.

Do you think those are the only problems with this medication category? No. **Calcium channel blockers also poison a crucial vitamin for diabetes control called biotin** which you'll learn more about in the next chapters (Vilches-Flores). **Biotin is needed to make insulin and regulate diabetes.** Calcium channel blockers also increase your risk of cancer and much more (to save space here, the evidence from scientific references for these facts are in *The High Blood Pressure Hoax*, prestigepublishing.com or 1-800-846-6687). In fact one of the simple remedies for normalizing the blood pressure of many folks described in there is merely arginine. Why?

Because **arginine** can not only **lower the blood pressure** but can **rev up or boost the peroxisomes**, which is exactly how diabetes medications like Avandia and Actos work. But as opposed to the drugs, the natural amino acid arginine not only does not create obesity (as the drugs do), but it elevates insulin, decreases fat, heals blood vessels, and improves metabolism thereby promoting normal weight (Tan). And of course many fatty acids that you will learn about such as DHA (a component of cod liver oil) can repair high blood pressure as well as a fast heart rate and more (Mori).

I could go on with the multitude of benefits of other nutrients versus categories of blood pressure medications loaded with side effects, but you get the gist. Studies show that blood pressure medications whether beta blockers (like atenolol, metaprolol, etc.), diuretics (like HCTZ), or ACE inhibitors (like Lisinopril, enalapril) can make diabetes worse, and at the very best do not prevent diabetes or death or improve insulin resistance or beta cell function (Taylor, The DREAM Trial Investigators, Nathan). **If you have high blood pressure, get rid of it once and for all by curing it.** If you choose to drug it for the rest of your life, you guarantee going on to other diseases while you accelerate your diabetes.

References:

- Tan B, et al, Dietary **L-arginine** supplementation differentially **regulates** expression of **lipid** metabolic **genes in** porcine adipose tissue and skeletal muscle, *J Nutr Biochem* 22:441-45, 2011

- Mori TA, et al, **Docosahexaenoic** acid but not eicosapentaenoic acid **lowers** ambulatory **blood pressure and heart rate** in humans, *Hypertension* 34:253-60, 1999

- Vilches-Flores A, et al, Biotin increases glucokinase expression via soluble guanylate cyclase/protein kinase G, adenosine triphosphate production and autocrine action of insulin in pancreatic rat islets, *J Nutr Biochem* 21:606-12, 2010).

- Taylor E, et al, Antihypertensive medications and the risk of incident type II diabetes, *Diabetes Care* 29:1065-70, 2006

- Nathan DM, Navigating the choices for diabetes prevention, editorial, *New Engl J Med,* 362; 16: 1533-5, 2010

- The DREAM Trial Investigators. Effect of ramipril on the incidence of diabetes, *New Engl J Med*, 355:1551-62, 2006

"I Need Medications for My High Cholesterol"

Wrong again! The **cholesterol statin medications cause serious brain deterioration leading to sudden amnesia which is most often misdiagnosed as a TIA or transient ischemic attack, also called a mini-stroke**. If you continue on the medications even if you don't have episodes of amnesia, statins can lead to full-blown Alzheimer's in years to come. Plus, as shown even in the *Journal of the American Medical Association* over a decade ago, **statins lead to cancers**. And if you don't get cancer, statins can lead to many other diseases and problems because they lower vitamin E, selenium, carnitine, detoxification sulfation, CoQ10, and many other nutrients. Just lowering CoQ10, as one tiny example, can bring on any disease from heart failure, high blood pressure, angina, exhaustion, and tooth loss to depression, and even cancers. Plus as the CoQ10 goes lower it increases your chance of dying of fatal muscle pain and damage, rhabdomyolysis, the scariest immediate symptom of statin use.

There are dozens of examples that statins lower vitamin E that is necessary to prevent Alzheimer's (Yatin). And drugs accelerate aging and decay of mitochondrial which are two things that can trigger diabetes or become the complications of diabetes and accelerate aging (Sugiyama). In fact you will learn later of the studies that show for example, **cod liver oil reduces death rate 23% in folks with high cholesterol, whereas the statins only reduce it 13%,** plus bring on a litany of side effects (Studer).

But the damage of **statins** does not end there. They also **damage the mitochondria** which are little organelles inside every cell **where energy is made**. Their deterioration determines whether or not you get any and every disease including premature aging, cancers and of course, even diabetes (Lowell, Wallace). To quote "all members of the two most popular classes of lipid lowering drugs (the fibrates and the **statins**) **cause cancer** in rodents, in some cases **at levels** of animal exposure **prescribed to humans**." Furthermore, the authors conclude HMG CoA reductase inhibitors or **statins and fibrates should *just* be used short-term** (Newman). Why **they even raise your risk of bone fractures** (Maier, Wang, Chan).

Obviously you're better off reading *The Cholesterol Hoax* (prestigepublishing.com or 1-800-846-6687) and getting rid of your high cholesterol, LDL, triglycerides, lipoprotein(a) and other cardiovascular risk factors of hyper-lipidemia. Meanwhile, a common cholesterol-lowering drug, Vytorin® (which is a combination of Zocor and Zetia) increases the cancer risk 70%. By the way, **statins also increase diabetes** (Sattar). And recall arginine was needed to heal high blood pressure. Well it is also needed to stop abnormal clotting, which is the focal worry of folks with high cholesterol. But it also needs the right combination of fatty acids, magnesium, and anti-oxidants, depending on the individual (Wolf). Arginine also is crucial to heal the inside of blood vessels, and diabetes is essentially a disease of blood vessels.

On one of the radio shows where I was a guest I met a unique man who was not only a medical doctor specialized in internal medicine, but a pilot, a NASA researcher, and an astronaut! Talk about credentials and accomplishments! On his way home from a walk one morning he had a sudden attack of amnesia for the first time in his life. He didn't know he was a doctor, didn't know his home, didn't know his wife of 40 years.

When he cleared in a few days, he figured out it was caused by Lipitor, prescribed by the flight physician to prevent heart disease, even though he did not even have high cholesterol. When his medical colleagues refused to believe his thoughts about the cause, he investigated and found thousands of folks similarly affected, researched the biochemical evidence, and wrote *Lipitor, Thief of Memory* plus *Statin Side Effects and the Misguided War on Cholesterol*. Meanwhile did you ever stop to wonder in how many bizarre accidents were cholesterol-lowering drugs involved? We don't know because it is rarely reported what drugs the pilot, air traffic controller, surgeon, toxic tanker driver, subway engineer, bus driver, or nuclear reactor technician was taking.

References:

- Wolf A, et al, Dietary L-**arginine supplementation normalizes platelet aggregation** in hypercholesterolemic humans, *J Am Coll Cardiol* 29:479-85, 1997

- Lowell BB, et al., Mitochondrial dysfunction and type II diabetes, *Sci* 307:384-7, 2005

- Wallace DC, A mitochondrial paradigm of metabolic and degenerative diseases, aging, and cancer: a dawn for evolutionary medicine, *Ann Rev Genet* 39:359-407, 2005

- Newman TB, **Carcinogenicity of lipid lowering drugs**, *J Am Med Assoc* 275; 1:55-60, 1996

- Sattar N, et al, **Statins and risk of incident diabetes**: a collaborative meta-analysis of randomized statin trials, *Lancet* 375; 9716:735-42, Febr. 27, 2010

- Meier CR, et al, **HMGCoA reductase inhibitors and the risk of fractures**, *J Am Med Assoc* 283:3205-10, 2000

- Wang PS, at all, HMGCoA reductase inhibitors and the risk of hip fractures in elderly patients, *J Am Med Assoc* 283:3211-16, 2000

- Chan AK, et al, Inhibitors of hydroxymethylglutarylcoenzyme A reductase and the risk of fractures among older women, *Lancet* 355:2185-88, 2000

- Studer B, et al, Effect of different anti-lipidemic agents and diets on mortality, *Arch Intern Med* 165:725-30, 2005

- Sugiyama S, **HMGCoA reductase inhibitor accelerates aging** effect and diaphragmatic mitochondrial respiratory function in rats, *Biochem Molec Biol Internat* 46:923-31, 1998

- Yatin SM, et al, Vitamin **E prevents amyloid** beta-peptide (1-42)-induced neuronal protein oxidation and reactive oxygen species, *J Alzheim Dis* 2; 2:1 to 3-31, 2000

"I Have to Take a Medication to Raise My Good Cholesterol, the HDL"

HDL, the "good" cholesterol, acts like a wheelbarrow carrying unwanted cholesterol and plaque away from arteries. HDL (high density lipoprotein) also is **a major detoxifier and protects against unwanted clots**. Over a dozen different nutrients can raise your levels of HDL (like gamma tocopherol, niacin, carnitine, taurine, DHA, tocotrienols, magnesium, phosphatidylcholine, vitamins D and C, and more).

And don't think that just diabetics have to raise their HDL. Everyone needs to. It has been proven for decades that **having a**

high HDL is more important than lowering the bad cholesterol or LDL. The only reason you didn't hear much about it was because there wasn't a drug in the earlier years for the HDL. But since there was one for cholesterol the focus was shifted to cholesterol, even though unoxidized cholesterol (cholesterol that is protected from destruction by antioxidants) is not a cause of cardiovascular disease or death.

Having a normal HDL, however, is a cause of early heart attacks. "What?!", you say. You see, many people have died from heart attacks that had normal cholesterol levels and a *normal* HDL. The problem was that the definition their doctors used for "normal HDL" was not in the "optimal" range, and there's a big difference between the two. The "normal" level of HDL for many labs begins around 30 ng/dL. So if your doctor is not reading *TW* (*Total Wellness* monthly referenced newsletter) he falls for this and he will tell you you're fine. That's not true. The good **protective level of HDL has to be above 60 ng/dl,** as I have referenced in *TW* (I can't make his education any cheaper than a dollar a week!). Remember many people are dead because they had no risk factors, but only had a "normal" (but not optimal) HDL around 30-40.

But it turns out there's more to the story than we realized. **Folks with diabetes have an HDL that doesn't work properly.** You might say *the diabetic's wheelbarrow* (remember HDL is like a wheelbarrow carrying oxidized cholesterol off the vessel wall) *is broken* or missing a wheel. Because the diabetic's wheelbarrow doesn't work properly, this then leads him to have earlier heart attacks. Fortunately, a recent study in *Circulation* (the American Heart Association's medical journal) has shown that niacin, as in the best form, **Niacin-Time, not only increases HDL, but it brings it back to normal function, even in diabetics**. This is extremely important because it means that **all diabetics should be on Niacin-Time twice daily.** What a simple and inexpensive solution! And yet I wonder how many diabetics will actually be recommended this. Instead they'll be placed on a prescription niacin med which has been proven to not be as effective as Niacin-Time, as well as causing B12 and zinc deficiencies, and more.

Furthermore, niacin has many other benefits. For example, it cut lipid peroxidation (a major indicator and cause of early aging) by 75%. Lipid peroxidation means free radicals from the thousands of unavoidable chemicals in our daily environments are burning holes in cell membranes (oxidizing them), causing the cells of organs to prematurely die. Lipid peroxidation actually makes cells spill their guts and die sooner, as well as develop abnormal function along the way, which doctors label as disease. Of course, all of this is measurable in a blood test you will learn about. The bottom line is **Niacin-Time actually repairs the HDL as well as raises the level of HDL.   That means we all need it**, diabetes or not. And tar and feather the diabetologist who doesn't recommend it! As well, it improves blood flow, **decreases the chance of unwanted clots and heals the inside of blood vessels**.

So if your wheelbarrow (to carry the bad cholesterol off your arteries) has lost its wheels, don't worry. A little **Niacin-Time** can fix your HDL, and it has been proven to also slow down the progression of coronary artery disease in anyone. Please don't be foolish enough to take **statins (cholesterol-lowering medications).** As you recall they **literally rot the brain as well as deplete many nutrients propelling you toward other diseases** in addition to brain loss. You deserve better. If Niacin-Time isn't enough for your particular total load then refer back to the protocols in *The High Blood Pressure Hoax* followed by *The Cholesterol Hoax* (even if you don't have the diseases in the titles). Remember we're focusing in this book on diabetes, since we have covered the associated problems like high blood pressure and cholesterol previously. Meanwhile, we certainly are all lucky to have the knowledge to fix what's broken. And let me remind you first time readers: You are doing a fantastic job. For this is written at a higher level for my faithful long-time readers. So let's continue to soar.

References:

- Rogers SA, *Total Wellness*, July 2010, prestigepublishing.com, 1-800-846-6687

- Parker J, et al, Levels of vitamin D and cardiometabolic disorders: systemic review and meta-analysis, *Maturitas*, 225-36, 2010

- Ashen MD, et al, Clinical practice: low HDL cholesterol levels, *N Engl J Med* 353:1 252-60, 2005

- Miller NE, et al, The Tromso Heart Study: high density lipoprotein and coronary heart disease: a prospective case-control study, *Lancet* 309:965-68, 1977

- Barger P, et al, HDL cholesterol, very low levels of LDL cholesterol, and cardiovascular events, *N Engl J Med* , 357:1301-10, 2007

- Sorrentino SA, et al, Endothelial-vasoprotective effects of **high-density lipoprotein are impaired in patients with type 2 diabetes mellitus but are improved after extended release niacin therapy,** *Circulation*, 121:110-22, 2010

- Lombardo YB, et al, Effects of dietary polyunsaturated **n-3 fatty acids** on dyslipidemia and **insulin resistance** in rodents and humans, A review, *J Nutr Biochem,* 17:1-13, 2006

"Well, I Have to Take a Drug for My Arrhythmia"

If you have arrhythmia (irregular heartbeat) you're in even worse shape. For one arrhythmia drug (amiodarone) the *PDR* tells doctors they had better make sure the patient is prepared to die, because this drug greatly increases the probability of death. Yet many arrhythmias can be absolutely totally cured with pennies of nutrients. However, when I reviewed the records of readers consulting with me on the phone who have been to the most prestigious cardiology clinics over the globe, never have I seen them checked for any of the curable causes. But what I did observe was that the bigger the clinic, the more different types of specialists the patient was referred to. Yet still no one looked for the curable causes that you'll learn about here.

Meanwhile, once you have an arrhythmia like atrial fibrillation, as an example, folks are usually put on Coumadin (Warfarin), a blood thinner, to prevent clots. Did you know that Coumadin pulls calcium out of bone and dumps it into the heart vessels and valves? So it nearly guarantees that you will eventually need a heart valve replacement or have a heart attack plus osteoporosis, if you live that long! Yet as shown in *The Cholesterol Hoax*, vitamin E's eight

21

parts (as in 2 **E Gems Elite**, 1 **Gamma E Gems**, and 2 **Tocotrienols**) are just a few of the nutrients that protect against hypercoagulability (increased clots), and far better and more safely. Plus if you insist on Coumadin, folks should at least be on 4000 IU of vitamin D3 (**Solar D Gems**) and 1- 5 mg of vitamin K2 (**Vitamin K2**) and adjust the prothrombin times accordingly. For these are part of the nutrients needed to rip calcium off the arterial wall and put it back in the bone where it belongs. Whereas coumadin does the opposite. It rips calcium off the bones and dumps it into coronary arteries and valves, leading to heart surgery. Coumadin also poisons vitamin K, which you need for cancer prevention as well as healthful longevity (McCann).

And if you are contemplating ablation for arrhythmias, please learn more! Even the *Journal of the American College of Cardiology* showed inexpensive **Arginine Powder** can normalize excessive clotting (references page 118, *Is Your Cardiologist Killing You?*). Ablation is a procedure where a cardiologist slips a catheter into your vessels and up into the heart, watching it through x-ray guidance. When he thinks he's in the electrical spot that your arrhythmia is originating from, he turns on the "juice" and literally electrocutes that part of the heart and its nerves, destroying them forever. This is in spite of the fact that pennies of nutrients often cure the arrhythmias. Yet I have never seen a cardiology report where the patient had had the blood tests to look for the curable causes before they had the permanent destruction of ablation.

I have even consulted on cases where ablation was recommended for young folks in their 30s and even children as young as 10. This is utterly disgusting, because the records showed no "specialist" looked for the curable causes. Fortunately, the parents were wiser than the cardiologists, because they read, got the tests, and we found that pennies of minerals and fatty acids cured their children of years of "intractable arrhythmias". More on this later.

Oh, and by the way, do you want to know the worst part? Even though ablation has been done for over a decade, **ablation is not**

FDA approved for arrhythmias (references in *Total Wellness* 2010). These physicians are arrogantly out of control. And the sad part is if you question them about any of the science, they are utterly clueless about the causes and cures of the very diseases that they treat every day as leading "specialists". If you need further details on how to find the causes and cures of arrhythmias plus how to get off Coumadin, start with *Is Your Cardiologist Killing You?* (prestigepublishing.com or 1-800-846-6687) and subsequent *TW's*. Remember, heart disease is the number one cause of death in folks with or without diabetes.

References:

- Rogers SA, *Total Wellness 2010*, prestigepublishing.com, 1-800-846-6687

- Price EA, et al, **Warfarin causes rapid calcification** of the elastic lamellae in rat **arteries and heart valves**, *Arterioscler Thromb Vasc Biol* 18:1400-07, 1998

- Singer-Vine J, The Research Report/New Medical Findings, *Wall Street J*, B8, June 2, 2009

- Schurgers LJ, et al, **Regression of warfarin induced medial elastocalcinosis by high intake of vitamin K** in rats, *Blood* 109:2823-31, 2007

- Gast GCM, et al, **A high menaquinone intake reduces the incidence of coronary heart disease**, *Nutr Metab Cardiovasc Dis*, 2008

- Essahili R, et al, A new model of isolated systolic **hypertension induced by chronic warfarin** and K-1 treatment, *Am J Hypert* 16:103-10, 2003

- Spronk HMH,, et al, Tissue-specific utilization of menaquinone-4 results in the **prevention of arterial calcifications** in warfarin-treated rats, *J Vasc Res* 40:531-7, 2003

- Geleijnse JM, et al, Dietary intake of menaquinone is associated with a reduced risk of coronary heart disease: the Rotterdam Study, *J Nutr* 134:3100-05, 2004

- Schurgers LJ, et al, Vitamin K-containing dietary supplements: comparison of synthetic vitamin K1 and natto-derived menaquinone-7, *Blood* 109:3279-83, 2007

- Tanko LB, et al, Relationship between osteoporosis and cardiovascular disease in postmenopausal women, *J Bone Min Res* 20:1912-20, 2005

- McCann JC, et al, Vitamin K, an example of triage theory: is micronutrient inadequacy linked to diseases of aging? *Am J Clin Nutr*, 90:899-907, 2009

"I Need Medications for My Stent"

No you don't. You need to cure those imbalances as well as what caused you to need a stent in the first place. Whether you have high blood pressure, high cholesterol, arrhythmia, angina, congestive heart failure, or have had a stent, learn how to get rid of the medications prescribed for these as well. Start with *Is Your Cardiologist Killing You?* (prestigepublishing.com or 1-800-846-6687). Subsequent *TW* and book in progress have more details.

For example, if you think **a stent** was the answer to your angina or coronary calcifications, first be aware that a stent **becomes a magnet for clots**. After all it's merely a hunk of chicken wire-like metal that is recognized by the body as foreign. So when the body cannot get rid of it, it does the next best protective thing. It tries to put a fence around it by coating it in fiber and clot to wall it off from the rest of the body. Folks are usually put on Plavix at $4 a capsule, but it was shown to be no better than aspirin. In fact the *PDR* says you have to take aspirin with it, because it is so ineffective. Plus there is no standard hospital test to see if you are among the 44% for whom it doesn't work (*TW*). And bear in mind many people are running around with half a dozen stents in them, but **the FDA only approved stents one per customer, and *not* after a heart attack, since drugs do a better job** (*TW* 2011-13). You can learn about nutrients that are many times better than drugs in protecting you after a stent.

And as the *New England Journal of Medicine* showed in 2007, **4 out of 5 stents were not needed. In fact, a stent "did not reduce the risk of death, heart attack** or other cardiovascular events when added to optimal medical therapy" (volume 356, page 5003, 2007). And for folks who choose the new drug-coated stent, there is an 18-30% increase risk of death in the next six months to three years according to the *New England Journal of Medicine* (page 1009). And why shouldn't there be since it is coated with chemotherapy. Furthermore, **folks with drugs only and with no stents did better than those with stents and angioplasty**. And as long ago as 1995 the *Journal of the American Medical Association* showed that **nutrients arrest plaque progression**. More later.

So where are the cardiologists who should be teaching you this? Hundreds of other journal articles that I've documented in our books and newsletters have shown that nutrients like cod liver oil, vitamin D and magnesium, as examples, can cut the death rate by more than half. No drug has that power. I've even cited studies on folks who were in intensive care and about to die after they had exhausted everything that medicine has to offer. As I detailed in *TW*, when researchers gave these near death patients only two nutrients, they cut the death rate in half! Yet I have not seen records from an ICU that routinely prescribes these 2 inexpensive and harmless vitamins (C and E), much less measures them.

To quote from the already cited *Wall Street Journal* article that brought to light many facts that even most cardiologists don't know (and I quote directly from the paper): **"stents did no better than cheaper treatments at preventing deaths, heart attacks or strokes in a large study of diabetics** with heart disease".

In fact, in the words of one epidemiologist, a five-year study of over 2000 diabetics showed "that **it really didn't matter at all which treatment you had** in terms of deaths, heart attacks and strokes". He went on to state "We're a little disappointed that **there was not a clear mortality benefit for any of the treatments"**. "Patients who had an immediate stenting angioplasty, a $15,000 procedure to open a clogged artery, had the same death rate over a five-year study as those who took generic medicines". And a 2007 study "concluded that **aggressive stenting didn't save lives or avert heart attacks compared with cheap pills"**, plus "24% of the patients who were immediately stented required a second operation". (Much more on this topic in 2013 *Total Wellness*.)

Does science matter to physicians? Do they read their own medical journals? Do they think about the consequences? I leave it to you to decide. Dr. Boden's study (called the Courage study) published in the prestigious *New England Journal of Medicine* in 2007 showed that **the $15,000 stent is not any better than using drugs**. And they followed over 2,287 patients for five years, **proving stents did not affect the rate of deaths or heart attacks.** But do you think this changed the way American cardiologists practice? No way. To quote the *Wall Street Journal*, "as the headlines about Courage faded, stentings soon began to rise again and are now back at peak levels at about 1 million a year". After all if your only tool is a stent, that's apparently what you're going to keep using, especially when it is much more profitable than an office visit where you have to spend time teaching the patients.

The article went on to show that the $15 billion that the U.S. spends on stent procedures each year could be reduced by more than a third. Plus it went on to show that even fundamental diagnostic procedures are thrown to the wind as cardiologists stampede to insert stents. As an example of how out of control many interventional cardiologists are, "Post-stent patients never received the cardiovascular stress test to verify the clogged artery is the cause of the chest pains, despite professional guidelines that urge such a test before stenting". As one cardiologist remarked, "nothing has been done to put some checks and balances into the stenting decision". You think?

So how can the world of medicine that folks depend on to keep them alive ignore the scientific evidence? What has replaced the cardiologist's quest for knowledge and ethics and doing the best for his patients? As the *WSJ* article pointed out, interventional cardiologists "have a financial incentive to use stents -- -- they **receive about $900 per stenting procedure, roughly 9 times the amount they get for an office visit**". And oddly enough under federal law, **the government's Medicare insurance program is legally barred from considering a treatment's benefits when deciding how much to pay doctors**. In other words, even if it doesn't work Medicare still pays for it. For example, the more expensive drug-coated stent (called DES or drug-eluting stent since it secretes chemotherapy) is not as good as the bare metal stent. After 3 years, the chance of restenosis is triple for the DES versus bare metal one (Weisz, Pfeister). But I'll show you how to compensate for it.

So a $15,000 stent (that takes less than an hour) sure brings more profit than a quickie $100 office visit (which they can only cram about 4 of into an hour). Plus, as referenced in *TW*, from the *Wall Street Journal*, the more money an insurance company pays out for high tech medicine, the more money the insurance company makes. They get a commission on payments. And this is regardless of whether studies show the procedure or medication is not in the best interest of the patient.

The solution for you and those you love? Devour *Is Your Cardiologist Killing You?* and subsequent *TW*s to learn how to actually cure your condition, and then to keep yourselves as healthy as possible. We literally have an epidemic now of young people in their 40s and 50s who have no problems except they've suddenly had a heart attack and were scared into a stent. Clearly, even if you do not have a cardiac problem, the nutrient guidelines in there are indispensable for all of us in this era. Plus the odds are you will eventually need this information....yet you are far better off to learn how to avoid the problems or at least be very prepared *before* you are coerced into a treatment that may not be in your best interest.

Meanwhile, once someone has had a stent then they are automatically put on Plavix (clopidigrel). But Plavix (the $8 billion annual world-wide drug to supposedly reduce clots) actually boosts your risk of a heart attack a gigantic 50% if you also take an acid inhibitor, like Prilosec, Nexium, Tagamet, etc. And guess what? Half the folks taking the $4 capsules of Plavix are already on one of these acid inhibitors (Singer-Vine, Mundy).

But even worse, Plavix has been shown to be no better than an aspirin, which is far cheaper. To quote right out of the *New England Journal of Medicine*, "clopidogrel **(Plavix) plus aspirin was not significantly more effective than aspirin alone in reducing the rate of myocardial infarction, stroke, or death**" (Bhatt). Some of these things I have to quote directly from the journals for you because I know otherwise you would find it too

27

hard to believe, as I did. Plus Plavix does not work in one out of three people (*TW* 2013 explores Plavix resistance).

My question is, what doctor would prescribe something that costs you $4 a day that's no better than an aspirin? And for which there is no blood test to see if you are among the 44% in whom it doesn't work? Only one who does not keep up with *TW*. And the *NEJM* journal is not alone. Here's an example of a quote from the *American Journal of Medicine*: "Current evidence does not support increased efficacy of clopidogrel relative to aspirin in patients following myocardial infarction." (Schleinitz). Translation? Don't give Plavix, give aspirin. Furthermore, as evidenced in *TW*, the action of Plavix is compromised by many medications that are simultaneously prescribed or taken OTC (over-the-counter), like acid inhibitors and NSAID (like Motrin) pain relievers.

And as for the **aspirin**, the American Heart Association's primary journal says it **increases your chance of having another heart attack 6%** (Gislason). As well, as referenced in *TW*, **aspirin increases your chances of macular degeneration, stroke, ulcers, hearing loss,** and much more. So how did this aspirin business get started anyway? Everything dates back to a 1983 *New England Journal of Medicine* study that by its own admission up front in the summary "was not statistically significant" and had many additional flaws. Furthermore, the authors of the paper admitted that none of the 6 previous studies (that were cited in the paper) were statistically significant. As you will figure out when you read further, damaged blood vessels and damaged platelets and damaged chemistry produce abnormal clots. They need to be fixed.

But if you have a foreign body, such as a stent, that changes the rules. **Folks need to stay on the medications prescribed once they have a stent, at least until they fully repair their chemistry.** 2011-14 *TW* has much more information and evidence as it explores the pros and cons of medications used with stents and how to get off them. *My purpose here is to (1) show you there is another side to medicine, and (2) that just because a doctor tells* *you something does not mean it's true, nor that he has kept up-to-date by reading to improve his knowledge.*

Reference:

- Winstein, KJ, A simple health-care fix fizzles out, *Wall St J*, 2/11/10, A1, A18

- Mundy A, et al, FDA Plavix warning, *Wall St J*, D5, Nov. 18, 2009

- Gislason GH, et al, Risk of death or reinfarction associated with the use of selective cyclooxygenase-2 inhibitors and non-selective nonsteroidal anti-inflammatory drugs after acute myocardial infarction, *Circulation* 113:2906-13, 2006

- Bhatt DL, et al, Clopidogrel and aspirin versus aspirin alone for the prevention of atherothrombotic events, *New Engl J Med* 354;16:1706-17, 2006

- Schleinitz MD, et al, Clopidogrel versus aspirin for secondary prophylaxis of vascular events: a cost-effectiveness analysis, *Am J Med*, 116:797-806, 2004

- Lewis HD, et al, Protective effects of aspirin against acute myocardial infarction and death in men with unstable angina, *New Engl J Med* 309:396-403, 1983

- Winslow R, et al, **Plavix plus aspirin shows few benefits**, *Wall Street Journal*, B3, March 13, 2006

- Pfeister M, et al, Late clinical events after clopidigrel discontinuation my limit the benefit of drug-eluting stents, *J Am Coll Cardiol* 18;12:2584-91, 2006

- Weisz G, et al, Late stent thrombosis in sirolimus-eluting versus bare-metal stents in for randomized clinical trials with 3-year follow-up (abstr), *J Am Coll Cardiol* 47 supple B:8B, 2006

"My Pain Medication Won't Have Any Bearing on My Diabetes"

If you are on medications for chronic pain (a category called non-steroidal anti-inflammatory drugs or NSAIDs, like Motrin, Aleve, Naprosyn, Tolectin, Celebrex, aspirin, etc.) these also have a litany of side effects, not the least of which is to **cause you to need a joint replacement in a few years, since they deteriorate the chemistry of cartilage repair**. Plus they **cause high blood pressure.** So any doctor treating your blood pressure who is not first helping you get rid of pain medications may be destined for failure. Yet in 3 out of 4 people **chronic pain and arthritis of any type is completely cured just by eliminating the nightshades** as described in detail in the book *Pain Free In 6 Weeks* (prestigepublishing.com or 1-800-846-6687).

And these pain drugs do a lot more than just guarantee you will need a joint replacement in the future. They cause over 16,000 deaths by intestinal hemorrhage each year, over 100,000 cases of congestive heart failure (which has a median survival of only five years), and they damage the gut by creating ulcers, irritable bowel syndrome, and colitis, as well as auto-immune diseases like thyroiditis, multiple sclerosis, rheumatoid arthritis, lupus, plus fibromyalgia, chronic fatigue, irritable bowel syndrome, and much more. And these medications interfere with the anticipated anti-clot benefits of aspirin (Catella-Lawson), an important fact for those with stents and taking expensive Plavix.

I could go through **every category of prescription and over-the-counter medicine to show you how they all lead to new diseases and make the one that you're treating worse.** How? For starters, they allow the under-educated dinosaur physician to ignore finding the cause and permanent cure for your problem. Instead physicians quickly get you out of the office with a prescription that needs very little instruction. Second, all drugs work by poisoning a pathway to turn off a particular symptom. But in doing so they also have to be metabolized by the body in order to work and also for the body to get rid of them. Both of these use up and deplete nutrients that should have been used to heal your diabetes.

References:

- Rogers S, *Pain Free In 6 Weeks, The Cholesterol Hoax, The High Blood Pressure Hoax, Is Your Cardiologist Killing You?*, all at prestigepublishing.com or 1-800-846-6687

- Rogers SA, Solonaceae (Nightshade) sensitivity as a reversible cause of juvenile and adult rheumatoid arthritis, chronic degenerative disc pain, and osteoarthritis, *J Appl Nutr* 52;1:2-11, 2002

- Hippisley-Cox J, et al, **Risk of myocardial infarction in patients taking** cyclooxygenase-2 inhibitors or conventional **non-steroidal anti-inflammatory drugs:** population-based nested case-control analysis, *Brit Med J*, 330:1366, 2005

- Galarraga B, et al, **Cod liver oil (n-3 fatty acids) as a non-steroidal anti-inflammatory drug-sparing agent in rheumatoid arthritis**, *Rheumatol* 47:665-69, Mar 2008

- DeMaria AN, Relative risk of cardiovascular events in patients with rheumatoid arthritis, *Am J Cardiol*, 89;6(Supple 1):33-38, 2002

- Joint meeting of the Arthritis Advisory Committee and the Drug Safety and Risk Management Advisory Committee of the US Food and Drug Administration, Feb 16-18, 2005. 2006

- Hernandez-Diaz S, et al, Epidemiologic assessment of the safety of conventional non-steroidal anti-inflammatory drugs, *Am J Med* 110;9 (supple 3A): S20-27, 2001

- Catella-Lawson F, et al, Cyclooxygenase inhibitors and the antiplatelet effects of aspirin, *New Engl J Med*, 345:1809-17, 2001

The Un-ending Dangers of Aspirin and Other Pain Relievers

Over a decade ago in *TW* 2000 I showed you the evidence right out of the *Journal of the American Medical Association* from 1980 where **aspirin increases your risk of stroke 200%**. Then in further issues as well as in more detail in *The High Blood Pressure Hoax* and *The Cholesterol Hoax* I detailed why it's a sign of an ignorant physician who recommends a daily aspirin. And then I showed other evidences of how it increases damage to the eye, hearing, and more.

So what else does a better job? In 2000 *TW* I gave you the evidence right out of the *American Journal Cardiology* showing **vitamin E can cut your heart attack rate as much as 70%**. Yet the majority of cardiologists, internists and family practitioners in the United States still recommend a daily aspirin. In fact, it is part of nearly every emergency room, intensive care unit and cardiovascular care unit's pre-printed order sheets. Doctors merely have to check it off to have it ordered. They don't even have to write it out. Yet only those who are totally unschooled in the chemistry of healing the body would ever think of something so ludicrous. Yet if they just recommend plain old vitamin E, it's just as bad, because that amounts to synthetic alpha tocopherol, which actually negates the good effects of natural vitamin E. More importantly, **real vitamin E is eight entities or parts and you have to have all 8 of them in concert**.

"What about the negative articles on vitamin E?" you ask. Those studies were designed with incredible ignorance, because they only used one of eight parts of E. For example, by just omitting gamma tocopherol (that you will learn more about), you lose the ability to control not only the abnormal clotting that leads to heart attacks, but the bad inflammatory gastric ulcer-type symptoms that aspirin produces (Jiang).

In previous *TW* issues I've shown you how the NSAIDs (non-steroidal anti-inflammatory drugs like aspirin, Motrin, Aleve, Celebrex, and even acetaminophen (Tylenol®), which is not technically an NSAID) all have serious side effects. Yet the FDA's job appears to be to protect the pharmaceutical industry, since it has made many NSAIDs available without a prescription as soon as their patents expired. I warned you (half a decade before it was finally taken off the market) in 2000 *TW* that the popular NSAID prescription Vioxx® quadrupled the heart attack rate. But stalling any FDA action enabled the manufacture to make billions annually. This is in marked contrast to nutrients that have literally been hauled off the shelves of health food stores within one week with far less evidence or danger. Don't forget the poison control units report over 100,000 folks die from medications a year, as opposed to none from nutrients.

In a short summary, the **NSAIDs including aspirin had been shown to increase the risk of stroke 200%, are a major cause of high blood pressure, congestive heart failure, kidney damage, liver damage, macular degeneration, deplete glutathione leading to cancers, irritable bowel disease, GERD, heartburn, and create leaky gut which leads to allergies, autoimmune diseases like rheumatoid arthritis, lupus, and multiple sclerosis.** In fact, they can contribute to just about every disease or condition that is associated with aging (with long-term use). But that's not all. There's more.

It turns out that in the study of over 27,000 men the longer they used NSAIDs, the **greater their risk of going deaf in old age** (defined as over age 60!). It's really sad to see people who are healthy at any age become socially isolated because they can't hear. This government-supported study was done by physicians at the Massachusetts Eye and Ear Infirmary as well as the Harvard School of Public Health. The published results in the *American Journal of Medicine* showed that folks who use **aspirin** (foolishly recommended by their physicians to prevent heart attacks) **increase their chance of going deaf 33-99%.** And **the odds of becoming deaf increase the longer you take it.** And these stats go for all the NSAIDs as well as the non-NSAIDs like acetaminophen (known as Tylenol, which has been investigated for many manufacturing problems in 2010-11). But does that stop this universal recommendation? No way.

In fact there are constant articles touting the use of aspirin, even now for cancer patients, which is ridiculous. Inflammation is part of the mechanism for cancer protection. And to give you an idea of how poor the evidence was, even though the title of the article in the *Wall Street Journal* was "Aspirin found to aid cancer patients", I'll quote how *un*convincing it was. The article went on to clearly state that (and I quote) "the study didn't prove aspirin contributed to the women's survival advantage". Furthermore "an earlier report... didn't find any link between aspirin use and reduced incidence of breast cancer". Yet they had the gall to flaunt this blatantly misleading article title. So for those who don't read the details, but only the headlines, they would think that this was one more reason to take that aspirin every day.

Why do reporters act with such irresponsibility? Everyone in the medical reporting media and those practicing medicine should know the mechanism of how a daily aspirin (as a cyclo-oxygenase inhibitor) increases medical problems. Taking even one medication inevitably leads to further medical problems which require more prescription medications. I wonder how many folks diagnosed with GERD or reflux blamed on a hiatus hernia really have it because of their daily aspirins. Then they take Prilosec (or worse Nexium, over 8 times more expensive) to quell the symptoms. But these inhibit their absorption of B12 which leads to brain destruction, it encourages the growth of H. pylori in the stomach which leads to coronary artery disease, and inhibits the absorption of minerals needed to prevent not only diabetes, but cancers, Alzheimer's, heart disease and in fact all the chronic diseases associated with "aging".

So if you don't want to be deaf when you grow up, correct your deficiencies, then cut that aspirin out. And if you are still convinced that you need it to prevent a heart attack, get a grip and get smarter. Also catch up on the multitude of reasons why it merely fosters new diseases. If your doctor still insists that you take a daily aspirin, ask him if he has ever read even one shred of evidence against aspirin, much less read about **all of the nutrients that do an infinitely better job than aspirin at preventing heart attacks, cancers, and all the chronic diseases** including accelerated aging. If he cups his ear with his hand and says "What did you say?", you already know the answer. Move on.

References:

- Curhan SG, et al, Analgesic use and the risk of hearing loss in men, *Am J Med*, 123:231-7, 2010

- Singer-Vine J, Say what? New risk in pain-reliever use, *Wall Street Jl*, D6, Mar 9, 2010

- Sataline S, Aspirin found to aid cancer patients, *Wall Street J*, D8, Feb 17, 2010

- Jiang Q, et al, Combination of aspirin and gamma tocopherol is superior to that of aspirin and alpha-tocopherol in anti-inflammatory action and attenuation of aspirin induced adverse effects, *J Nutr Biochem* 20:894-900, 2009

"I Need My Diabetes Medicine to Prevent Kidney Damage Leading to Dialysis"

I wish there were a drug that could do this, but they are proven to be impotent. Likewise the advice for a low protein diet, with or without adding fatty acids, has not been curative either, since it still allows the doctor to ignore fixing what caused it. However, the good news is there is much data (as you will learn) proving that once you fix the chemistry of diabetes, you also can actually turn off the albuminuria (the leaking of a protein called albumin into the urine, one of the first signs of the death of the kidneys).

And albumin loss is more important than you think because 2 out of 5 diabetics get kidney disease (Gross). Yet its cure (the earlier the better) is sometimes as simple as pennies of **Vitamin B6** (pyridoxamine) or **Vitamin B1** (thiamine) as you will learn. But where are the diabetologists who give thiamine (B1), much less even measure to see how much you need? Instead dialysis (over $60,000/year) tanks the person up with aluminum which then can lead to Alzheimer's. In addition, chemicals from the dialysis tubing, cyclohexanone and phthalate plasticizers, insidiously damage the heart and other organs (Thompson-Torgerson, *TW*).

References (many more later on in subsequent chapters):

- Nakamura S, et al, **Pyridoxal phosphate prevents progression of diabetic nephropathy**, *Nephrology Dialysis Transplantation*, 22:2165-74, 2007

- Thompson-Torgerson CS, et al, **Cyclohexanone contamination** from extracorporeal circuits **impairs cardiovascular function**, *Am J Physiol Heart Circul Physiol* 296: H1926-32, 2009

- Gross JL, et al., Diabetic nephropathy: diagnosis, prevention and treatment, *Diabetes Care* 28:164-76, 2005

- Babaei-Jadidi R, et al, **Prevention** of the incipient **diabetic nephropathy by high-dose thiamine** and benfotiamine, *Diabetes,* 52; 8:2110-20, 2003

"What About Meds for My Painful Legs?"

Folks with incredibly painful legs are prescribed Lyrica® for their peripheral neuropathy from diabetes, possibly because this drug has sported full-page advertisements for diabetic nerve pain in major magazines. But when you look at the *PDR,* it makes you wonder how it was ever approved. It has "an unexpectedly high incidence of hemangio-sarcoma" which is a **cancer of blood vessels.** It raises your creatinine kinase (leads to kidney disease), lowers your platelet count, causes changes in the EKG that can lead to heart block, causes weight gain, swelling of the ankles and has caused life-threatening angioedema (swelling of the throat and face inhibiting breathing). Many of the symptoms it causes as side effects are things that the diabetic is trying to avoid anyway. This drug just hastens it.

But the scariest thing is that **Lyrica causes retinal atrophy as well as corneal inflammation and calcification. Translation? You can go blind from it** as it progresses to macular degeneration or you at least get cataracts. And to top that, any improvements in pain often wear off after a year. Peripheral neuropathy is a serious disease of blood vessels that supply the nerves as well as the nerves themselves. They must be relieved of their heavy metal, pesticide and other toxic loads and then repaired and regenerated, as you will learn.

But don't despair. The chances are that with the nutrients you will learn about here you may cure your peripheral neuropathy and you may not need to go further with more aggressive detoxification. Just look at a smattering of the evidence below for nutrients that have actually reversed or cured diabetic neuropathy such as acetyl-L-carnitine, lipoic acid, vitamin E (Quatraro, Scarpini, Zeigler,Tutuncu). Although **one in three diabetics develops peripheral neuropathy** (Fedele), seldom does a diabetologist cure it. In fact I have not seen any records from a diabetologist who even looked at the adequacy of any of the above nutrients. This is in spite of numerous studies from their very own journals proving that you can reduce or even get rid of peripheral neuropathy by fixing what's broken.

What diabetologist would prescribe Lyrica when he has not measured and corrected something as simple as ALC (acetyl-L-carnitine) for nerve regeneration (Ido, Onofrij, Lowitt, DeGrandis, Sima)? In fact there is evidence for just about every nutrient from biotin to riboflavin (vitamin B2); depending on the individual (*Am J Clin Nutr* 71:1676-81 S, 2000). Sometimes it is as simple as the diabetic neuropathy being totally cured with just vitamins B1 or B6. It all depends on what the person is low in (Abbas). But of course, the more alcohol you drink, the more you lower things like your vitamin B1 and B6 which then can lead to brain damage (Thomson). And don't think only nutrients (biotin, fatty acids, etc.) can reverse diseases. Diets, like a vegetarian diet have caused **regression of diabetic neuropathy** (Crain). Later *I'll be mapping out a plan for you regarding what nutrients to take, their sources, doses and forms.*

References:

- Sima AA, et al, Acetyl-L-Carnitine Study Group, **Acetyl-L-carnitine improves pain, nerve regeneration**, and vibratory perception in patients with chronic diabetic neuropathy: an analysis of two randomized placebo-controlled trials, *Diabetes Care* 28; 1:89-94, Jan 2005

- Quatraro A, et al, **Acetyl L-carnitine for symptomatic diabetic neuropathy,** *Diabetologia* 38:123, **1995**

- Scarpini E, et al, Effect of **acetyl-L-carnitine in the treatment of painful peripheral neuropathy** is in HIV-positive patients, *J Peripher Nerv Syst* 2: 250-2, 1997

- Zeigler D, et al, **Alpha-lipoic acid in the treatment of diabetic peripheral and cardiac autonomic neuropathy**, *Diabetes* 46 suppl. 2: s 62-6, 1997

- Nakamura J, et al, Polyol pathway hyperactivity is closely related to **carnitine deficiency in the pathogenesis of diabetic neuropathy** of streptozotocin-diabetic rats, *J Pharmacol Exp Ther*, 287:897-902, 1998

- Tutuncu NB, et al, **Reversal of defective nerve condition with vitamin E supplementation in type 2 diabetes**, *Diabetes Care* 21:1915-18, 1998

- Fedele D, et al, Peripheral diabetic neuropathy. Current recommendations and future prospects for its prevention and management, *Drugs* 54:414-21, 1997

- Ido Y, et al**, Neural dysfunction** and metabolic imbalances **in diabetic rats. Prevention by acetyl-L-carnitine.** *Diabetes* 43:1469-77, 1994

- Onofrij M, et al, **Acetyl-L-carnitine as a new therapeutic approach for peripheral neuropathies with pain,** *Int J Clin Pharmacol Res* 15:9-15, **1995**

- Lowitt S, et al, **Acetyl-L-carnitine corrects the altered peripheral nerve function** of experimental **diabetes,** *Metab* 44:677-80, 1995

- DeGrandis D, et al, **Acetyl-L-carnitine in the treatment of diabetic neuro**pathy. A long-term randomized, double-blind placebo-controlled study, *Drugs R D*, 3: 223-31, 2002

- Abbas ZG, et al, Evaluation of the efficacy of **thiamine and pyridoxine in the treatment of** symptomatic **diabetic peripheral neuropathy**, *East African Med J,* 74:803-8, 1997

- Thomson AG, Mechanisms of vitamin deficiency and chronic alcohol misuse is in the development of Wernicke-Korsakoff's syndrome, *Alcohol Alcohol Suppl*, 35:2-7, 2000

- Crain MG, et al, Regression of diabetic neuropathy with total vegetarian diet, *J Nutr Med* 4:431-9, 1994

- Koutsikos D, et al, **Biotin for diabetic peripheral neuropathy**. Biotin may also reduce pain, *Biomed Pharmacother* 44:511-4, 1990

"If Nothing Else, I Should Take Diabetes Medicines to Reduce the Damage to My Eyes From Cataracts and Macular Degeneration"

You have been hoodwinked again. There's no proof that diabetes drugs slow down any disease. But multiple nutrients have not only prevented, but then slowed down and even reversed serious eye conditions. In fact, when you look at the enormous amount of evidence (that I have detailed in past issues of the *Total Wellness* newsletter of over 24 years) it should be malpractice to fail to prescribe nutrients to prevent the eye complications of diabetics (Packer, Weisberger, Taylor, Robertson, Jacques). As one tiny example, a Harvard study showed **DHA** (docosahexaneoic acid) as **found in cod liver oil** (and also available separately that you will learn about) **cuts the risk of macular degeneration** a walloping 38%! (Christen).

The same goes for the even worse condition, macular degeneration. At least with cataracts you can have lenses implanted. But with macular degeneration there are only two ways to go: (1) you can believe the ophthalmologist that you will be blind in 5 years and that there's nothing that can be done about it, or (2) you can identify the nutritional deficiencies and toxicities that caused it and reverse them. Many people have done so. As with any disease, **it is much easier to prevent it than wait until it has gotten much worse** and then attempt to reverse it (Seddon, Mozaffariah). Many of the nutrients you will learn about here are also important in reversing macular degeneration.

References:

- Mozaffarieh M, et al, The role of the carotenoids and lutein and zeaxanthin in protecting against age-related macular degeneration: a review based on controversial evidence, *Nutr J* 2; 1:20, Dec 11, 2003

- Jacques PF, et al, Epidemiologic evidence of the role for antioxidant vitamins and carotenoids in cataract prevention, *Am J Clin Nutr* 53:352s-355s, 1991

- Robertson JA, et al, The possible role of vitamins C and E in cataract prevention, *Am J Clin Nutr* 53; 1 suppl: 346S-351S, 1991

- Taylor A, Role of nutrients in delaying cataracts, *Ann NY Acad Sci*, 669; 1:11-23, 1992

- Seddon JM, et al, Dietary fat and risk for advanced age-related macular degeneration, *Arch Ophthal* 119; 8:1191-99, 2001

- Packer L, Antioxidant properties of **lipoic acid** and its therapeutic effects in **prevention** of **diabetes** complications and **cataracts**, *Ann NY Acad Sci* 738: 257-64, 1994

- Weisberger J, Scientific basis for medical therapy of cataracts by antioxidants, *Am J Clin Nutr* 53; 1 supple) 1992

- Christen WG, et al, Dietary omega-3 fatty acid and fish intake and incident age-related macular degeneration in women, *Arch Ophthalmol*, 2011

Why Do Insurance Companies Only Cover Drugs?

Great question. This, too, was a puzzle for me. Why are they not interested in doing what is best for the patient, or at least interested in saving money? Why would they ignore saving money and actually curing folks as opposed to expensively drugging them forever? By endorsing the type of medicine you will learn about here, actually curing folks (as we and others have done for decades), they could save enormous amounts of money, as well as stop the inevitable avalanche into other diseases. The answer came from *The Wall Street Journal.* It showed that **insurance companies make money on the claims they pay out,** sort of like a sales commission. So there is no incentive to cure folks. **This continual income is the essence of their business.** I couldn't believe that I was totally unaware of this incentive to keep folks sick.

If you find this as difficult to believe as I did, let me quote the *WSJ*, "<u>**insurers generally earn a profit by charging a premium on claims they pay**</u>", so "**they don't necessarily have an incentive to crack down on excess spending**" nor on **bad medicine** (Winstein). Yes, I was as surprised by this as you probably are. **Insurance companies make money on handling the claims they pay for, sort of like a sales commission**, but at your and my expense. And premature death is the ultimate price paid.

So it should be no surprise that in spite of all of our "modern" medicine and the billions of dollars spent by people each year on their drugs, that recent research proves it is all for naught. For poisoning the body with medications does not change the rate of developing new diseases nor forestall the inevitable consequences of failing to cure a disease. To reiterate the findings of the *New England Journal of Medicine*, **the U.S. medical system has been a failure for diabetics. Years of the most highly recommended medications and doctor visits didn't result in fewer heart attacks or fewer strokes or fewer heart related deaths.** The study clearly showed that **drugs are nearly useless for chronic diseases. They just make blood tests look better and symptoms temporarily improve or stabilize. They don't cure nor prolong life.** You deserve better than that ruse. I can't think of any disease that is a deficiency of the latest drugs. Can you?

References:

- Winslow R, Search for better **diabetes therapy falls short. Current treatments,** while effective, **fail to also help prevent heart attacks and stroke,** in blow to researchers, patients, *Wall Street Journal*, A5, March 15, 2010

- Pelton R, et al, *Drug-Induced Nutrient Depletion Handbook*, 2nd Ed, 1-877-837-LEXI (5394), 2001

- Winslow R, **Study questions evidence behind heart therapies**, *Wall Street Journal*, D1, Feb. 25, 2009

- Winstein, KJ, **A simple health-care fix fizzles out**, *WSJ*, 2/11/10, A1, A18

If You Still Think the FDA is Pro-Consumer, Consider This:

One of the **most recent diabetes drugs** is Avandia® (or generic rosiglitazone). You'll find it as unbelievable as I did that in 2007 it was published in one of the most prestigious and high profile medical journals that this popular diabetes drug **increases the heart attack rate a devastating 43%** (Nissen). Then on top of that the impropriety and lack of scientific ethics from the industry-controlled clinical trial was documented (Nissen). Yet even though there are **over 700 lawsuits from folks injured by the drug, totaling more than $60 million, and even though the trials on it** had to be ended because it was so dangerous, the FDA was still deciding its fate as of 2012. Does that stalling have anything to do with the fact that this drug brings in over \$3 billion in a single year (Mitka)?

In fact over four years ago studies showed that not only did **Avandia triple the death rate over placebo, but it increased congestive heart failure, raised the bad cholesterol, LDL, 18%, damaged genes and promoted cancer.** As in many other documented incidences, **the FDA has continued to stall to allow huge billion dollar/year profits to accrue for pharmaceutical companies** while a patent is still in place. Meanwhile innocent Americans continue to take the drug and trust other drugs related to it (Nissen).

References:

- Nissen SE, et al, Effect of **rosiglitazone on the risk of myocardial infarction and death** from cardiovascular causes [published correction appears in *New Engl J Med*, 2007; 357 (1): 100] *New Engl J Med* 356; 24:2457-71, **2007**

- Mitka M, **Critics press FDA to act on evidence** of rosiglitazone's cardiac safety issues, *J Am Med Assoc*, 303;23:2341-2, 2010

- Nissen SE, Setting the RECORD straight, *J Am Med Assoc*, 303; 12:1194-1195, 2010

Just How Many Millions of Dollars and Hundreds of Doctors Does it Take to Prove That Diabetes is Not a Deficiency of the Latest Drug?

Remember the old jokes about "How many (choose any ethnic group your best friend represents that you want to jokingly mock) does it take to screw in a lightbulb?" Well it is no longer a joke, because millions of taxpayer dollars and hundreds of physicians across the United States have proven that the current focus on drugs for diabetes is worthless….but how many physicians does it take to change our focus from drugs to cure? **Drugs do not improve longevity, in fact they increase the death rate, sometimes doubling and tripling it**. Do you still find it as hard as I did to believe? Then let me help you review the pertinent evidence right out of the latest and most prestigious medical journals.

Back in 2008, the prestigious *New England Journal of Medicine* published a study called **ACCORD (the Action to Control Cardiovascular Risk in Diabetes Study Group).** Using the latest drugs for diabetes for intensive lowering of the sugar and using the glycosylated hemoglobin A1C as a measure of their success, they studied over 10,000 patients for over 3 1/2 years. The result of focusing on the lab values rather than fixing what's broken? **Lowering the glycated hemoglobin for over three years actually increased the death rate 22%.** And that's not all. It **increased retinopathy** (the chance to go blind) and **renal failure 37%.** This leads to dialysis which ushers in more medical problems, like aluminum toxicity which leads to Alzheimer's. And it **increases swelling, weight gain, congestive heart failure, heart attack rates and cancers.** But did that stop U.S. doctors from trying to bludgeon every patient's hgb A1C into a normal level with the drug? No way. And it gets worse.

The ACCORD study group went further and in 2010 published another study again in the prestigious *New England Journal of Medicine*. In this one they gave nearly 5000 diabetics **the best blood pressure medicines for nearly 5 years**. The results? It **didn't make one bit of difference in the amount of strokes, heart attacks or death.** Again why not? Because **they're only treating laboratory numbers. They are not fixing what's broken**. They are not finding and repairing what caused the disease.

But wait! It gets worse. They then decided to see if lowering the cholesterol made any difference in folks with type II diabetes. So once more they now treated over 5000 patients for nearly 5 years. The results were that adding another type of cholesterol-lowering drug, fibrates, to a statin drug did not reduce the rate of death. And of course, they did this *knowing* that there were already published studies showing that when you combine these two drugs you increase kidney damage and the chance of dying from fatal rhabdomyolysis from the statin drug. This really defies explanation and yet it was supported by the United States government's National Heart, Lung, and Blood Institute (that we support with tax dollars) as well as five other institutes, while dozens of doctors were involved. The amazing thing is that they never really realized what they had actually proven: that **diabetes and its related diseases are not the deficiency of any drugs**. You have to find the cause and fix what's broken in order to bring about cure.

Meanwhile, how many millions of our tax dollars and useless hours of scores of clinicians' research time do we have to waste until they see the light? They **have proven that you can throw all the best drugs at a patient for diabetes, blood pressure and cholesterol, etc., and it makes no difference in death rate compared with doing nothing**. And in some cases **drugs** *increased* **the death rate**, as they should since you have added a drug that further depletes nutrients, ushering in a myriad of side effects and new diseases.

Just watch any educational TV show and see the incredible things that man can do in. So why don't we cure diseases like diabetes? There is no excuse, since thousands of researchers have devoted their lives to proving how it is done. But mainstream medicine is somehow able to turn a blind eye to all this. Does it have anything to do with the fact that came from the *Wall Street Journal* that **the average office visit is 7 minutes and the average time a patient gets to tell their symptoms is 18 seconds? You can't teach anything in that time. You can only write a script and bolt to the door.** We need people power to change medicine.

And if you really want to recall the true colors of medical deceit, remember this study. The ADVANCE Collaborative Group studied over 11,000 patients for 5 years. Then **the ACCORD Study was stopped before it was completed because of increased deaths. The ADVANCE** results? **Intensive lowering of glucose** (monitored again by **hemoglobin A1C) did not lower**

deaths, did not reduce blindness, and did not reduce heart attacks. **But it did increase the number of strokes, vision loss problems, nerve damage, and hospitalizations.** And that is not all! It **increased dementia (severe memory and brain function loss) by 50%.** Oddly enough, none of these worse effects were mentioned in the front page summary, which is the only part of a study that many physicians, medical reporters and newscasters read.

And not to be outdone, another group of researchers wasted more of our tax money by studying another diabetes drug. The NAVIGATOR Group looked at over 9000 patients for 5 years and found....you guessed it. **No help from drugs.** The researchers used a blood pressure diuretic like Diovan, and an angiotensin receptor blocker and Valsartan. Although these reduced the sugar levels, this drug combo **made no difference in the number of deaths, heart attacks and other diabetes-related problems.** But they must be slow learners. Unbelievably, they did another study using yet another blood sugar-lowering drug (an insulin secretogogue, neteglinide, like Starlix) again with over 9000 patients for over 5 years, and with the same negative results. I think only People Power can change medicine.

So back to my original question: *Just how many docs does it take to prove diabetes is not a drug deficiency?* But I guess it pales in comparison to other medical deceits. Just look for example at the millions of women who for decades were brow-beaten into taking Premarin® by their doctors, in spite of research showing it raised the death rate from cancers and cardiovascular disease. It actually did the opposite of what their doctors authoritatively told them it would protect them from, while they continually assured women they were ignorant not to follow their doctors' advice.

References:

- The ACCORD Study Group, Effects of **intensive blood-pressure** control in type 2 diabetes mellitus, *New Engl J Med*, 362;17:1575-85, 2010

- The ACCORD Study Group, Effects of **combination lipid therapy** in type 2 diabetes mellitus, *New Engl J Med*, 362;17:1563-74, 2010

- The ACCORD Study Group, Effects of **intensive glucose lowering** in type 2 diabetes mellitus, *New Engl J Med*, 358; 24:2545-59, 2008

- Dluhy RG, et al, **Intensive glycemic control** in the ACCORD and ADVANCE trials, *New Engl J Med,* 358;24:2630-3, 2008

- The ADVANCE Collaborative Group, **Intensive blood glucose control** and vascular outcomes in patients with type 2 diabetes, *New Engl J Med*, 358:2560-72, 2008

- The NAVIGATOR Study Group, Effect of Nateglinide on the incidence of diabetes and cardiovascular events, *New Engl J Med* 362;2:1463-76, 2010

- The NAVIGATOR Study Group, Effect of Valsartan on the incidence of diabetes and cardiovascular events, *New Engl J Med* 362;16:1477-90, 2010

- Krumholz HM, et al, Redefining quality—Implications of recent clinical trials, *N Engl J Med* 358;24:2537-9, 2008

Is Your Diabetes Doc a Danger to Your Health?

It depends on whether he's a tinker or a thinker, a dinosaur or a dynamo. If he tinkers in medicine and uses drugs for everything, he is merely a legalized drug pusher and chooses to keep his mind unencumbered with the evidence of how to cure medical conditions like diabetes. If on the other hand, he is a thinker, he studies continually to do the best for his patients. Even if he prescribes drugs, with your help by introducing him to this book, he may be ready to start to do "real" medicine, where we find the causes and cures of conditions. And don't be too rough on him, for he suffers from pressures you wouldn't believe. For example, realize that the definition of malpractice is not that you are doing harm to your patients, but that you are not doing what the rest of the "herd" is doing. **So you can be doing the worst medicine in the world, but if the majority of the rest of the docs are doing it, the current tort system finds you "not guilty".**

Government statistics conservatively show there are well over 120,000 deaths per year caused by our 700,000 physicians, leaving a death rate of 0.171 per doctor. The FBI reports there are 1500 deaths from guns per year and 80 million gun owners, leaving 0.000188 deaths per gun owner. Therefore *doctors are 9000 times more dangerous than gun owners*. Since not everyone has a gun but everyone has at least one doctor, this makes it over **900 times more likely you will be killed by a doctor than a gun**.

45

Have You Had Enough Evidence?

I could go on, you know, and fill volumes with the evidence that taking drugs (prescription medications) is the wrong way to go for chronic conditions. On the flip side, **for emergencies or acute situations, drugs are great and can't be beaten.** Plus **you in no way should stop any drugs yet.** First, you haven't learned how to isolate and repair the underlying causes. Once you have enough of them to get rid of your symptoms (or blood abnormalities), then you and your doctor can decide when it is prudent to wean off.

The bottom line is **drugs simply do not fix what is broken, and have a litany of side effects guaranteeing the sick will get sicker, quicker.** Our medical education, practice and reimbursements are strongly influenced by the pharmaceutical world in spite of the overwhelming proof that most conditions are curable with nutrient corrections and through getting rid of the other underlying correctable accumulated toxic causes. But assuming this short sample of the overwhelming body of evidence is convincing you, **don't stop what your doctor has ordered until you have cured yourself.** Instead, use this evidence and knowledge to help you find a doctor worthy of your investment (your life!).

I am not recommending you blindly stop any medications, for I have never examined you, I'm not your doctor, and there is much more that I will never know about you as an individual. Furthermore, some drugs cannot be abruptly stopped but have to be systematically weaned off over months. At least what was prescribed was done so by someone who has examined and studied you, which is more than I can claim. And clearly **before you and your chosen physician make any changes you need to become a lot more knowledgeable.** In fact *you need to become a dynamo.* Why? Because your knowledge (and lack thereof) is the most important determinant of your future and its health. Having clarified that, are you ready for the next step of *your healing adventure*? Let's go.

Chapter II

Diabetes Dinosaur Docs Deny Disparity

I know you learned about the dangers of prescription drugs in chapter 1. As I begin to show you how to cure, in this chapter let's also crack just a few of the many **medical myths of diabetes that are perpetrated and defended by dinosaur** docs. Let's make sure you know there is a huge disparity, and more than one way to treat. To begin with, watch out for the doc who checks the wrong tests. As you started to learn in Chapter 1, if the level is elevated, then the knowledge-challenged diabetologist will merely increase your medications. He is treating a lab value, not a live person. So let's crack some medical myths and misconceptions.

"My Doctor Says I'm Fine as Long as My Hgb A1C is Normal".

An elevated hgb A1C is not a deficiency of any drug. Instead, it indicates that the nutrients which *control* **glycosylation are deficient**. Remember from Chapter 1, **folks who kept their glycosylated hemoglobin A1C perfectly normal did not live any longer.** In fact the startling outcome of the study showed that despite just taking medication to make a blood test look normal and by-passing fixing what's broken, **medications actually increased the death rate 22%.**

The correct treatment which is actually healthful for you is to restore these nutrients that control glycosylation. For by merely increasing your medication, he is actually lowering many nutrients, like your level of vitamin C (as an example of one of many drug side effects). But **vitamin C is one of the nutrients needed to stop glycosylation, or premature destruction** of body cells (Davie). Many other nutrients correct the Hgb A1C, like **vitamin D** (Ceriello), **lipoic acid** (Jain, Bierhaus), **P-5-P** (a metabolite of vitamin B6) (Nakamura), **Magnesium, ALC** (chapter 1), and more that I will tell you about (and give you their sources and doses for

47

later). But first I want you to see how much sense all of this makes and **how surprisingly clueless much of medicine is in terms of the actual curing of diabetes**.

As an example, **vitamin B6** doesn't work right away in the body to lower Hgb A1C. First it **has to be changed (metabolized) into P5P** (pyridoxal-5-phosphate). How does the body change B6 to its active form, P5P? With an enzyme that must have zinc. But most diabetics are not only low in B6 but are also low in zinc. Consequently, **many diabetics will never get better unless someone is checking for the metabolite of B6 or even knows how**, as I will show you later on (Goepp). Sadly, P5P isn't even considered a necessary supplement by the FDA, while many prescription drugs also deplete B6 and zinc, thus poisoning the conversion of B6 to P5P (Laines-Cessac).

Meanwhile, P5P actually traps glycated or fried (aged) proteins and guides them out of the cell, plus prevents the classic protein loss of kidneys (albuminuria) for which years of expensive and damaging dialysis are done (references include *J Am Soc Nephrol* 16; 1:144-50, Jan. 2005, *Nephrol Dial Transplant* 22; 8:2165-74, Aug. 2007). No wonder there are tens of thousands of diabetics getting over $60,000 a year of damaging dialysis when a simple correction of deficiencies could have prevented the death of their kidneys. Instead they get tanked up with disease-producing chemicals from the IVs and dialysis machine plastic tubes, which then actually create worse diabetes, high cholesterol, and that's just for starters! Dialysis loads you with aluminum, which is one of the heavy metals triggering Alzheimer's senile brain deterioration.

P5P is absolutely essential for a normal Hgb A1C. Furthermore, adequate B6 is crucial in preventing cataracts, blindness from diabetic retinopathy (flame haemorrhages that are treated by burning the retina with a laser!), Alzheimer's heart disease, and many other side effects of diabetes. Yet where are the diabetologists who even know how to check for the organic acids that show if you are silently deficient in P5P (much less zinc), and whether or not it's deficiency is already destroying your brain (elevated quinolinate, see *TW*), heart, kidneys, eyes or anywhere else? **In this book you will learn how to not only put your doctor to the test, but how to cure medical problems in spite of his lack of knowledge.**

Clearly, B6 is needed to stop the accelerated deterioration of diabetes. Fortunately, this can be measured in a variety of ways, such as the measurement of damage to your genes (via 8-OHdG) and destruction of your cell membranes (lipid peroxidation). And these are all reversible with adequate B6 (as just one nutrient example). But remember the gene and cell membrane damages that are the precursors to all the lethal side effects of diabetes are not averted by the common diabetes medications (*Horm Metab Res* 36; 3:183-7, Mar 2004).

And are you worried about Alzheimer's, a common side effect of diabetes? Alzheimer's disease patients were 12 times more likely to have a low P5P level (*Neurol* 58; 10:1471-5, May 28, 2002). In fact it is so important that it turns out that **the level of P5P is an identifier for Alzheimer's disease with 100% reliability** (*J Nutr Health Aging*, 8; 5:407-13, 2004)! Clearly, studies have overwhelmingly proven for over a decade that P5P is crucial for anti-glycation (*Biochim Biophys Acta* 126; 3:286-90, Jul 18, 1994 *Nutr Sci Vitaminol* (Tokyo) 41; 1:43-50, Feb 1995).

Are you beginning to appreciate why with our epidemic deficiencies, many people have an elevated hemoglobin A1C, even if they're not diabetic? In fact even researchers who don't understand glycation is a deficiency of antioxidants are stumped when they see it in non-diabetics (Yudkin). Consequently many docs don't appreciate that everyone should be tested for hgb A1C, since it is an indicator of serious deficiency and hidden accelerated deterioration. Usually doctors who do not read this literature are not programmed to check hgb A1C unless the person has diabetes. Furthermore, many other nutrients control this (some you already learned about in Chapter 1, like Acetyl-L-Carnitine, B1 and magnesium, as examples). I will show you later how to know if you have enough.

Another powerful way to reduce the damage from sugars is with one of the 8 forms of vitamin E, **gamma tocopherol**. It actually **revs up the control of A1C** (by regulating its precursor methylglyoxal), preventing the rise in A1C that leads to mitochondrial damage, glucose intolerance, accelerated aging, endothelial dysfunction (arteriosclerosis, high blood pressure, angina, etc.).   Unfortunately, when I look at the Cardio/IONs the vast majority of folks are low in gamma tocopherol, while most folks are never even ever measured. And studies bear this out.

So whether or not you have diabetes I would make sure you add one **Gamma E Gems** to your daily two **E Gems Elite** and 2-4 **Tocotrienols** (in split doses). And of course in all of the studies that denigrated vitamin E, those researchers were too ignorant to include gamma tocopherol, which is why their studies ended up "proving" that vitamin E doesn't help any chronic diseases like diabetes, heart disease and cancer.   For to make matters worse, as I've shown, a-tocopherol (the only E they use in those studies) actually lowers the level of any gamma that you did get from food! So they made folks even worse and didn't even know why. So be it. You are smarter (and probably healthier) than they are.

With just these tiny examples I trust you are getting jolted into an infinitely more honest, a new but truer picture of how the "practice" of medicine works, and how much healing power is totally ignored at the expense of drug profits. So let's continue to crack some other myths about diabetes as we continue to expose and explore the incomparable healing power of nutrients.

References:

• Masterjohn C, et al, γ-**Tocopherol abolishes postprandial increases in** plasma **methylglyoxal** following an oral dose of glucose in healthy, college-aged men, *J Nutr Biochem* 23:292-8, 2012

• Jiang Q, Ames BN, **Gamma-tocopherol, but not a-tocopherol, decreases pro-inflammatory eicosanoids and inflammation damage** in rats, *FASEB J* 17:816-22, 2003

- Saldeen T, et al, **Differential effects of alpha-and gamma-tocopherol** on low-density lipoprotein oxidation, superoxide activity, platelet aggregation and arterial thrombosis, *J Am Coll Cardiol* 34:1208-15, 1999

- Ford ES, et al, Distribution of serum concentrations of alpha-tocopherol and gamma-tocopherol in U.S. population, *Am J Clin Nutr* 84:375-83, 2006

- Bierhaus A, et al, Advanced **glycation**-induced activation of NF-kappa B is **suppressed by a-lipoic acid** in cultured endothelial cells, *Diabetes* 46; 9:1481-90, Sept 1997

- Davie SJ, et al, Effect of **vitamin C** on glycosylation of proteins, may **reduce glycosylation**. *Diabetes* 41:167-73, 1992

- Ceriello A, et al, **Vitamin E reduction of protein glycosylation** in diabetes. New prospect for prevention of diabetic complications, *Diabetes Care* 14; 1:68-72, 1991

- Jain SK, et al, **Lipoic acid decreases** lipid peroxidation and protein **glycosylation** and increases (Na++ K+)- and Ca++-ATPase activities in high post-treated red blood cells (RBC). *Free Rad Biol Med* 29; 11:1122-28, 2000

- Nakamura S, et al, **Pyridoxal phosphate prevents progression of diabetic nephropathy,** *Nephrol Dialysis Transplant,* 22:2165-74, 2007

- Goepp J, **B6 vitamins: natural protection against the complications of diabetes and accelerated aging,** *Life Extension, Collector' s Edition 2010,* 99-107, 2010, 1-800-544-4440

- Depeint F, et al, Mitochondrial function and toxicity: Role of B vitamins, one-carbon transfer pathways, *Chemico-Biologl Interact* 163:113-32, 2006

- Jain SK, et al, **Pyridoxine** and pyridoxamine inhibit superoxide radicals and **prevents** lipid peroxidation, protein **glycosylation** and (Na+ + K+)-ATPase activity reduction in high glucose-treated human erythrocytes, *Free Rad Biol Med* 30:232-37, 2001

- Onarato JM, et al**, Pyridoxamine, an inhibitor of glycation reactions**, also inhibits lipid peroxidation reactions, *J Biol Chem,* 275:21177-84, 2000

- Metz TO, et al, **Pyridoxamine** traps intermediates in lipid peroxidation reactions in vivo: evidence on the role of lipids and chemical modification of protein **and development of diabetic complications**, *J Biol Chem* 278:42012-19, 2003

- Booth AA, et al, **Thiamine pyrophosphate and pyridoxamine inhibit** the formation of antigenic advanced **glycation** end-products: comparison with aminoguanidine, *Biochem Biophys Res Commun,* 220:113-19, 1996

- Stitt A, et al, The **AGE inhibitor pyridoxine inhibits development of retinopathy** in experimental diabetes, *Diabetes* 51:2826-32, 2000

- Laines-Cessac P, et al, Mechanisms of the **inhibition of human erythrocyte pyridoxal kinase by drugs,** *Biochem Pharmacol* 54:863-70, 1997

- Yudkin JS, et al, Unexplained variability in glycated hemoglobin in non-diabetic subjects not related to glycemia, *Diabetologia* 33; 4:208-15, 1990).

51

"If My Sugars Go Up in Spite of a Good Diet, I Need Diabetes Medications"

Wrong! If your sugars are out of whack, you are deficient in nutrients that regulate sugars in the body. This can start with (1) how insulin is produced, or (2) how sugars are processed, or (3) how insulin inserts itself into the cell membrane receptor, or (4) how the cell mitochondria fail to make energy even when supplied with glucose. For example, as you'll learn in the next chapter, chromium is absolutely essential for the cure of diabetes. After seeing the evidence from decades of brilliant researchers, I feel any diabetologist who doesn't check red blood cell chromium levels shouldn't even be practicing. For chromium has been known for over three decades to not only control the metabolism of sugar, but triglycerides, cholesterol, and arteriosclerosis, but much more. As I showed in much more detail in *The Cholesterol Hoax*, it's crucial for many other aspects of cardiovascular health.

And of course, this is not the only nutrient that is missing when your body cannot control your sugar levels. For example, **vitamin K is essential for control of diabetes** (Sakamoto). Yet how often does a diabetologist prescribe it? In addition vitamin C, vitamin D, magnesium, vitamin E (which includes all of its eight parts), and much more are also crucial. And then besides acetyl-L-carnitine, and R-lipoic acid that you began earlier learning a little bit about, there are nutrients that you may not hear much about like one of the B vitamins, biotin. But there's much more to know (Mingrone, Konrad, Anderson, Paolisso, Knekt, Salonen). However, don't worry, I won't give you the evidence for every nutrient here. For I want this book to be light enough for you to be able to carry it to the beach. And I'll map out later what to take.

Are you beginning to get the picture? **Medicine is failing you miserably if you're just prescribed a drug. For don't forget that drugs continually lower even more nutrients** in the work of being detoxified by the body. Not only that, they are doubly dangerous because they've enabled you to ignore fixing what's

52

actually broken. By not addressing the above nutrients you set yourself up for a major heart attack, cancers, accelerated aging and every chronic disease you can think of. Yet these are merely considered the "expected" consequences of having diabetes. Does anyone ever blame the doctor who prescribed the drugs without looking for the curable causes? Yet it has been proven repeatedly that **when you take drugs, the sick get sicker, quicker**. Do you still think you're getting a fair shake by taking a medicine rather than repairing your body?

References:

• Mingrone G, et al, **L-carnitine improves glucose** disposal and type II diabetic patients, *J Am Coll Nutr* 18; 1:77-82, 1999

• Konrad T, et al, Alpha **lipoic acid** treatment **decreases serum lactate and pyruvate** concentrations and **improves glucose** effectiveness in lean and obese patients with type II diabetes, *Diabetes Care*, 22:280-87, 1999

• Paolisso G, et al, Pharmacological doses of **vitamin E improved insulin action** in healthy subjects and non--insulin-dependent diabetics, *Am J Clin Nutr* 57; 5:650-56, 1993

• Anderson RA, Elevated intake of supplemental **chromium improved glucose and insulin** variables in individuals with type II diabetes, *Diabetes* 46:1786-91, 1997

• Knekt P, et al, **Low vitamin E status is a potential risk factor for type insulin-dependent diabetes mellitus,** *J Intern Med* 245:99-102, 1999

• Abram A, et al, The effects of **supplementation on serum glucose** and lipids in non-insulin-dependent diabetics, *Metab* 41; 7:768-71, 1992

• Riales R, et al, Effect of **chromium** chloride **supplementation on glucose** tolerance and serum lipids including high-density lipoprotein of adult men, *Am J Clin Nutr* 34:2670-78, **1981**

• Anderson RA, **Chromium, glucose intolerance and diabetes**, *J Am Coll Nutr* 17:548-55, 1998

• Anderson RA, **Chromium in the prevention and control of diabetes**, *Diabetes Metab* 26:22-27, 2000

• Offenbacher EG, et al, Beneficial effect of **chromium**-rich yeast **on glucose tolerance** and blood lipids in elderly subjects, *Diabetes* 29:919-25, **1980**

• Maebashi M, et al, Therapeutic evaluation of the **effect of biotin on hypoglycemia** in patients with non-insulin-dependent diabetes mellitus, *J Clin Biochem Nutr*, 14:211-18, 1993

• Coggeshall JC, et al, **Biotin** status and plasma **glucose in diabetics**, *Ann N Y Acad Sci* 447:389-92, 1985

• Eriksson J, et al, **Magnesium and ascorbic acid** supplementation in diabetes mellitus may **improve glucose tolerance**, *Ann Nutr Metab*, 39:217-23, 1995

• Bierenbaum ML, et al, The effect of supplemental **vitamin E** on serum parameters in diabetics, post coronary and normal subjects, **improved glucose** tolerance, *Nutr Rep Int*, 31:1171-80, 1985

- Salonen JT, et al, Increased risk of non-insulin-dependent diabetes mellitus at low plasma vitamin E concentrations: a four year follow-up study in men, *Brit Med J*, 311:1124-27, 1995

- Boucher BJ, An adequate vitamin D status: does it contribute to the disorders comprising syndrome "X'?, *Br J Nutr* 79:315-27, 1998

- Albarracin CA, et al, **Chromium picolinate and biotin combination improves glucose** metabolism in treated, uncontrolled overweight to obese patients with type 2 diabetes, *Diab Metab Res Rev* 24; 1:41-51, Jan 2008

- Kent H, **Vanadium for diabetes**, *CMAJ*, 160; 1:17, 1999

- Labriji-Mestaghanmi H, et al, **Vitamin D and pancreatic islet function**, *J Endocrine Invest* 11:577-84, 1988

- Salonen JT, et al, **Increased risk of non--insulin-dependent diabetes mellitus at low plasma vitamin D concentrations**: a four year follow-up study in men, *Brit Med J* 311:1124-27, 1995

- Sakamoto N, et al, **Low vitamin K intake effects on glucose tolerance** in rats, *Internat J Vit Nutr Res* 69:27-31, 1999

- Sakamoto N, et al., Relationship between acute insulin response and vitamin K intake and healthy young male volunteers, *Diab Nutr Metab* 12:37-41, 1999

- Sakamoto N, et al, Possible effects of one week or vitamin K (menaquinone-4) tablets intake on glucose tolerance in healthy young male volunteers with different descarboxy prothrombin levels, *Clin Nutr* 19:259-63, 2000

"I Have Incurable Insulin Resistance or Metabolic Syndrome X"

Metabolic syndrome or Syndrome X is not incurable. It is merely a constellation of risk factors that leads to early heart death. They **include (any or all): obesity, high triglycerides and low HDL, elevated blood pressure, weight gain that won't budge, and elevated sugars and/or elevated insulin (insulin resistance).** The only reason insulin resistance (also called metabolic syndrome, also called Syndrome X) is called "incurable" is because there's no medication for it. But you will learn you can cure it yourself.

What do you think insulin resistance really means? Normally when insulin comes knocking at the cell door it fits into the cell membrane receptor like a key in a lock. It opens the cell "door" so sugar can enter the cell and be used to create energy. But when the lock on the outside of the cell is broken, the key doesn't work. That's called **insulin resistance**. Insulin comes knocking at the door but the cell is deaf, dysfunctional, in a state of disrepair. It

54

doesn't respond. So the pancreas sends out even more insulin. As your insulin level rises, the knowledge-challenged doc diagnoses insulin resistance or metabolic syndrome X and it automatically becomes a deficiency of a drug. How do you repair this lock or docking site or receptor (use whatever analogy that helps you conceptualize this)? Simply **by repairing the insulin receptors on the surface of the cell**. **The membrane of every cell contains** all sorts of receptors or **docking sites**, including those **for insulin**. To further oversimplify **the cell membrane** (or coating or cell envelope), you can think of the cell membrane (which holds the docking site) as a sandwich, **a double-layered lining for every cell**. The "bread" of the sandwich is cod liver oil, and the "meat" of the sandwich is phosphatidyl choline, with the eight forms of vitamin E being the salt and pepper. This information is not new. I described it in detail in *Detoxify Or Die* and it has been **known for a quarter of a century that mere cod liver oil in many people can stop them from getting insulin resistance** (Storlien). But where are the doctors who should be recommending this?

There are many other "spices" that are needed in this cell membrane envelope or "sandwich", like magnesium, zinc, vanadium, chromium, etc., but you get the picture. In fact, as one example, you will notice from the references that **magnesium deficiency has been known for over 20 years to be a curable cause of insulin resistance. So there is no excuse for a diabetologist who fails to check it.** Plus when magnesium goes lower it can lead to sudden death by heart attack. You don't have to be a molecular biochemist to know that you can repair all of this chemistry and bring it back to normal or to where you were before you got sick. And for most folks (like myself), once they repaired nutrient deficiencies, they actually got better than they had ever been in their entire lives. Don't fret. We'll go through these nutrients in more detail later with their doses and sources.

As you will learn there are many other causes for metabolic syndrome, because like every disease, **it depends on each**

individual person's deficiencies and toxicities. For example, **vitamin K is crucial in many pathways needed to cure diabetes or syndrome X.** Yet a surprisingly significant portion of the populace is deficient in vitamin K (Pan), and especially those on coumadin (it literally poisons vitamin K synthesis).

Yet how many diabetologists ever check your vitamin K level? Or for that matter, how many even know what test to check? In fact this would make *a quick little test* of whether or not the doctor you have chosen to manage your diabetes is capable of helping you cure it or if he's just a legal drug pusher. Innocently asked him "Are you going to check my vitamin K level, Doctor?", and see what kind of response you get. If you get a denigrating look suggesting you don't know anything, you are in the wrong office. Or if he thinks it is only for clotting blood and suggests that is not something you want, he's a dinosaur. If he actually says he plans on it, then ask "And what test are you going to use?". If he says he will check a vitamin K level, he has failed and doesn't know that the **best test is the undercarboxylated osteocalcin**. It's a very sad era when you have to learn the molecular biochemistry of healing and **you even have to test your physician**. But so be it. Consider yourselves lucky that you know how to do it.

And if he does order a mere vitamin K level, don't fall for being told you're okay if your level is in the normal range. Look at it this way. Since there is a high degree of unrecognized deficiency of K in many folks, you don't want to be compared with whatever their levels are. Unfortunately labs are forced to define "normal" as where 95% of random population's blood test results fall. But you don't care where everyone else is, especially someone who eats junk food, takes drugs, has several diagnostic labels, is in ICU or on death's doorstep and knows nothing about health. You only want to know if *your* body has a high enough vitamin K to perform optimally. This type of test is called *a functional assay*. It is the most useful test for you and your doctor to determine how much vitamin K your system actually needs to make you healthy, not just how you stack up next to the "average" person. We don't all just look different. Each has an individual chemistry inside as well, that differentiates us from others. Therein lies a huge difference.

The test called an **undercarboxylated osteocalcin is high when there is not enough vitamin K.** And K is not just for syndrome X, but other diabetic complications. It makes a hormone in our bodies called osteocalcin that is not only needed to make our bones strong, but keep calcium from building up in the lining of blood vessels ("hardening of the arteries" or arteriosclerosis or coronary artery disease) and calcifying heart vessels.

In essence, as I showed in *Is Your Cardiologist Killing You?*, **vitamin K is crucial for preventing the main calcium deposits or plaque** in arteries and heart valves. This is pivotal for everyone, not just those with metabolic syndrome or diabetes. **Vitamin K has even caused regression (melting away) of plaque** (Schurgers). But as you learned in the first chapter, without sufficient vitamin K (as poisoned by coumadin, also called warfarin), calcium gets pulled from the bone and dumped into heart valves and arteries (much more detail and references are in *The Cholesterol Hoax)*. Not only that but **osteocalcin regulates the pancreas, insulin response and even the genes that make us fat; but only if there is enough vitamin K** (Ferron, Lee, Sakamoto). Again the evidence is overwhelming. In fact it's so overwhelming that **vitamin K adequacy is actually a marker for whether or not you die of early heart disease** (Erkkila, Jie). How can any diabetologist neglect checking your functional vitamin K adequacy?

The focus of this book is not to show you how to get off Coumadin. But I mention it since many diabetics have atrial fibrillation and other symptoms that lead to Coumadin prescriptions which then needlessly lead to accelerated calcification of their heart valves and coronary arteries. Clearly, no one is going to cure your metabolic syndrome until they also include enough **Vitamin K2**, and much more. Also studies show that vitamin K2 and not K-1 is the preferred form to protect

57

vascular health and decrease calcifications (Beulens). Remember, **one in five Americans between age 20 to 45 in the U.S. now have metabolic syndrome**. Furthermore, there's also a crucial need for balancing of vitamin K with other vitamins like D and minerals like zinc, as you will learn further on (Braam, Pan).

References:

• Sakamoto N, et al, Relationship between acute **insulin response and vitamin K** intake and healthy young male volunteers, *Diab Nutr Metab* 12:37-41, 1999

• Ferron M, et al**, Osteocalcin differentially regulates beta cell and adipocyte gene expression** and affects the development of metabolic diseases in wild-type mice, *Proc Nat Acad Sci USA* 105:5 to 66-70, 2008

• Lee NK, et al, Endocrine regulation of energy metabolism by the skeleton, *Cell* 130:456-69, 2007

• Erkkila AT, et al, Phylloquinone intake as a marker for coronary heart disease risk but not stroke in women, *Euro J Clin Nutr* 59:196-204, 2005

• Jie KS, et al, Vitamin K intake and osteocalcin levels in women with and without aortic atherosclerosis: a population-based study, *Atherosclerosis* 116:117-123, 1995

• Schurgers IJ, et al, **Regression of warfarin-induced medial elastocalcinosis by high intake of vitamin K** in rats, *Blood* 109:2823-31, 2007).

• Beulens JW, et al, High dietary **menaquinone** intake is associated with **reduced coronary calcifications**, *Atherosclerosis* 203:489-93, 2009).

• Braam LA, et al, Beneficial effects of **vitamin D and K on the elastic properties of the vessel** wall in postmenopausal women: a follow-up study, *Thrombosis Hemostasis* 91:373-80, 2004

• Pan Y, et al, Dietary **phylloquinone intakes and metabolic syndrome** in U.S. young adults, *J Am Coll Nutr* 28; 4:369-79, 2009

• Lombardo YB, et al, Effects of dietary polyunsaturated **n-3 fatty acids** on dyslipidemia and **insulin resistance** in rodents and humans, A review, *J Nutr Biochem,* 17:1-13, 2006

• American Diabetes Association, Magnesium supplementation in the treatment of diabetes. Connection between **magnesium deficiency and insulin resistance**, *Diabetes Care* 15:1065-67, **1992**

• Paolisso G, et al, **Improved insulin response and action by chronic magnesium** administration in aged NIDDM subjects, *Diabetes Care* 12:265-69, 1989

• Popp-Snidjers C, et al, Dietary supplementation of **omega-3 polyunsaturated fatty acids improves insulin sensitivity** in non-insulin-dependent diabetes, *Diabetes Res*, 4 141-7, 1987

• Halberstam M, et al, Oral **vanadyl sulfate improves insulin sensitivity** in NIDDM but not in obese non-diabetic subjects, *Diabetes* 45:659-66, 1996

• Faure P, et al, **Zinc and insulin sensitivity**, *Biol Trace Elem Res*, 32:305-10, 1992

• Lombardo YB, et al, **Metabolic syndrome: effects of n-3** PUFAs on a model of dyslipidemia, insulin resistance and adiposity, *Lipids* 42; 5:427-37, May 2007

- Storlien LH, et al, **Fish oil prevents insulin resistance** induced by high-fat feeding in rats, *Sci* 237; 4817:885-88, **1987**

- Anderson RA, **Chromium** and polyphenols from **cinnamon improves insulin sensitivity**, *Proc Nutr Soc* 67; 1:48-53, Feb 2008

"My Doctor Says It's Dangerous and Foolish Not to Take a Diabetes Drug to Lower My Sugar"

Remember from the preceding chapter that **after being perfect patients and taking 5 years of the leading prescribed diabetes drugs**, plus even taking drugs for related conditions like high blood pressure or high cholesterol, that there was NO IMPROVEMENT, NO ADVANTAGE. **Patients did not live longer**. Nor did taking meds reduce the number of heart attacks, strokes, etc. And if you think that is a waste of money and body metabolism, the two leading diabetes drugs, Avandia (generic rosiglitazone) and Actos (pioglitazone), more than double your rate of heart attack!! Dr. Nissen of the Cleveland Clinic published in 2007 that **Avandia resulted in a 43% greater risk of a heart attack. Yet it has remained on the market for well over 5 years** after this. And this is even after an FDA drug-safety official also publicly warned of this drug (Whalen). There is no protection from the power of the drug industry. We are on our own.

Let's take a look at a smattering of the evidence for the importance of just some nutrients that are necessary to lower your blood sugar. A substance similar to the body's **CoQ10 dropped sugar levels 31% in diabetics** (Shigeta). This has been known for over 50 years. You make your own coenzyme Q10 inside your mitochondria.....if they are healthy. They are little kidney bean-shaped organelles inside our cells where God's miracle of converting a molecule of food into a molecule of energy occurs. And this energy is what we define as "life".

If I were suddenly dead in front of you, I am the same mass of chemicals that I was as a live person. The only difference is my electricity that creates energy has stopped flowing. Likewise, if your mitochondrial CoQ10 is poisoned from environmental toxins, nutrient deficiencies, or medications like blood pressure drugs like metaprolol or cholesterol-lowering statin drugs like Lipitor, Crestor, Vytorin, etc., then your diabetes can go out of control for lack of CoQ10 (Ghirlanda, Bliznakov). And even though the **lowering of CoQ10 from statin cholesterol-lowering drugs** has been known for over 20 years, it is not checked or supplemented by the majority of physicians who prescribe statins. But as the deficiency continues, it leads to not only diabetes, but fatal heart failure, tooth and hair loss, depression, high blood pressure and more.

Later you will also learn that **a mineral like vanadium or a vitamin like biotin can act as insulin mimics** in the body. Multiple other nutrients as well are needed. You have seen only a smattering of the decades of enormous evidence proving nutrients control the body's sugar. That's how the body was designed to work. It was not designed as a Metformin or Avandia deficiency. **Foods and nutrients harmonize to orchestrate not only wellness, but healing against all odds**. Our bodies possess an unfathomable and magnificent molecular biochemistry beyond description that scientists have unsuccessfully tried to duplicate. So my question is where are the diabetologists who know and use this?

References:

- Whalen J, Mundy A, **FDA scientist attacks Avandia safety**, *WSJ*, B4, Jun 11, 2010

- Shigeta Y, et al, Effect of coenzyme Q7 treatment on blood sugar and ketone bodies of diabetics, *J Vitaminol* (Kyoto) 12:293-8, **1966**

- Ghirlanda G, et al, Evidence of plasma CoQ10-lowering effects of HMG-CoA reductase inhibitors, *J Clin Pharmacol*, 33; 3:226-9, 1993 (for 20 years this has been known!)

- Bliznakov EG, et al, Biochemical and clinical consequences of **inhibiting coenzyme Q10 biosynthesis by lipid lowering** HMG-CoA reductase inhibitors (**statins**): a critical overview, *Adv Ther*, 15; 4:218-28, 1998

- Paolisso G, et al, Pharmacological doses of **vitamin E improved insulin action** in healthy subjects and non-insulin-dependent diabetics, *Am J Clin Nutr* 57; 5:650-56, 1993

"My Doctor Says I Must Take Medicines to Prevent Kidney Damage"

What's the first thing that happens when a diabetic goes to his doctor for a check up? The nurse usually runs away with a sample of your urine to check for albumin, a protein that kidneys lose when they are starting to die. Yet sometimes preventing and/or **curing the kidney disease that kills diabetics, called diabetic nephropathy, can be as simple as repairing a deficiency of thiamine (vitamin B1) or Pyridoxal-5-Phosphate** (the metabolite of vitamin B6, if you have enough zinc), as just two examples of extremely inexpensive yet powerful and neglected nutrients. Yet medications like angiotensin converting enzyme inhibitors are prescribed, even though they have disappointing results.

As one example, pyridoxal-5-phosphate (**P5P**), a metabolite of vitamin B6, **can stop albumin loss** that leads to dialysis. But P5P does a lot more. It also lowers HGB A1C as well as the risk for blindness, amputations, heart attacks, and Alzheimer's, which are also common side effects of diabetes. In fact in view of the evidence, it looks like anyone whose diabetes has progressed to blindness, amputations, heart attacks or kidney disease requiring dialysis has been treated by someone who does not read and study the very disease he's licensed to treat. I could actually fill this book just with the evidence for P5P alone, much less all the other nutrients that are needed as well. But don't worry, I won't.

One out of every three diabetics develops serious and potentially fatal kidney disease Since **anyone with kidney disease usually also has heavy metals** (like aluminum, cadmium, lead, arsenic, mercury, etc.) on board contributing to it, hooking them up to a dialysis machine which further raises the levels of aluminum is eventually counterproductive. The safest, non-prescription, and least expensive ways of removing heavy metals from the body will be in chapter 6.

Albumin is the protein that is the blood stream carrier or transporter for most medications as well as nutrients. When its **level starts going down** in the standard blood tests that all doctors do (chemical profile) and starts going up in the urine, this shows that the kidneys are damaged and leaking. **This can a subtle early sign that the person will potentially be dead in a few years.** That's when dialysis comes to the "rescue" as it becomes a substitute kidney. The diabetic is hooked up to IVs weekly and sometimes daily depending on the severity. Plastic intravenous lines connect him to a dialysis machine that does the work that the kidneys are no longer able to do, cleaning the blood. But at the same time dialysis machine and tubes fill him with chemicals (cyclohexanone, phthalates, etc.) that make diabetes' complications worse, as you will learn (Thompson-Torgerson).

Yet just to show how dangerously misguided drug-focused medicine is, literal pennies a day of **Vitamin B-1 (thiamine)** given three times a day in just three months has **lowered the albumin loss more than 40%** in patients. In fact in 35% of diabetics **just pennies a day of thiamine (B1) literally reversed or cured this common diabetic complication that invariably leads to death.** Even vitamin C has lowered the albumin and improved diabetic kidney disease (Lee). Because of this, you can appreciate what little value I place on a dangerous diabetologist who chooses instead to medicate with expensive side effect-laden drugs which have never cured the problem and lead to dialysis. Yet this is the standard or norm in medicine.

Needless to say, just measuring the thiamine level is for amateur physicians who do not understand that **a blood level in the "normal" range does not mean it is in the "optimal" range for** *that* **person. Far superior tests are what we call functional,** such as the pyruvate and lactate levels (as found on the **Cardio/ION** that you will learn about later). These **show whether the person needs more thiamine (B1) than the average person** and not just whether or not he has the same levels as the "average" overly-medicated "walking wounded" sick person.

References:

- Nakamura S, et al, **Pyridoxal phosphate prevents progression of diabetic nephropathy,** *Nephrology Dialysis Transplantation,* 22:2165-74, 2007

- Thompson-Torgerson CS, et al, **Cyclohexanone contamination** from extracorporeal circuits **impairs cardiovascular function,** *Am J Physiol Heart Circul Physiol* 296: H1926-32, 2009

- Ritz E, Diabetic nephropathy in type II diabetes, *J Intern Med,* 245: 111-126, 1999

- Rabbani N, et al, **High-dose thiamine therapy for patients with type II diabetes and microalbuminuria**: a randomized, double-blind placebo-controlled pilot study, *Diabetologia,* 52:208-12, 2009

- Baylis C, et al, Peroxisome proliferated-activated receptor gamma agonist provides superior renal protection versus angiotensin converting enzyme inhibition in a rat model of type II diabetes with obesity, *J Pharmacol Exper Therapeut,* 307; 3:854-60, 2003

- Lee EY, et al, Blockade of oxidative stress by **vitamin C ameliorates albuminuria** and renal sclerosis and experimental diabetic rats, *Yonsei Med J,* 48; 5:847-55, 2007

"My Doctor Says Nutrients Have No Place in Diabetes"

I'm embarrassed for him. This is the true mark of a dinosaur. If I put all the evidence for nutrients in this book, it would be well over 6 feet thick. Let's look at just one example, vitamin D, since there is a huge hidden epidemic deficiency of this in the United States, the land of plenty. How does the diabetic die? Usually of a sudden heart attack. But the right amount of **minerals like magnesium, selenium, vanadium, zinc, chromium, manganese, and much more are absolutely crucial for not only healing diabetes but for preventing a sudden cardiac arrest.** Likewise you need the right fatty acids like the omega-3s, as found in cod liver oil and the "oil change", plus other antioxidants, and to repair nutrient deficiencies, as identified in the Cardio/ION.

OK, let's look at one vitamin, D. In one study of over 100,000 people who had **higher than average levels of vitamin D, these folks had a 43% lower risk of any heart or vascular or metabolic disease.** For starters, folks with high levels of vitamin D in their blood had 33% less cardiovascular disease and **55% less of**

type II diabetes (adult onset) and **51% had less metabolic syndrome** (inability to lose weight, high blood pressure, elevated triglycerides, and more).

And remember (1) this is only one nutrient, (2) most doctors don't measure it, (3) and when they do they often prescribe a weekly synthetic one that doesn't work as well in the human body, plus (4) the cut-off for the lowest permissible level of vitamin D in most labs is too low, leaving most folks deceivably "normal", when in reality they are deficient. The optimal level should be over 60 ng/mL, whereas most labs mandated by government advisers using antiquated data, cut off at around 30. Most folks need at least 1-2 **Solar D Gems** 4000 I.U. a day to attain a blood level of over 75 ng/mL (or 150 nmol/L). Unfortunately, due to the arbitrary **government definition of "normal" as any living being** who can send a specimen to a lab, many labs erroneously report results over 60 as too high (Aloia, Holick, Hollis).

As with any nutrient won't he be surprised if other things are improved? For example, as we've shown in *TW*, vitamin D is crucial for reversing depression and reversing coronary artery plaque, plus you cannot heal osteoporosis without it. And even more importantly, you can't heal cancers without it since it causes re-differentiation (making cancer cells go back to normal). As one example, **there is a 50% drop in the rate of prostate cancer (as well as bowel and other cancers) if your vitamin D level is even at rock bottom of the pathetically inferior "normal" (20 ng/mL).** Just imagine what benefit there is with the right dose!

Lack of knowledge like this has contributed to astronomical epidemics. For example, now more than **20% of Americans have non-alcoholic fatty liver disease (NAFLD or NASH) which then can proceed to cirrhosis or cancer of the liver** and a high percentage of folks share this with their insulin sensitivity and/or diabetes (Fernandez-Real). Yet they are all curable.

As several prominent researchers have suggested, it should be malpractice for a diabetologist to fail to at least prescribe, much less fail to actually measure how much you need of such nutrients as vitamin **D3, R-Lipoic Acid, Acetyl L-Carnitine, DHEA, DHA, Vanadium, Chromium, Manganese, Moly B** (molybdenum), and *much* more. Meanwhile, when you have diabetes, you must **think of "D for diabetes"**. Could **D** also warn you to *distance yourself from dinosaur diabetologists who are dangerous dullards disinterested in destroying disease*? Begin your search for your **Dr. Dynamo!**

References:

• Fernandez-Real JM, et al, Circulating soluble CD36 is a novel marker of liver injury in subjects with altered glucose tolerance, *J Nutr Biochem* 20:477-84, 2009

• Parker J, et al, Levels of vitamin D and cardiometabolic disorders: systemic review and meta-analysis, *Maturitas*, 225-36, 2010

• Aloia JF, et al, Vitamin D intake to attain a desire to 25-hydroxy vitamin D concentration, *Am J Clin Nutr* 87:1952-58, 2008

• Holick MF, Vitamin D deficiency, *New Engl J Med,* 357;3:266-81, 2007

• Hollis BW, Circulating 25-hydroxy D levels indicative of vitamin D deficiency: **implications for establishing a new effective dietary intake recommendation for vitamin D,** *J Nutr* 135;2:317-22, 2005

• Chen TC, et al, **Vitamin D and prostate cancer prevention and treatment,** *Trends Endocrinol Metab* 14:423-30, 2003

• Whitlatch LW, et al, 25-Hydroxy **vitamin D-1-a-hydroxylase activity is diminished in human prostate cancer cells** and is enhanced by gene transfer, *J Steroid Biochem Molec Biol* 81:135-40, 2002

• Schwartz GG, et al, Human prostate cells synthesize 1,25-dihydroxy-vitamin D3 from 25-hydroxyvitamin D3, *Cancer Epidemiol Biomarkers Prev* 7:391-95, 1998

• Aydemir-Koksoy A, et al, **Antioxidant treatment protects diabetic** rats from **cardiac dysfunction** by preserving contractile protein targets of oxidative stress, *J Nutr Biochem* 21:827-833, 2010

Ayez M, et al, **Prevention of diabetes-induced alterations in [Zn2+]** and metallothionein level of the rat **heart** by a restoration of cell redox cycle, *Am J Physiol,* 290:H 1071-80, 2006

• Morris CD, et al, **Routine vitamin supplementation to prevent cardiovascular disease: a summary of the evidence for the U.S. Preventive Services Task Force,** *Ann Intern Med* 139:56-70, 2003

• McNeill JH, et al, **Insulin-like effects of sodium selenate** in stretozotocin-induced diabetic rats, *Diabetes* 40:1675-8, 1991

- Berg EA, et al, **Insulin-like effects of the vanadate and selenate** on the expression of glucose-6-phosphate dehydrogenase and fatty acid synthase in diabetic rats, *Biochimie*, 77:919-24, 1995

- Tuncay E, et al, Gender related different effects of **omega-3 treatment on diabetes-induced left ventricular dysfunction,** *Mol Cell Biochem* , 304:255-63, 2007

- Bjelackovic G, et al, **Antioxidant supplements for prevention of mortality** in healthy participants and patients with various diseases, *Cochrane Database Syst Rev* 16; 2: CD007176, 2008

- Jude S, et al, Dietary long-chain **omega-3 fatty acids** of marine origin: a comparison of their **protective effects of coronary heart disease and breast cancers,** *Progr Biophys Mol Biol*, 90:299-325, 2006

- Turan B, et al, Oxidative **effects of selenite on** rat **ventricular contractility and Ca+2** movements, *Cardiovasc Res*, 32:351-61, 1996

- Bloch-Damti A, et al, Proposed mechanism for the **induction of insulin resistance by oxidative stress,** *Antiox Redox Signal* 7:1553-67, 2005

"I Need Medications for My Heart Failure"

Ask any cardiologist if severe congestive heart failure is completely reversible, completely curable, and ….. (the hooker) all without drugs. He will tell you, "Absolutely not". Then ask him then if there has ever been anything to rejuvenate the failing heart muscle and actually bring it back to normal. He will probably answer "Never", but he kindly tells you he wishes there were.

Let's look at one tiny example, the mineral copper. Years ago researchers decided to study the adequacy of copper in the healthiest men on the planet they could find, U.S. Navy SEALS. And even though the researchers used the least sensitive test there is for copper adequacy, **over a third of the supposedly healthiest specimens were deficient in copper.** This deficiency is even more rampant nowadays because diets are more depleted, folks are eating more processed foods, the soils are more depleted as well, plus medications use up nutrients.

Yet researchers in medical schools in the United States have shown that, **you can actually cure congestive heart failure by repairing a copper deficiency,** as just one nutrient example. Of course, it always depends upon the total deficiencies that each individual brings to the table. Meanwhile, **the failing heart muscle was**

literally regenerated. This is something that's unheard of in medicine, because they rarely cure anything, much less heart failure. The rule in congestive heart failure (CHF) is to progressively pile on more drugs. Many end-stage heart failure patients are on well over $10,000 of medications each year, and the median time of death is 5 years after diagnosis.

But **copper can even make heart cells regenerate or revert back to being entirely normal**. The same goes for zinc, magnesium, chromium, and many other minerals that are important in the body, *depending on the individual's deficiencies*. I'll show you how to determine your needs later. The sad thing is that this has been known for over a quarter of a century that **people who die from heart attacks, heart failure and cardiomyopathy have much lower levels of copper, as well as lower levels of other nutrients in their hearts.** Yet show me a diabetologist or cardiologist who ever checks your RBC (red blood cell or erythrocyte) copper, and I'll show you a dynamo cardiologist you should keep.

Just remember: **no disease is the deficiency of some drug or device**. If you care about a physician and want him to give you the best care, start him with *Is Your Cardiologist Killing You?*. If he doesn't have time, move on, since it's highly referenced, extremely concise and a quick read (10 minutes a day in two weeks!). It has condensed years of research into the most concise and practical way to cure heart disease that exists. If he doesn't have time for this quick read, he is closed for learning, has no interest in curing your problems and does not care to move beyond the comfort of the drug- and device-orientation of medicine. If you have a serious disease, you must know what tests to insist your doctor order, and then how to proceed with the most common cures for your symptoms (and *TW* 2012 tells you how to *order your own tests* if he won't).

I've seen heart failure folks who were scheduled for ablation go from barely able to walk across the room because of shortness of breath to completely reversing their heart disease. And they went back to tennis, golf, dancing, etc., and they were able to shed their drugs and avoid damaging ablation! Fortunately once you are over the ignorance hump you can never be fooled again.

References:

•   Zhou Z, et al, **Regression of copper-deficient heart hypertrophy**: reduction in the size of hypertrophic cardiomyocytes, *J Nutr Biochem* 20:621-28, 2009

•   Zhou Y, et al, **Copper reverses cardiomyocytes hypertrophy** through vascular endothelial growth factor-mediation reduction in the cell size, *J Molec Cell Cardiol* 45:106-17, 2008

•   Jiang Y, et al, Dietary **Copper supplementation reverses hypertrophic cardiomyopathy** induced by chronic pressure overload in mice, *J Exp Med* 204:657-66, 2007

•   Medeiros DM, et al, Newer findings on a unified perspective of copper restriction and cardiomyopathy, *Proc Soc Exp Biol Med*, 215:299-313, 1997

•   Elsherif L, et al, **Regression of** dietary copper restriction-induced **cardiomyopathy by copper** repletion in mice, *J Nutr* 134:855-60, 2004

•   Mancini DM, et al. Low incidence of myocardial recovery after left ventricular assist device implantation in patients with chronic heart failure, *Circulation* 98:2883-89, 1998

•   Zama N, et al, Cardiac copper, magnesium, and zinc in recent and old myocardial infarction, *Biolog Trace Elem Res* 10:201-8, 1986

•   Webster PO, Trace elements in human myocardial infarction determined by neutron activation analysis, *Acta Scand Med*, 178:765-88, 1965

•   Chipperfield B, et al, Differences in metal content of the heart muscle in death from ischemic heart disease, *Am Heart J* 95:732-7, 1978

"I've Had All the Right X-rays"

Three out of four diabetics die from a heart attack (Anderson, Fava). And diabetics have more severe coronary artery disease with more ulcerated plaques and more clots and more vascular complications than the average person their age. As well, they have poisoning of the autonomic nervous system of the heart which can confuse a diagnosis of a heart attack. Most importantly diabetes is an independent predictor of death, heart attack and re-admission to the hospital. Yet **one out of three folks who have a heart attack get little or no warning**. Sometimes they might just feel short of breath or feel fatigue as the only signs. Sadly **folks can have a silent heart attack with no chest pain**. And remember, **half of folks who have a heart attack did not have the standard risk**

68

factors, nor did they make it to a second attack. The first one was fatal. One out of two die immediately.

One of the best crystal ball tests is the ultrafast CT heart scan which gives a calcium score. The Agatston coronary calcium score gives a better idea of when to expect your heart attack. And better yet, then you know that you had better get busy learning how to reverse it (*TW* 2012-13) or schedule bypass. For example, one cardiologist (Budoff) has shown you can dramatically slow down the progression with something as simple as non-prescription **Kyolic Liquid**, two squirts twice a day. Much more directions in *The Cholesterol Hoax.*

Meanwhile, you can get an ultrafast CT heartscan with coronary calcium score without a prescription for around $200 and it takes less than five minutes and you don't even take your clothes off. Furthermore, as opposed to the angiogram in the hospital, you're not injected with anything that can kill you. If any of your business or leisure travel takes you to Florida, you might want to get one in Orlando or St. Petersburg/Tampa from DOC (Diagnostic Outpatient Center), 1-727-896-0000 or 1-800- 890-4452.

References:

• Fava S, et al, Outcome of unstable angina in patients with diabetes mellitus, *Diabetes Med* 14:209-13, 1997

• Greenland P, et al, ACCF/AHA 2007 clinical expert consensus document on coronary artery calcium scoring by computed tomography in global cardiovascular risk assessment and evaluation of patients with chest pain, *J Am Coll Cardiol*, 49; 3:378-402, 2007

• Budoff MJ, et al, Rates of progression of coronary calcium by electron beam tomography, *Am J Cardiol*, 86:8-11, 2000

• Anderson JL, et al., ACC/AHA 2007 guidelines for the management of patients with unstable angina/non-ST-elevation myocardial infarction: executive summary: a report of the American College of Cardiology/American Heart Association Task Force on Practical Guidelines (writing committee to revise the 2002 guidelines for the management of patients with unstable angina/non-ST-elevation myocardial infarction): developed in collaboration with the American College of Emergency Physicians, the Society for Cardiovascular Angiography and Interventions and the Society of Thoracic Surgeons: endorsed by the American Association of Cardiovascular and Pulmonary Rehabilitation and the Society for Academic Emergency Medicine, *Circulation*: 116:803-77, 2007

"My Doctor Says He's a Specialist in Diabetes and Knows All There is to Know About the Medical Management of It"

Specialist or not, how can you tell if your doctor is smart enough to help you *cure* your diabetes? Easily. **Test him** with anything in this book, for your life depends on it. In fact, if he hasn't read this, I don't know of another book that has all of these facts and directions complete with the scientific back-up. That is why I took years out of my very happy life to collate the evidence *for you.* I don't need to write another book, I don't want fame, I'm very happy with Luscious in my semi-retirement. But the fact is I can't stand to see folks suffering and dying needlessly.

A simple test might be to ask him how he's going to test your biotin. He may not even know what **biotin is**. It's **an extremely important vitamin that regulates the genes to control insulin and sugar metabolism**. Without adequate levels, you cannot hope to cure anybody's diabetes. Along with vanadium, cinnamon and other agents, it also **acts as an insulin mimic**. It even improves the diabetes of experimental animals whose pancreases have been poisoned in order to create diabetes. It has been proven essential along with chromium and other nutrients in folks whose diabetes was poorly controlled. And for folks who don't even have diabetes, they need it for regular energy production. And for those who haven't gotten the message yet, **we *all* need the information in this book** and these nutrients for regular energy as well as prevention of diseases, even if we don't have diabetes.

So back to your question, merely ask him how he's going to test your biotin. If you get a quizzical look which suggests he doesn't even know what it is or wasn't planning on it or a denigrating assertation that you don't need it (to cover up for his ignorance), you know you're in the wrong place. If he knows right away that the test is your **beta-hydroxy iso-valerate**, you have hit the jackpot. Most likely he is a dynamo, not a dinosaur. If he doesn't know but is at least interested in growing, in being a part of 21st century medicine and helping you cure your diabetes, then share this book with him.

References:

- Vilches-Flores A, et al, Biotin increases glucokinase expression via soluble guanylate cyclase/protein kinase, adenosine triphosphate production and autocrine action of insulin in pancreatic rat islets, *J Nutr Biochem* 21:606-12, 2010

- Zhang H, et al, **Biotin administration improves the impaired glucose tolerance** of streptozotocin-induced diabetic Wistar rats, *J Nutri Sci Vitaminol* 43:271-80, 1997

- Singer GM, et al, The effect of **chromium picolinate and biotin** supplementation on glycemic control **in poorly controlled patients with type II diabetes** mellitus: a placebo-controlled, double-blinded, randomized trial, *Diabetes Technol Therap* 8:636-43, 2006

- Fernandez-Meija C, Pharmacologic effects of biotin, *J Nutr Biochem* 16:424-7, 2005

- If not convinced, check out other evidences in *Biomed Pharmacother* 44; 10:511-4, 1990

Drugs Can't be Beat

Wrong. It's almost as if there is prize for whomever gets to heaven with the most drugs. The majority of folks over 50 have a pocket full of pills which increase yearly. You saw **the evidence in chapter I that just drugging diabetes, blood pressure and cholesterol did not increase longevity**. An equally revealing study looked at **the most commonly prescribed drugs for adults** which included a statin (like Lipitor to lower cholesterol), three blood pressure drugs including a diuretic (like hydrochlorothiazide or HCT, also amiloride), a beta blocker (like metoprolol or atenolol, carvedilol), and an angiotensin converting enzyme inhibitor (like lisinopril, enalapril). They noted that some researchers even wanted to make a "poly-pill" that contained all of these plus add a little bit of folic acid and aspirin. They actually believed that this was pure genius and thought that it could reduce cardiovascular deaths. Of course they were apparently clueless about the combined nutrient deficiencies that these drugs induce.

Then something interesting happened. This unique researcher knew enough about the molecular biochemistry of healing to realize that if you merely check all of the actions of membrane-essential fatty acids (as in cod liver oil), they actually fill the role of the "poly-pill". In fact **nature' s fatty acids do a <u>better</u> job at correcting these broken biochemical pathways than the leading drugs**. And because fatty acids are molecules that are present in almost all of our tissues, they have no side effects, and could be taken for long periods of time and even by pregnant women, lactating mothers, infants and children (classes of patients that are often not included in drug testing protocols). The bottom line was **God's essential fatty acids can do a better job at preventing cardiovascular diseases (high blood pressure, diabetes, stroke, heart attacks, peripheral vascular disease, kidney disease) than a basket-full of the leading drugs.**

Then, this brilliant researcher went one step further and showed that **the right combination of fatty acids will also protect people from other things like depression, schizophrenia and Alzheimer's, and a host of inflammatory diseases** (Das). He gave the rationale for recommending that fatty acids (like cod liver oil) should be given from childhood throughout life. And other researchers have confirmed these findings and have explained why taking the right balance of fatty acids protects us from everything from coronary heart disease to breast cancers…..and diabetes.

So why is this so important? Most disease begins in the cell membrane. But **we have literally changed the chemistry of the human body in this era.** The ratio of n-3 fatty acids (like cod liver oil) to n-6 fatty acids (as in grocery store vegetable oils, dairy products and meats) should be 4:1. Instead in this era it has been flipped around to as much as 1:15. **This change in the ratio of fatty acids from 4:1-1:15 makes a dramatic change in the electrical activity of the cell membrane which governs every action in the human body and all disease.** Think about it. **There's a potentially 60-fold difference in the balance between the two major fatty acid categories that determine every disease**. It's a flagrant example of the idiocy of trying to treat any disease without first examining and repairing the cell membrane. For oftentimes that's all that is needed.

So how do you repair the cell membrane and put it back to the beneficial ratio? Remember the cell membrane is like a sandwich (yes, I've repeated this because I want you to *memorize* this for life): the bread (cod liver oil), the meat (phosphatidylcholine powder), and the salt and pepper (the 8 forms of vitamin E). So you would begin by using a daily 1-3 teaspoonsful of each, Lemon-Flavored **Cod Liver Oil** (not in capsules) and a heaping tsp. of **Phosphatidyl Choline Powder,** and 2 **E Gems Elite**. There's a lot more to creating healthy membranes and hormone receptors, but this is a great start for many, and in fact may be the only thing they need to repair. After a while you can cut the doses to every other day or less, since **you can also get an imbalance of too many omega-3 oils** as well.

References:

•   Das UN, Essential fatty acids and their metabolites could function as an endogenous HMG CoA reductase and ACE enzyme inhibitors, and anti-arrhythmic, antihypertensive, anti-atherosclerotic, anti-inflammatory, cytoprotective, and cardioprotective molecules, *Lipids in Health and Disease*, 7:37-55, 2008

•   Jude S, et al, Dietary long chain omega-3 fatty acids of marine origin: a comparison of their protective effects on coronary heart disease and breast cancers, *Prog Biophys Molec Biol*, 90:299-325, 2006

•   Chajes K, et al, Omega-6/omega-3 polyunsaturated fatty acid ratio and cancer, *World Rev Nutr Diet* 92:133-51, 2003

•   Leaf A, et al, **Clinical prevention of sudden cardiac death by n-3** polyunsaturated fatty acids and mechanism of **prevention of arrhythmias** by n-3 fish oils, *Circulation* 107: 2646-52, 2003

Arrest Arrhythmias Without Drugs

I'll never forget when I knew I was leaving this world. I passed out when my heart raced over 250 beats per minute (supra-ventricular tachycardia), pounding like it was going to burst out of my chest. There's nothing like your heart beating wildly fast with chaotic irregularity, or pounding like it's going to slit your chest to get your attention. And cardiac arrhythmias now are literally epidemic. But when you show up panicked at the ER, the cardiologist's options include (1) drugs, (2) cardioversion, (3) ablation, and/or (4) implanted pacemaker or defibrillator. They sound so high tech and since you are desperate and pretty much unprepared for this emergency, you leave it to the specialist to make the choice. Wrong! He neglected to give you the most important option, (#5) CURE. As just one example, merely raising the magnesium or selenium levels has been the cure, costing mere pennies to completely eradicate an arrhythmia. For others, repair of the fatty acids in the cell membrane (as you just learned) have been an inexpensive cure with far-reaching other benefits.

Are you developing an appreciation for the legions of myths perpetrated by medicine? And this is in spite of decades of infallible proof from the most respected journals.

References:

• Pepe S, et al, **(n-3)** Long chain PUFA dose-dependently increase oxygen utilization efficiency and **inhibit arrhythmias** after saturated fat feeding in rats, *J Nutr*, 137:2377-83, 2007

• Leaf A, et al, **Prevention of fatal arrhythmias** in high-risk subjects **by fish oil n-3 fatty acid** intake, *Circulation* 112:2762-8, 2005

• Kromhout D, et al, The inverse relation between fish oil consumption and 20-year mortality from coronary heart disease, *New Engl J Med*, 312:1205-9, **1985**

• Billman GE, et al, **Prevention of sudden cardiac death by** dietary **pure omega-3** polyunsaturated fatty acids in dogs, *Circulation* 99:2452-57, 1999

• Charmock JS, et al, **Omega-3 PUFAs reduce** the vulnerability of the rat to ischemic **arrhythmia** in the presence of a high intake of saturated animal fat, *Nutr Res* 11 1025-34, 1991

• Leaf A, et al, **Clinical prevention of sudden cardiac death by n-3 polyunsaturated fatty acids and mechanism of prevention of arrhythmias by n-3 fish oils**, *Circulation* 107:2646-52, 2003

• McLennan PL, et al, **Dietary fish oil prevents ventricular fibrillation** following coronary artery occlusion and reperfusion, *Am Heart J*, 116:709-17, 1988

• McLennan PL, et al, **Reversal of the arrhythmogenic effects of long-term saturated fatty acid intake by dietary n-3** and n-6 polyunsaturated fatty acids, *Am J Clin Nutr*, 51:53-8, 1990

• Pepe S, et al, Dietary **fish oil confers direct antiarrhythmic properties** of the myocardium of rats, *J Nutr* 126:34-42, 1996

• Zaloga GP, et al, (n-3) Long chain polyunsaturated **fatty acids prolong survival following myocardial infarction** in rats, *J Nutr* 136:1874-8, 2006

• McLennan PL, et al, Membrane basis for **fish oil** effects on the heart: linking natural hibernators to **prevention of human sudden cardiac death**, *J Memb Biol* 206:85-102, 2005

• Pepe S, et al, **PUFA** and aging modulate **cardiac mitochondrial membrane** lipid composition and activation of PDH, *Am J Physiol*, 276: H149-58, 1999

Heart Ablation is FDA Approved....or is it?

This is not a myth, but the truth. Permanent destruction of heart nerve and muscle, done "blindly" through a catheter is not FDA-approved for that indication. Please don't fall for ablation. As I started to tell you in chapter I, for over a decade, interventional cardiologists have employed a technique called ablation to treat such things as **atrial fibrillation, congestive heart failure** and other cardiac conditions. As I showed in a previous *TW*, the dozen top prominent medical textbooks for physicians on ablation disappointingly do not contain even one chapter on looking for the curable causes. There is not even mention of the most rudimentary cures, which in some folks can be as simple and inexpensive as magnesium and the oil change with **Cod Liver Oil** and **Phosphatidyl Choline Powder** and **E Gems Elite.**

I became particularly concerned when I started phone consulting with some of you readers in your 30s and 40s who have had ablation for arrhythmias at prestigious cardiac clinics. For in reviewing your records not one physician had even looked for anything as rudimentary as deficiencies of your RBC magnesium, EPA/DHA fatty acids, or any of the other **totally curable causes of arrhythmia.** Hence I wrote *Is Your Cardiologist Killing You?* to educate and protect folks, enabling them to cure themselves, regardless of cardiac label. And although the title might seem over the top, evidence from *The Wall Street Journal* and the *Journal of the American Medical Association* have proven me even more right on than I had believed. For subsequently the article was published in the *New England Journal of Medicine* showing that in examining over 2,700 **recommendations by American cardiologists, less than 11% are based on scientific evidence.** The rest are merely practice guidelines dictated by "authorities" with financial pharmaceutical ties. Hence every symptom is a drug deficiency!

So what is ablation? It involves slipping a catheter with a high-powered laser tip into the blood vessels and up into the heart.

When the interventional cardiologist *thinks* he is in the area of the heart that will benefit from permanent destruction of its nerves, the device is activated. When the laser is turned on it permanently burns and destroys heart nerve and muscle. There's no going back. There is also another version that permanently freezes the tissue instead. Over 25,000 procedures are done yearly as it brings in over $100 million dollars annually. What blew my mind was this extremely damaging procedure, **ablation, is not FDA approved.**

To quote from the *Wall Street Journal* article, "The devices widely used for this operation (to fix the most common type of faulty heartbeat, atrial fibrillation) **haven't been approved by the U.S. government to treat** that condition." "**The Justice Department is investigating** whether companies that make these surgical-ablation devices have been **violating the law by actively marketing them for non-FDA-approved uses such as treating atrial fibrillation.**" And companies unabashedly promote it as "the best growth market in the medical device space for the next 5-7 years." Does it sound like cardiologists are out of control?

In fact, still after years of use, the FDA does nothing about it. What the device is approved for is to stop bleeding that is *visually* seen (and caused) by the surgeon during open heart surgery. It's much like the dentist or the dermatologist using laser to stop bleeding with cautery that they have created and can *actually see*. It is not OK'ed for permanently and blindly destroying nerve and muscle in the heart.

The bottom line is that **cardiac ablation is not and never has been an FDA approved procedure**. Yet cardiologists continue it unabashedly to the tune of over $25,000 each, and even more depending on complications over the year. And after calling a cardiology office plus a local hospital and the local medical school, it turns out that many insurances don't cover it. Plus there can be roughly another $25,000 incurred in the first year in office visits, blood tests, medications, and further radiologic tests. Plus more than **one in ten patients suffers permanent heart failure,**

shortness of breath, and more from too aggressive a killing of heart nerves. And now it's being recommended for children with arrhythmias. Fortunately kids that I've consulted on had mothers who were smarter than the cardiologists. For when we looked at the childrens' chemistries we were able to totally cure their arrhythmias with pennies of nutrients, and usually within just a few weeks. They never had ablation, thanks to their mothers.

Ablation is done blindly via x-ray guidance, not direct visualization. And **the ablation procedure doubles the rate of stroke and increases the chance of a heart attack, !** And don't forget one of the medicines prescribed after it has been done is usually Coumadin (warfarin). This rips calcium out of bone and dumps it into heart valves and arteries, necessitating clot-attracting stents or surgical replacement of heart valves. Once you enter the medical system of drugs and devices, it becomes an endless merry-go-'round of more drugs and devices, medications and machines.

This is all in spite of the fact that **most arrhythmias and heart failures can be cured by finding and correcting the underlying nutrient deficiencies and toxicities, sometimes with literally pennies of nutrients**. No wonder **92% of arrhythmia patients treated with cardiac drugs fail to respond.** That's easy to understand. It is not a deficiency of any drug or permanently destructive procedure. Cardiologists who have failed to assay and correct the true underlying causes that you will learn about here are inexcusable. The nutritional evidence is undeniable and some even decades old. There is no excuse for such irreparable harm.

References:

- Burton TM, Fix for a faulty heartbeat, *Wall St J*, Mar 16, 2010
- Burton TM, **Surgical-device firms walk a fine line**, *WSJ,* A1, A8, Mar 11, 2010
- Mundy A, et al, Third-party reviews of **devices come under scrutiny at the FDA**, B1-2, *Wall St J*, Mar15, 2010

"I Must Take Nitroglycerin for Angina"

Nearly every man on the street knows the signs of an impending heart attack. Chest pain, shortness of breath, "heartburn" symptoms, a tightness in the chest that radiates up into the neck or to the left ear or left arm can be signs that you should get checked out in an emergency room right away. Once you have been released, then your cardiologist, as a diagnostic tool and precautionary measure, often gives you a trial prescription for nitroglycerin. Nitroglycerin, a vasodilator, opens up the arteries so that more blood flow gets to the heart. It certainly sounds logical, doesn't it? The problem is if that's all you were given is drugs, your cardiologist has failed you miserably.

Let's take a look at one example out of many nutrients that are able to literally cure the problem, solo or in combination, depending upon the individual person. **D-Ribose Powder**, the rate limiting sugar in the production of heart energy is one of several nutrients that can in some folks take the place of nitroglycerin, since **often folks no longer get angina once they are making enough energy in the heart muscle.** And research shows that once the storage pool of ATP (energy) has been stressed enough to cause a symptom, just because the symptom disappears in a few minutes with a medicine like nitroglycerin, does not mean that the pool has been replenished. **It takes days for the heart to rally and get its energy chemistry back.** Yet that is assuming you have the right chemistry to do that.

This heart energy chemistry also needs **R-Lipoic Acid, Vitamin B1, Arginine Powder, Niacin-Time** (long-acting B3, proven better than the prescription Niaspan, see *The Cholesterol Hoax* for evidence), and more. Plus as you know **the energy for every heart cell is made in the mitochondria**. If you slit the mitochondria lengthwise and look inside them they are a mass of membranes, folded back and forth on each other, resembling Christmas ribbon candy. Luckily you already know how to begin to fix these cell membranes with the membrane oil change.

So if you're out gardening, shoveling, exercising or doing anything that brings on chest pain or angina (called ischemia) and you've only been given nitroglycerin and other drugs, you've been cheated out of curing your heart problem. What's even worse is you are being cheated out of a longer life, since **ribose is absolutely essential as part of the real treatment for angina**. The discouraging part? All this has been known for over three decades but is ignored, because (un-patentable natural) nutrients don't make the money that prescription drugs do.

Clearly folks with angina, heart failure, diastolic hypertension (the low blood pressure number is above 90, an early sign that you may be going into heart failure) and especially after having a heart attack, heart surgery or any other heart problem like **cardiomyopathy** deserve to be on D-Ribose. And bear in mind, that impressive-sounding diagnostic labels, like cardiomyopathy merely mean "We haven't the slightest idea of what the cause or treatment is". *The High Blood Pressure Hoax* gives much more detail on how we can make our own nitroglycerine-type of vasodilator in vessels with arginine, magnesium, etc.

Take at least 3 gm (3 grams equals 3,000 milligams or mg) of **D-Ribose Powder** twice a day to make sure your heart has enough energy while you find the causes. In *TW* other uses of D-Ribose include shortening the recovery time from a multitude of maladies from having physically over-exerted by running a marathon or from fibromyalgia or having just had a heart attack. And if taken right away, it even makes the area of heart damage from a heart attack smaller. Remember, heart disease is the number one cause of death in everyone. Diabetics are just on a greatly accelerated roll.

References:

• St. Cyr JA, et al, Enhanced high-energy phosphate **recovery with ribose** infusion after global **myocardial ischemia** in a canine model, *J Surg Res* 46:157-62, 1989

• Sami H, et al, The effect of **ribose** administration on contractile recovery following brief periods of **ischemia,** *Anesthesiol,* 67; 3A: A74, 1987

- Pliml W, et al, Effects of **ribose on exercise-induced ischemia** in stable coronary artery disease, *Lancet,* 340:507-10, 1992

- Wallen JW, et al, Pre-ischemic administration of **ribose to delay the onset of irreversible ischemic** injury and improve function: studies in normal and hypertrophied hearts, *Canad J Physiol Pharmacol*, 81:40-47, 2003

- Pauly D, et al, **D-Ribose as a supplement for cardiac energy** metabolism, *J Cardiovasc Pharmacol Therap* 5; 4:249-58, 2000

- Pasque M, et al, **Ribose-enhanced myocardial recovery following ischemia** in the isolated working rat heart, *J Thorac Cardiovasc Surg*, 83; 3:390-98, 1982

- Seifert J, et al, The effects of ribose ingestion on indices of free radical production during **hypoxic exercise**, *Free Rad Biol Med* 33 (supple 1): S269, 2002

- Neilan TG, et al, Persistent and **reversible cardiac dysfunction among amateur marathon runners**, *Europ Heart J* 27; 9:1079-84, 2006

- Zimmer HG, et al, **Ribose accelerates the repletion of ATP** during recovery from reversible **ischemia** of the rat myocardium, *J Mol Cell Cardiol,* 16:863-66, 1984

- Tveter KJ, et al, **Ribose enhanced recovery of diastolic function after global myocardial ischemia,** *Ped Res* 23:226 a, 1988

- Ingwall JS, et al, Is **the failing heart energy starved**? On using chemical energy to support cardiac function, *Circul Res* 95:135-45, 2004

- Illie S, et al, **D-Ribose improves myocardial function in congestive heart failure** , *FASEB J,* 15; 5:A 1142, 2001

- Omran H, et al, **D-Ribose improves myocardial function and quality of life in congestive heart failure patients**, *J Mol Cell Cardiol*, 33;6: A173, 2001

"Plavix and Aspirin are a Must for Me"

As I started to show you in the preceding chapter, Plavix (clopidogrel is the generic or non-patented name used in research) is prescribed for nearly everybody after a heart attack, ostensibly to prevent them from clotting unnecessarily and having another heart attack. It works by poisoning the platelets. Once they are poisoned they ostensibly cannot produce blood clots as well.

But recall that **in at least one out of three people Plavix doesn't even work at all.** Plus **diseased platelets abnormally produce clots**. Normal healthy platelets (with enough taurine, magnesium, phosphatidyl choline, EPA, etc.) do not make abnormal amounts of clots. They only produce clots to stop bleeding. But **unhealthy platelets and blood vessels that are lacking important nutrients foster clots.** As well, **foreign objects like stents, implants, and**

infection can become a trigger and magnet for clots, since one of the roles of platelets is to also protect the body against foreign invaders. We'll continue to build on what you started to learn earlier (and *TW* 2013 will expand in this even further).

You've probably been told that aspirin is necessary as well. But recall that **after you've had a heart attack, taking aspirin increases your chance of having another heart attack 6%** (Gislason). And if you take something like Motrin or other NSAIDs (non-steroidal anti-inflammatory drugs, like the over-the-counter pain relievers) while you're on aspirin it also stops aspirin from working (Catella-Lawson). Furthermore, **NSAIDs, of which aspirin is one, are known for causing increased size of the damaged area after a heart attack, plus rupture of the heart,** edema (swelling of the body) and more clots (Timmers, Jugdutt). If that weren't enough, **NSAIDs increase blood pressure and congestive heart failure** (Solomon, Lewington). Even though folks become resistant to Plavix, as you will learn, nutrients do a better job anyway. At this point in time I'm just wondering who reads the cardiovascular journals any more, because it doesn't look as though cardiologists do and certainly not the "authorities" who make the practice guidelines (recommendations for doctors) advising them to use drugs and shun nutrients.

References:

• Antman EM, et al, Use of nonsteroidal anti-inflammatory drugs: an update for clinicians: a scientific statement from the American Heart Association, *Circulation* 115:1634-42, 2007

• Jaremo P, et al, **Individual variations of platelet inhibition after loading doses clopidogrel**, *J Intern Med*, 252:233-38, 2002

• Gurbel PA, et al, **Clopidogrel for coronary stenting**: response variability, **drug resistance**, and the effect of pretreatment platelet reactivity, *Circulation* 107:2908-13, 2003

• Matetxky S, et al, **Clopidogrel resistance** is associated with **increased risk** of recurrent atherothrombotic events in patients with acute myocardial infarction, *Circulation* 109:3171-75, 2004

• Wiviott SD, et al, **Clopidogrel resistance**. A new chapter in a fast moving story, *Circulation* 109: 3064-67, 2004

• McKee SA, et al, **Aspirin resistance** and cardiovascular disease: a review of problems, mechanisms and clinical significance, *Thromb Haemost* 88:711-15, 2002

- Gislason GH, et al, **Risk of death** or reinfarction associated with the use of selective cyclooxygenase-two inhibitors and non-selective nonsteroidal anti-inflammatory drugs after acute myocardial infarction, *Circulation* 113:2906-13, 2006

- Catella-Lawson S, et al, Cyclooxygenase inhibitors and the antiplatelet effects of aspirin, *New Engl J Med* 345:1809-17, 2001

- Timmers L, et al, **Cyclooxygenase (Cox)-2 inhibition increases mortality**, enhances left ventricular remodeling and impairs systolic function **after myocardial infarction**, *Circulation* 115:326-332, 2007

- Jugdutt BI, et al, **Cyclooxygenase inhibition and <u>adverse remodeling during healing</u>** after **myocardial infarction**, *Circulation* 115:288-91, 2007

"I Must Take Drugs to Lower My Cholesterol"

I had to chuckle. Four years after *The Cholesterol Hoax* was published, the *Wall Street Journal* warned us, the "FDA warns on statin drugs: labels on popular **cholesterol medicines may cite risk of diabetes, memory loss**". And even though this #1 prescribed drug in the country is part of the epidemic rise of diabetes as well as Alzheimer's, it's still on the market. In fact the FDA was going to add a warning that *cholesterol-lowering drugs also damage liver enzymes.* But they decided not to because putting the warning on didn't bring about any prevention of the side effect, they said! And why not? Because doctors prescribing cholesterol-lowering drugs are too ignorant to check for deficiencies of the very nutrients that the drug lowers that trigger liver disease. As well, the cholesterol-lowering drugs can trigger liver cancers, too. And that certainly will never make the labels!

Of course, you folks who have read *The Cholesterol Hoax* are on top of this and have seen the evidence. But isn't it sad *that more than 20 million Americans are ignorant enough to take cholesterol-lowering drugs*? I guess they think it's a fair trade to get diabetes and mental disease for saving one person from a heart attack. Yes, you heard right, because for every 200 people who take a statin drug one will develop diabetes and two *may* avoid a heart attack. And they haven't even begun to calculate how many will develop Alzheimer's, cancers, accelerated heart disease, and more. Plus these projections are only for the first few years. It takes longer to develop most diseases from the serious hidden deficiencies that drugs continually induce.

Also, remember from the evidence presented there that the 26% fewer heart attacks for **statin** users was a wash, because there were 26% more deaths from other causes, as there should be. This drug category is extremely dangerous since **it lowers CoQ10 which leads to premature heart attacks, depression, congestive heart failure**, and much more, while it **lowers selenium which raises your risk of cancer, elevated PSA**, strokes, and it **lowers vitamin E and poisons fatty acids which raise your risk of cardiovascular disease, Alzheimer's, cancers**, etc. There just is not a knowledgeable person who would take this drug category. Oh, and don't forget the least known common side effect, **sudden amnesia**. Yet most pilots are on it!

And then of course, the most telling fact was that most people can normalize their lipids (cholesterols) by correcting their biochemistry and/or getting rid of the toxins that created it to begin with. Sometimes cure can be as simple as a few nutrients known to normalize cholesterol, for example, **Tocotrienols** or **Magnesium** or **Niacin-Time** or **Solar D Gems** or **Phosphatidyl Choline Powder** (I'll give you doses and sources plus harmonizing nutrients later). So if you do have high cholesterol (or triglycerides, Lp(a), LDL, etc.) make sure you *cure* it, since you sure don't want diabetes, brain loss and the other symptoms that statins invariably bring on.

Reference:

• Burton TM, Winslow R, **FDA warns on statin drugs:** labels on popular cholesterol medicines may cite **risk of diabetes, memory** loss, *Wall St J*, A3, Feb 29, 2012

How Prescription Drugs Create the Very Diseases
They are Designed to Treat

I frankly don't know whether to laugh or cry. The medical field is exhibiting such flagrant ignorance of the chemical mechanisms of healing that I continually find it harder to believe. For example, millions of folks are prescribed the combination of statin drugs (like Lipitor, Crestor, Zocor, etc.) for high cholesterol or "staving off a heart attack", a diuretic (like HCT or hydrochlothiazide, etc.) to reduce blood pressure or fluid, and a beta blocker (like Toprol, Coreg, Corgard, etc.) for blood pressure or angina, arrhythmias, heart failure, migraine, panic, or even eye problems.

The problem is **all three categories of these common drugs dramatically deplete, as one example, the nutrient CoQ10**. Then **an undiagnosed deficiency of CoQ10 in turn can lead to** diabetes, heart failure, heart attack, high blood pressure, arrhythmia, angina... **the very things the drugs were prescribed to prevent**. Clearly, if you don't yet have the diseases, you will....or instead exhaustion, depression, or cancer!

Clearly it doesn't stop here. CoQ10 deficiency can lead to tooth loss, insomnia, impotency, exhaustion, memory loss, Parkinson's Disease, and many other problems. Yet in reviewing records from high profile U.S. medical clinics, I have never seen a medical record where CoQ10 adequacy was checked for, even in patients on statins. These cholesterol-lowering drugs directly poison CoQ10 synthesis in the body. At least use 1-3 **Q-ODT** under the tongue twice daily if you are on any of these. The sublingual absorption by-passes the gut (which may not be healthy yet), hence sparing you one more capsule (details in *The Cholesterol Hoax*). Anytime you can use a sublingual (absorbed under the tongue like nitroglycerin) or powder or liquids, I'm all for it since we have too many capsules that are needed to thwart our deficiencies.

To my way of thinking there is no excuse. A physician is responsible for doing the best for his patient, not just feathering the coffers of the pharmaceutical industry. Any physician can bring his practice, regardless of specialty, into the 21st century by merely reading this monthly referenced newsletter at a dollar a week and a few of the books. And these pale in price compared with expensive medical journals (some of the ones I subscribe to are well over $400 a year) and courses (most are well over $2000 when you add up course fee, airline, cabs, hotel, meals, etc. not to mention time away from the practice) where they only focus on drugs. Put your doc on notice. Let him know you deserve better and your goal is awesome drug-free health and vitality. **Does his M.D. stand for "Master of Drugs" or "Master of Discovery" for causes and cures?**

So these were just a few of the myths and deceptions I frequently hear folks parrot from their dinosaurs. And diabetics often have more of these conditions and drugs than the non-diabetic population. That is why I feel compelled to digress and protect you (yes, even with repetition, which makes learning easier). Hopefully these misconceptions will no longer be a part of your belief system. Now let's get on with empowering you by showing you the awesome power of some crucial nutrients.

References:

- Pelton R, et al, *Drug-Induced Nutrient Depletion Handbook*, www.lexi.com or 1-800-837-5394

Chapter III

Dinosaur Diabetes Docs Don't Diagnose Deficiencies

Nutritional Evidence is Undeniable

You'll find this as hard to believe as I did. Researchers studied people who were dying in intensive care units. They were riddled with infections that no antibiotics could cure, and all the fancy specialists had run out of options. There were no other medications left to give these folks who were on death's doorstep. At that point they were **given pennies worth of two ordinary vitamins. The results?** Over half of them, yes **54% of these near-death ICU patients, rallied and survived**. Yet to this day I don't know of one ICU that even carries vitamins C and E, much less uses them. If nutrients can be that powerful, it should not come as a surprise to you that given the right nutritional repair (and usually detoxification to follow, as you will learn) can bring about healing of just about everything. So let's look at *just a few* examples of nutrients that are bare-bones indispensable for diabetics.

The Magnificent Minerals

Minerals come from the Earth's rocks. They are rich in plant-based foods as well as animal foods, but not in processed foods. They are the core or the engine for most enzymes, for without sufficient amounts we have disease. Let's look at three minerals that are crucial for both ends of the sugar spectrum, from healing hypoglycemia or low blood sugar (sudden headaches, cravings, irrational mood swings, sweating, dizziness, brain fog, inability to lose weight, and more) to diabetes. For remember, as we go through life a variety of factors serve to make our minerals progressively more depleted.

Chocolate, **van**illa or strawberry? As a kid, if there ever was ice cream, we had only 3 choices. My point? Maybe that will help you remember the 3 top over-looked trace mineral choices for diabetes: **chr**omium, **van**adium, and selenium.

Chromium

Car bumpers used to be chromium plated to protect them from rust, or oxidation (I know, I'm showing my age! I've been informed by my car-buff friends they no longer make them). But, likewise, you need chromium in your body to prevent rust, medically called oxidation (also called lipid peroxidation, another measurable indicator or warning of accelerated aging that you'll learn about). And no, the newer bumpers of fiberglass/plastic will not do the trick in your body. In fact, plastics are one of the chief causes of diabetes, as you will learn later. Chromium is so fundamental to the action of the pancreas and insulin that even in cases where insulin didn't improve the patient any further, chromium did (Wang, 2010). For starters, I suggest a daily 200 mcg **Chelated Chromium** to protect your cell membranes (where the insulin receptors reside) from oxidizing (deteriorating). Another form is **Kyo-Chrome**, which combines unique yeast-fighting patented Kyolic® with chromium (more in the next chapter).

References:

• Morris DW, et al, **Chromium supplementation improves insulin resistance in patients with type II diabetes mellitus**, *Diabetes Med,* 19; 9:684-5, 2000

• Cefalu WT, et al, Rule of chromium in human health and in diabetes, *Diabetes Care,* 27:2741-51, 2004

• Balk EM, et al, Effect of chromium supplementation on glucose metabolism and lipids: a systematic review of randomized controlled trials, *Diabetes Care,* 30;8:2154-63, 2007

• Albarracin CA, et al, **Chromium** picolinate and biotin combination **improves glucose metabolism in** treated, uncontrolled overweight to **obese** patients with type II **diabetes**, *Diab Metab Res Rev,* 24; 1:41-51, 2008

• Anderson RA, Chromium and polyphenols from cinnamon improve insulin sensitivity, *Proc Nutr Soc,* 67; 1:48-53, 2008

• Anderson RA, et al, Elevated intakes of supplemental **chromium improves glucose and insulin** variables **in** individuals with type II **diabetes**, *Diabetes* 46; 11:1786-91, 1997

• Wang ZQ, et al, **Chromium** picolinate enhances skeletal muscle cellular insulin signaling **in** vivo in obese **insulin resistant** JCR: LA-cp rats, *J Nutr* 136; 2:415-20, 2006

• Wang ZQ, et al, Current concepts about **chromium** supplementation **in** type II **diabetes** and **insulin resistance**, *Curr Diabetes Rep* 10; 2:145-51, 2010

• Vrtovec M,et al, **Chromium supplementation shortness QTc interval** duration in patients with type II diabetes mellitus, *Am Heart J*, 149:632-6, 2005

Vanadium

Diabetics are known to be at enormously higher risk for early heart attacks than folks without diabetes. As well, they are at much greater risk for strokes, kidney damage leading to a dialysis and early death, cataracts, blindness from retinal hemorrhages, neuropathies resulting in mysterious pain, numbness, loss of nerve function, impotency, and even gangrene and amputations. And that's just for starters. Yet as I've shown you in the book about blood vessel health, *The High Blood Pressure Hoax*, disease of your blood vessels is reversible, curable.

A variety of **minerals, chromium as one example, vitamins like vitamin D as an example, fatty acids like DHA, and various orphan nutrients like R-lipoic acid are so absolutely essential for getting rid of diabetes** that it should be considered malpractice not to check for them and then regulate the doses accordingly. So let's look at a less known mineral that is crucial for not only reversing high blood sugars in diabetes, but in prolonging life without medications and the plethora of medication complications.

Vanadium actually mimics the action of insulin and so it can **lower blood sugar**. And for proof, vanadium also lowers the test that shows if you have damaged your blood vessels in the last three months, the **Hgb A1C**. The difference in lowering hgb A1C with vanadium versus a diabetes medication is that vanadium actually helps promote healing elsewhere in the body, thereby promoting longevity. Whereas when you merely bludgeon a test result with more medication, you don't boost longevity, but silently deplete crucial nutrients (recall evidence in chapter I).

Taking sufficient **vanadium has also allowed folks to reduce their medications while reducing their sugars and the side effects of diabetes, like frequent urination, thirst, fatigue, sugar cravings**, and more. And vanadium deficiency has been the answer for many with hypoglycemia (a precursor warning of diabetes). Plus never lose sight of the fact that **every hypoglycemia episode has the power to contribute to overall brain deterioration and eventual dementia like Alzheimer's** (Whitmer). Furthermore, **vanadium even has anticoagulant activities**, thus decreasing the risk of not only clots causing heart attacks and strokes, but cancer metastases.

What's in it for folks without diabetes? A huge portion of the population has **Metabolic Syndrome X** which can do just about all the damage that diabetes does (increased risk of heart disease, etc.), and it is often a precursor to diabetes. As well, **folks without diabetes** but with Syndrome X also get cataracts, kidney disease, vascular damage from excessively high sugar levels and get early heart attacks. Plus no matter how hard they try, they cannot lose weight. Or if they do, it rapidly piles on again in a few months. They need nutrient protection just as much as the diabetic. Since the average diet supplies 6-18 mcg of vanadium, and most folks need 200-400 mcg, it's important to supplement it (but not with a sulfated kind that is less effective and counter-productive). I suggest a daily Carlson' s 200 mcg **Chelated Vanadium.**

References:

- Sakurai H, et al, Chemistry and biochemistry of **insulin-mimetic vanadium** and zinc complexes. Trial for treatment of diabetes mellitus, *Bull Chem Soc Jpn*, 79:1645-64, 2006

- Schamberger RJ, The **insulin-like effects of vanadium**, *J Adv Med*, 9:121-31, 1996

- Bosia S, et al, **Protective effect on nephropathy and on cataract** in the streptozotocin-diabetic rat of the **vanadium**-lazaroid combination, *G Ital Med Lav,* 17:71-75, 1995

- Funakoshi T, et al, **Anticoagulant action of vanadium**, *Chem Pharm Bull* (Tokyo) 40:174-6, 1992

- Whitmer RA, **Hypoglycemic episodes and risk of dementia** in older patients with type II diabetes mellitus, *J Am Med Assoc,* 301; 15:1599-1601, 2009

- Cam MC, et al, **Distinct glucose lowering and beta cell protective effects of vanadium** and food restriction **in** streptozotocin-**diabetes**, *Eur J Endocrinol* 141; 5:546-54, 1999

- Hamel FG, et al, The relationship between insulin and vanadium metabolism and insulin target tissues, *Mol Cell Biochem*, 153:95-102, 1995

- Kent H, Vanadium for diabetes, *Can Med Assoc J*, 160; 1:17, 1999

- Halberstram M, et al, Oral **vanadyl** sulfate **improves insulin sensitivity** in NIDDM **but not in obese nor diabetic subjects**, *Diabetes* 45:659-66, 1996

- Cohen N, et al, Oral **vanadyl** sulfate **improves** hepatic and peripheral **insulin sensitivity** in patients with non-insulin-dependent diabetes mellitus, *J Clin Invest*, 95:2501-09, 1995

- Anonymous monograph, Vanadium/Vanadyl Sulfate, *Alt Med Rev* 14; 2:117-80, 2009

- Tas S, et al, Vanadyl sulfate, taurine, and combined vanadyl sulfate and taurine treatments in diabetic rats: effects on the oxidative and anti-oxidative systems, *Arch Med Res* 38; 3:276-83, 2007

Selenium: The Destiny Mineral

What did a 7-year-old with five years of intractable seizures have in common with an 11-year-old with four years of cardiac arrhythmia? They were both cured by correcting their selenium deficiencies. How did a young woman get off her thyroid medication (that the endocrinologist assured her she would need forever, *TW* 2011), an executive stop having unexplained muscle pain and elevated PSA, or a middle-aged man get off his diabetes medication? They all repaired an unsuspected, long-standing undiagnosed selenium deficiency. Sure, these people had other concomitant deficiencies. Some had toxicities that needed addressing, but **before repairing selenium they had one thing in common. They were at a standstill**. Nothing worked, even medications, until finally someone assayed the RBC intracellular selenium.

A hidden selenium deficiency is a major reason why some folks will never rally from their cancers and why others are destined to get a cancer. Likewise an unsuspected undiagnosed selenium deficiency leads to increased clotting, also to a low potassium which then leads to arrhythmias and extreme weakness and fatigue. And in fact a low selenium increases the toxicity of our daily onslaught of environmental chemicals, raising the vulnerability for getting every disease from prostate, breast and other cancers to heart failure, arrhythmia and hypothyroidism, chemical sensitivity, cardiomyopathy, Barrett's esophagitis, intractable headaches, depression, NASH (non-alcoholic steatohepatitis, the most common liver disease), and much more.....including diabetes.

Without overloading you with its many biochemical attributes, let me just say that **selenium is needed for the electrical nature of the cell membrane where insulin attaches and does its magic.** So why are folks so deficient? Not only do industrial and vehicular exhausts create acid rain that depletes selenium from the soil (and foods), but unavoidable environmental toxins like the plasticizers (phthalates) deplete selenium (from our bodies), as do many common medications like the cholesterol-lowering statins such as Lipitor®, Zocor®, and Crestor®.

Once the sugar is elevated it is a well-known fact that **sugar causes changes in membrane function** *within days* **and also changes in the ability of heart muscles to contract** (Aydemir-Koksoy). And yet the simple antioxidant mineral, selenium, can prevent it (Ayaz). **Selenium deficiency makes it impossible to heal thyroid problems, or even heal damaged calcium channels** (Turan). But no worry, medicine bludgeons them with calcium channel blockers (like Norvasc) which can shrink the brain and rot the intellect within less than 5 years.

The bottom line? If you think you are locked into any medication or diagnosis, your destiny may be as simple as finding a hidden selenium deficiency. And if you enjoy great health at least make sure you have 200 mcg of **Chelated Selenium** plus an **ACES with Zinc** 3-7 times a week. Don't worry, I'll give you all the nutrients, doses, their sources, etc., later. I'm looking out for you and you are doing a great job in getting yourself this far. *Isn't it ironic that medicine has become so uninterested in healing that folks have had to learn the molecular biochemistry of healing in order to get what doctors should have provided decades ago?*

References:

- Papp LL, et al, From selenium to selenoproteins: synthesis, identity, and their role in human health, *Antioxidants & Redox Signaling* 9;7:775-810, 2007

- Ayaz M, et al, Effects of selenium on altered mechanical and electrical cardiac activities of diabetic rat, *Arch Biochem Biophys* 426:83-90, 2004

- Cooney CA, Dietary selenium and arsenic affect DNA methylation, *J Nutr* 131:1871-2, 2001

- Aydemir-Koksoy, et al. Antioxidant treatment protects diabetic rats from cardiac dysfunction by preserving contractile protein targets of oxidative stress, *J Nutr Biochem*, 21: 827-33, 2010

- Ayez M, et al, Selenium prevents diabetes induced alterations in [Zn2+] and metallothionein level of rat heart via restoration of cell redox cycle, *A J Physiol Heart Circul Physiol* 290: H1071-80, 2006

- Turan B, et al, Oxidative effects of **selenite on ventricular contractility and calcium** movements, *Cardiovasc Res* 32:351-61, 1996

Magnificent Magnesium

And of course anyone who has not been living under a rock for the last decade knows the importance of magnesium, which I have researched and written about extensively in the last four books. As far back as 1990 (over 2 decades ago) the *Journal of the American Medical Association* showed even using the most inferior test (the serum magnesium) that well over half of hospitalized patients were seriously low in magnesium. Just imagine how many were actually low in magnesium if the proper test were used. If that were not enough inexcusable tragedy, this magnesium was ordered by the researchers doing the study, not by the docs caring for hospitalized patients. Over **90% of these Boston physicians never ordered any magnesium. Consequently, their undiagnosed magnesium deficiencies were a major cause of in-hospital deaths.**

For starters today, the best oral form is magnesium citrate (Walker), as in **Natural Calm or Happy Bodies' Mag**. I would suggest you start a heaping teaspoonful (in divided doses) every day right now, since government studies prove **the average diet provides less than a third of the magnesium you need in a day and its deficiency is a major cause of sudden death** with no other discernible medical problems.

In a recent study, **77% of diabetics were deficient in magnesium**, which doesn't say much for their clinicians' awareness of how **magnesium deficiency heavily contributes to the worsening of diabetes** and accelerates getting all of its deadly complications (Sales). Even the most clueless of diabetologists should at least check the RBC magnesium, but **never rely on the grossly inferior serum magnesium**. Why? Because **as the magnesium inside the heart cell goes down, the body tries to compensate. So the serum magnesium actually goes up** (Nielsen). This is an extremely important fact for you to know: the serum magnesium (called simply "magnesium" when you see your lab test) can actually be high or even too high, when at that same moment your rbc magnesium (inside the heart cells) is so low you could have an instantaneous fatal heart attack. And when the magnesium is low enough, nothing, not even the dramatic paddles in the ER delivering cardioversion can rejuvenate the heart.

The **serum magnesium gives the unknowledgeable physician an unwarranted sense of security**. The result? The patient dies or has life-threatening arrhythmia from improperly diagnosed magnesium deficiency. Meanwhile, the physician thinks he has done a good job and that the (worthlessly opposite of reality and highly dangerous) serum magnesium is fine. He is clueless that his lack of knowledge could have been the cause of his patient's sudden death! I'll give you an even more potent magnesium form in chapter 5. For now, know that **manganese is also a crucial mineral in helping magnesium work,** as in one daily **Chelated Manganese** (more later).

References:

• Walker A, et al, **Mg citrate found more bioavailable** than the other Mg preparations in a randomized, double-blind study, *Magnes Res* 16; 3:183-191, 2003

• Sales CH, et al, Magnesium and diabetes mellitus: their relations, *Clin Nutr* 25; 4:554-62, 2006

• Sales CH, et al, Influence of magnesium status and **magnesium intake on the blood glucose control**, in patients with type II diabetes, *Clin Nutr*, 2011

- Nielsen FH, et al., Dietary **magnesium deficiency** *induces heart rhythm changes*, **impairs glucose tolerance** and *increases serum cholesterol* in postmenopausal women, *J Am Coll Nutr* 26; 2:121-32, 2007

- Whang R, et al, **Frequency of hypomagnesemia** and hypermagnesemia, requested versus routine, *J Am Med Assoc*, 2634:3063-4, **1990**

No "Complete Physical Exam" is Complete Without It

Over half the population is deficient in a vitamin that is rarely checked in a physical, in spite of the fact that its deficiency can be fertilizer for every disease. And **for kids under 21 it's 70% who are deficient;** that's over 2 out of 3 kids. D stands for diabetes but also dumb if you haven't been checked for a vitamin D deficiency, for **low levels are clearly linked to type II diabetes.** Studies confirm most individuals with auto-immune diseases of various types are deficient in vitamin D (Cantorna). Furthermore, when folks get an auto-immune disease, whether it's diabetes or another auto-immune disease, it is more likely to worsen and progress to full-blown status if they are vitamin D-deficient (Zold). In fact, in many studies **the lower the vitamin D levels, the greater the auto-immune disease activity** (Cutolo). Furthermore, **vitamin D has a role in insulin secretion** and in the action of insulin.

Vitamin D is so crucial to restoring health that many researchers have suggested that **no matter what a physician is treating someone for, vitamin D deficiency should be checked.** In fact many **researchers feel it should border on malpractice to fail to do so. Vitamin D is one of the most important hormones to regulate not only diabetes, but its sequelae like cancer, heart disease, infection, osteoporosis, and depression.** Many researchers have even proven that **getting the flu, or any infection for that matter, can be dramatically reduced by having adequate levels of vitamin D.**

But checking the level of vitamin D is not standard in spite of the data being over a decade old. Why? Because as I've referenced before from the *New England Journal of Medicine*, **87% of the physicians who make the practice guidelines have financial** connections with the pharmaceutical industry. **That's why every symptom turns out to be a mere deficiency of the latest drug**. Furthermore, many insurances only cover drug therapies while ignoring anything to do with finding the causes and the cures of symptoms.

Recall from chapter I that I never could figure out why insurance companies were not interested in covering cures versus life-long drugs that promote an avalanche of new diseases. But then the *Wall Street Journal* explained (2/11/10), **"insurance companies make a profit by charging a premium on claims they pay"**. *In other words, insurance companies make a lot more money keeping you using expensive drugs and devices than if you were well and not using their services.* Since (1) nutrients cure diseases, (2) require knowledge that is not taught in medical schools, (3) take time to explain, and (4) they don't promote the drug industry, wouldn't you say the insurance industry plus pharmacy-focused medical education are due for an overhaul?

When you do have your vitamin D level checked in this era of documented pandemic deficiency, remember that **folks with vitamin D in the lower end of "normal" range** (around the "accepted" 30-40) **were the most likely to have a heart attack within the next 5-8 years.** And since having diabetes already increases your risk of a heart attack as well, **an undiagnosed D deficiency is double jeopardy** (Kulie, Melamed). Your lab value must be above 60 ng/dL for your vitamin D (sorry for repetitions, but some things are just too important to your future, plus it facilitates learning). And remember a lot of lab "normal values" have been dumbed down, so be sure to see yours, and not settle for being told "It's O.K.", as for the antiquated current "norm" of many commercial labs in the 30 range.

Vitamin D is a hormone disguised as a vitamin. To fail to assay it and be sure the level is over 60 ng/dL (the modern current proven minimum level, as opposed to most laboratory cut-offs that are around 30) is the height of dinosaur diagnostics. Why? Because vitamin D has not only been shown to be deficient in most diabetics, but it is <u>crucial for pancreatic regeneration</u>. In fact, in many cases **restoring vitamin D has reversed not only insulin resistance and diabetes, but protected the brain from diabetic deterioration, protected the diabetic against osteoporosis, high blood pressure, fixed their calcium channels thereby protecting them against arrhythmias and again hypertension, as well as depression and increased infections** (Kumar). The sad part? **It's been known for nearly 30 years.** But where are the physicians who act upon it?

Regarding foods high in D, 3 1/2 ounces of sardines will give you about 400 IU of vitamin D as well as some omega-3 oils, four times more than an 8 ounce glass of milk (with synthetic D) or yogurt. How much D is too much? Studies have shown **10,000 units daily (and even more in some cases) are safe** and could be considered a normal daily intake for many folks, so certainly 4000 I.U. is not harmful (Garland, *TW*). Meanwhile, steer clear of docs who prescribe 50,000 I.U. of (synthetic) D weekly. This damages your system, as I've referenced before (*TW*). Meanwhile multiple studies confirm that government recommendations are about 10-fold too low, so we can expect epidemic diabetes to continually escalate (McCullough).

For extra **vitamin D to disease-proof your body,** start with at least 4000-8000 IU of **Solar D Gems** (vitamin D3) or think of supplementing 2000 of it with the new **Super D Omega-3**, Carlson's Cod Liver Oil which has an extra 2000 IU of vitamin D3 per teaspoon. Cod liver oils already have natural vitamins A and D in them, so avoid "fish oils" (unless you have no other options), which have been processed to lose the fishy taste (which is not a problem with **Lemon-Flavored Cod Liver Oil**), and in the process have been depleted of their natural vitamins A and D.

If anyone has not only diabetes, but is on pain medicines, or has osteoporosis, congestive heart failure, coronary artery disease, arteriosclerosis, multiple sclerosis, recurrent fractures,

pain syndromes, auto-immune disease, autism, arrhythmias, seizures, recurrent infections, psoriasis, prostate or breast cancers or colon cancers, myeloma or leukemia, learning disability, depression, or obesity, there is absolutely no excuse for neglecting to assay vitamin D. Why? Because all of these symptoms can stem from a vitamin D deficiency or it can be a major contributor. Food and nutrients like vitamin D (and toxins) talk to the genes and change them (Costa). It is that simple. Sadly in this high tech era, many folks will never get well until their hidden vitamin D deficiency is diagnosed and corrected. The body was miraculously designed to communicate with itself and figure out how to heal,.....that is, when all of its tools are present.

References:

• Garland CF, et al, Vitamin D supplement doses and serum 25-hydroxyvitamin D in the range associated with cancer prevention, *Anticancer Res* 31:607-12, 2011

• Cannell JJ, Hollis BW, et al, Diagnosis and treatment of vitamin D deficiency, *Expert Opin Pharmacother* 9; 1:1-12, 2008

• Holick MF **High prevalence of vitamin D inadequacy** and implications for health, *Mayo Clin Proc* 81; 3:353-73, 2006

• Holick M, Sunlight and **vitamin D** for bone health and **prevention of auto-immune diseases, cancer and cardiovascular disease**, Am J Clin Nutr 80:1678s-1688s, 2004

• Holick M, A **vitamin D deficiency pandemic** and consequences for non-skeletal health. Mechanisms of action, *Molec Aspects Med* 29:361-68, 2008

• Lappe JM, et al, **Vitamin D** and calcium supplementation **reduces cancer risk**: results of randomized trial, *Am J Clin Nutr, 85; 6:1586-91, 2007*

• Cantorna M, et al, Mounting evidence for **vitamin D** as an environmental factor **affecting autoimmune disease** prevalence, *Exper Biol Med* 229:1136-42, 2004

• Cantorna M, et al, Vitamin D status, 1, 25-dihydroxy vitamin D3 and the immune system, *Am J Clin Nutr*, 2440; 80: 1717s-1720s

• Costa V, et al, Nutritional genomics era: opportunities toward genome-tailored nutritional regimen, *J Nutr Biochem*, 21: 457-67, 2010

• Melamed M, et al, 25-Hydroxyvitamin D levels and the risk of mortality in the general population, *Arch Intern Med* 168; 15:1629-37, 2008

• Cutolo M, Vitamin D or hormone D deficiency in autoimmune rheumatic diseases, *Arthr Res Therapy*, 10:123, 2008

• Kulie T, et al, Vitamin D: An **evidence-based** review, *J Am Fam Pract* 22:698-706, 2009

• Zold E, et al, Vitamin D deficiency in undifferentiated connective tissue disease, *Arthr Res Therapy* 10:R123, 2008

- Hypponen E, et al, Intake of **vitamin D and risk of type I diabetes**: a birth-cohort study, *Lancet* 358:1500-03, 2001

- McCullough ML, et al, Vitamin D status and impact of vitamin D3 and/or calcium supplementation in a randomized pilot study in the southeastern United States, *J Am Coll Nutr* 28; 6:678-86, 2009

- Vieth R, et al, **The urgent need to recommend an intake of vitamin D that is effective**, editorial, *Am J Clin Nutr* 85:649-50, 2007

- Kumar PT, et al, **Vitamin D3 restores** altered cholinergic and **insulin receptor** expression in the cerebral cortex and muscarinic M3 receptor expression **in pancreatic** islets of streptozotocin induced diabetic rats, *J Nutr Biochem* 22:418-25, 2011

Vitamin K for Diabetes?

Most folks think vitamin K is just for blood clotting. But it's crucial, as you have been learning, in the control of metabolic syndrome, diabetes, high triglycerides, raising the good cholesterol HDL, protecting dialysis patients, and much more (Pan).

The sad fact? **One in five folks under 45 are already deficient.** Recall if they use **Coumadin (warfarin) for atrial fibrillation, that overtly poisons vitamin K. This leads to the body ripping calcium out of the bones and dumping it into the heart valves and coronary vessels,** exactly what you do not want to do. Can you see how **drug-driven medicine is like a freight train destined for destruction**? Meanwhile just ask your diabetes doc if you need to have your level checked. If he knows that it's important, he is an absolute jewel, a dynamo doc. If he doesn't, recall the test you want is the **undercarboxylated osteocalcin.**

References (see previous chapter for more):

- Pan Y, et al, Dietary phylloquinone intakes and metabolic syndrome in US young adults, *J Am Coll Nutr* 28; 4:369-79, 2009.

How Not to Die of Diabetic Heart Disease

How does the diabetic die? Usually of a sudden heart attack. In fact the average person without diabetes has a one in three chance of dying of heart disease while you more than double or **triple the chance once you have diabetes**. And this epidemic has only just begun. For example, **in the last 10 years diabetes has increased 33% and is escalating rapidly** (Mokdad).

I showed you the evidence proving that **giving all the best medications for diabetes, blood pressure, and cholesterol did not improve the death rate compared with taking nothing**. So what does the diabetic do? He learns how to protect and prevent a sudden heart attack. For research for decades has proven that the right amount of minerals like magnesium, selenium, vanadium, zinc, chromium, manganese, and the right fatty acids like the omega-3s (as found in cod liver oil and the "oil change"), plus other antioxidants like vitamin E (all of its 8 forms!) are absolutely crucial for not only healing diabetes, but preventing a sudden cardiac arrest. As always, **when you heal with nutrition, you get an avalanche of benefits in other organs** as well.

The bottom line? Just take a peek at a brief example of the overwhelming evidence from dedicated scientists and clinicians. If you have merely been put on diabetes medications, blood pressure or arrhythmia medications plus statins and/or aspirin and a "blood thinner" like Plavix to prevent a heart attack, these are **signs of a dinosaur diabetes doc**. As you are continuing to learn, if he hasn't sought cause, he hasn't a clue of how to heal you. You deserve better.

References:

• Aydemir-Koksoy A, et al, **Antioxidant treatment protects diabetic** rats from **cardiac dysfunction** by preserving contractile protein targets of oxidative stress, *J Nutr Biochem* 21:827-833, 2010

• Ayez M, et al, **Prevention of diabetes-induced alterations in** [Zn2+] and metallothionein level of the rat **heart** by a restoration of cell redox cycle, *Am J Physiol,* 290:H 1071-80, 2006

• Morris CD, et al, **Routine vitamin supplementation to prevent cardiovascular disease: a summary of the evidence for the U.S. Preventive Services Task Force,** *Ann Intern Med* 139:56-70, 2003

• McNeill JH, et al, **Insulin-like effects of sodium selenate** in stretozotocin-induced diabetic rats, *Diabetes* 40:1675-8, 1991

• Berg EA, et al, **Insulin-like effects of the vanadate and selenate** on the expression of glucose-6-phosphate dehydrogenase and fatty acid synthase in diabetic rats, *Biochimie,* 77:919-24, 1995

- Tuncay E, et al, Gender related different effects of **omega-3 treatment on diabetes-induced left ventricular dysfunction,** *Mol Cell Biochem* , 304:255-63, 2007
- Bjelackovic G, et al, **Antioxidant supplements for prevention of mortality** in healthy participants and patients with various diseases, *Cochrane Database Syst Rev* 16; 2: CD007176, 2008

- Jude S, et al, Dietary long-chain **omega-3 fatty acids** of marine origin: a comparison of their **protective effects of coronary heart disease and breast cancers,** *Progr Biophys Mol Biol*, 90:299-325, 2006

- Turan B, et al, Oxidative effects of selenite on-rat ventricular contractility and calcium movements, *Cardiovasc Res*, 32:351-61, 1996

- Bloch-Damti A, et al, Proposed mechanism for the **induction of insulin resistance by oxidative stress,** *Antiox Redox Signal* 7:1553-67, 2005

- Jain SK, et al, Effect of modest **vitamin E supplementation on blood glycated hemoglobin and triglyceride** levels and red cell indices in type I diabetic patients, *J Am Coll Nutr* 15:458-61, 1996

- Mokdad AH, et al, The continuing epidemics of obesity and diabetes in the United States, *J Am Med Assoc* 286:1195-2000, 2001

Disease and Death Begin in the Mitochondria

Mitochondria. Now don't let that word scare you. They are merely little kidney bean-shaped organelles inside our cells. The mitochondria is the place where *all* energy is made, where God's miracle of changing one molecule of food into a molecule of energy (that we call "life") occurs. Although mitochondria deteriorate after age 40, environmental toxins (like **plasticizers (phthalates, the number one pollutant in the human body) are a major destroyer of mitochondria (via destroying ALC, fatty acids,** as well as many other parts of the mitochondria). In addition, heavy metals (like aluminum from baked goods, deodorants, coffee makers, etc., plus cadmium, lead, mercury, etc.) plus our nutrient deficiencies (that sneak up on all of us) enormously speed up their demise. When enough mitochondria are damaged this is the beginning of any and every disease.

ALC (Acetyl L-Carnitine) you recall from chapter I works inside those little powerhouses inside of our cells. **ALC is the train that carries the fatty acids (food molecules) into the mitochondria so that they can be changed into energy**. The sad thing is that **as we age, the mitochondria deteriorate and the levels of ALC drop off dramatically**. What happens as ALC manufacture drops

100

off? You just become more tired, dull, and blame it on aging. Then as your energy supply continues to dwindle, you slide into a myriad of disease labels. Statins and phthalates damage carnitine.

ALC deficiency is often even the reason why thyroid replacement doesn't do the trick for many folks' energy. But for the person whose doc checks the chemistry of the mitochondria and repairs them, this is all reversible. In case you are thinking you might not need it, recall carnitine not only shuttles fats into mitochondria, but improves insulin sensitivity, lowers blood sugars, as well as improves abnormal lipid profiles, including lipoprotein (a), increases walking distance, has slowed down aging, has enabled folks to lower their medications, and has improved memory, as well as erectile dysfunction (Goepp).

Clearly, **diseases cannot be reversed until this energy crisis chemistry has been repaired** (you'll learn how to do it in subsequent chapters). Meanwhile, for the resurrection of your mitochondria, consider adding **ALC Powder** (500-1000 mg) to your daily detox cocktail (also coming later). Are we not lucky to know these things that the majority of medical professionals don't even know?

References:

• Ames BN, et al, Delaying the mitochondrial decay of aging with acetyl-L-carnitine, *Ann NY Acad Sci*, 1033:108-16, 2004

• Hagan TM, et al., **Acetyl-L-carnitine fed to old rats partially restores mitochondrial function and ambulatory activity**, *Proc Nat Acad Sci USA* 95:9562-66, 1998

• Paradies G, et al, The effect of **aging and acetyl-L-carnitine** on the **pyruvate** transport and oxidation in rat heart mitochondria, *FEBS Lett*, 454:207-09, 1999

• Paradies G, et al Effect of **aging and acetyl-L-carnitine** on the activity of **cytochrome oxidase** and adenine nucleotide translocation in rat heart mitochondria, *FEBS Lett* 213-15, 1994

• Savitha S, et al, **Mitochondrial membrane damage during the aging process** in rat heart: potential efficacy of l-carnitine and alpha lipoic acid, *Mech Aging Dev* 127:349-55, 2006

• Melnick RL, et al, **Mitochondrial toxicity of phthalate esters**, *Environ Health Persp* 45:51-6, 1982

• Winberg LD, et al, Mechanism of **phthalate-induced inhibition of hepatic mitochondrial** beta-oxidation, *Toxicology Letters* 76:63-69, 1995

- Chicco AJ, et al, Role of Cardiolipin and alterations in mitochondrial dysfunction and disease, *Am J Physiol Cell Physiol* 292:33-44, 2007

- Ames BN, et al, **Mineral and vitamin deficiency can accelerate the <u>mitochondrial decay of aging</u>**, *Molec Asp Med* 26:363-78, 2005

- Atamna H, Heme, iron and **the <u>mitochondrial decay of aging</u>**, *Aging Res Rev* 3:303-18, 2004

- Victor VM, et al, Targeting antioxidants to mitochondria: a potential new therapeutic strategy for cardiovascular diseases, *Curr Pharmaceut Design* 13:845-63, 2007

- Depeint F, et al, Mitochondrial function and toxicity: Role of B vitamins, one-carbon transfer pathways, *Chemico-Biological Interactions* 163:113-32, 2006

- Goepp J, Combating the "Diabesity" epidemic, *Life Extension* (www.lef.org), 39-48 Aug 2010

You are Only as Old as Your Mitochondria

So now you already know some cool facts about mitochondria. (1) These little bean-shaped packages inside of our cells are a mass of membranes folded back and forth upon themselves much like Christmas ribbon candy. (2) They are where God's miracle changes one molecule of food into the energy that we call "life". (3) And as we age the mitochondria loose carnitine which is needed to carry fatty acids into them. Now you can appreciate why researchers have **brought the chemistry of aging rat brains back to youthful levels and even repaired some degenerated brains** with ALC and lipoic acid. There's not a reason I can think of why anyone would not want to add at least 500-1000 mg of **Acetyl L-Carnitine Powder (ALC)** to their detox cocktail (R-lipoic acid is already in it) every night. Besides, you don't want any old lab rat being smarter than you, do you?

References:

- Liu J, Ames, BN, et al, Age-associated mitochondrial oxidative decay: **improvement of carnitine acetyltransferase substrate-binding affinity and activity in brain by feeding old rats acetyl-L-carnitine and/or R-a-lipoic acid**, *Proc Nat Acad Sci*, 99; 4:1876-81, 2002 (and pages 2356-61 in the same issue by these authors shows these nutrients improve brain function as well as reduce brain lipid peroxidation, Alzheimer's)

- Lee SJ, Effects of alpha-lipoic acid on transforming growth factor beta 1-p38 mitogen-activated protein kinase-fibronectin pathways in diabetic nephropathy, *Metabolism* 58; 5:616-23, 2009

Do You Have Leaky Mitochondria?

In *No More Heartburn* you learned how folks get leaky gut syndrome. Infections from overgrowth of yeasts like Candida from antibiotics can inflame the gut lining, as one example. This inflamed gut then can bring on anything from auto-immune diseases like diabetes, lupus and multiple sclerosis to rheumatoid arthritis or thyroiditis, and much more.

Well gut membranes are not the only membranes to get leaky. The mitochondria where we make the very energy we call "life" also develop leaky membranes. When this happens it becomes the basis for all disease since the very essence of life is created in the mitochondria. Luckily we know how to repair them beginning with your "oil change" that you are already versed in: **Phosphatidyl Choline Powder, Cod Liver Oil, E Gems Elite**, and other nutrients you will learn about.

Without this repair, diabetes worsens, and avalanches into deterioration of everything from vision to vessels, heart to brain (German, Jiang). In fact, a multitude of research clearly proves that **you cannot hope to cure diabetes without repairing the peroxisomes (organelles that control the mitochondria)**, and that begins with EPA and DHA, the components of cod liver oil (Yu). But even as powerful as cod liver oil is in repairing multiple damaged pathways in the diabetic and other diseases, don't forget that you can lower other important fatty acids or they can already be deficient. So precise measurement is crucial (Horrobin, Keen). So where are the diabetologists who are measuring and prescribing the proper doses?

Once you understand that the mitochondria must be assayed and repaired, it puts a whole new focus on every disease whether it's heart disease, Alzheimer's, cancers, or diabetes. **The label any physician gives your condition is inconsequential. What matters most is if mitochondria have been assayed and repaired.** **The only** possible way to measure this, to my knowledge, is with the 13-page assay I'll tell you more about, the **Cardio/ION**.

References:

- Victor VM, et al., Targeting antioxidants to mitochondria: a potential new therapeutic strategy for cardiovascular diseases, *Curr Pharmaceut Design* 13:845-63, 2007

- Stavrovskaya IG, et al, The powerhouse takes control of the cell: is the **mitochondrial permeability** transition **a viable therapeutic target against neuronal dysfunction and death**? *Free Rad Biol Med* 38:687-97, 2005

- Di Lisa F, et al, **Mitochondrial** function and myocardial aging. The critical analysis of the role of **permeability** transition. *Cardiovasc Res* 66:222-32, 2005

- Zhao K, et al, Cell-permeable peptide antioxidants targeted to inner mitochondrial membrane inhibit mitochondrial swelling, oxidative cell death and reperfusion injury, *J Biol Chem* 279:34682-90, 2004

- DeLa Asuncion JG, et al, AZT induces oxidative damage to cardiac mitochondria: protective effect of vitamin C and E, *Life Sci* 76:47-56, 2004

- Aleynik SI, et al, Alcohol-induced pancreatic oxidative stress: Protection by phospholipid repletion, *Free Rad Biol Med* 26 (5-6): 609-19, Mar 1999

- Lombardo YB, et al, **Metabolic syndrome**: effects of **n-3 PUFAs** on a model of **dyslipidemia, insulin resistance, and adiposity**, *Lipids* 42; 5:427-37, 2007

- German OL, et al, Docosahexaenoic acid prevents apoptosis of retina photo receptors by activating the ERK/MAPK pathway, *J Neurochem* 98:1507-20, 2006

- Jiang LH, et al, The influence of orally administered **docosahexaenoic acid on cognitive ability** in aged mice, *J Nutr Biochem* 20:735-41, 2009

- Storlien LH, et al **Fish oil prevents insulin resistance** induced by high-fat feeding in rats, *Science* 237:885-8, **1987**

- Rizzo MR, et al, Evidence for anti-inflammatory effects of combined administration of **vitamins E and C** in older persons with impaired fasting glucose: impact **on insulin action**, *J Am Coll Nutr* 27; 4:505-11, 2008

- Horrobin DF, **Essential fatty acids in the management of impaired nerve function and diabetes**, *Diabetes* 46(suppl 2):S 90-3, 1997

- Keen H., et al., Treatment of diabetic neuropathy with gamma linolenic acid. The Gamma-Linolenic Acid Multicenter Trial Group, *Diabetes Care* 16; 1:8-15, 1993.

- Yu YH, et al, The function of porcine PPAR gamma and dietary **fish oil and effect on** the expression of lipid and glucose metabolism related **genes**, *J Nutr Biochem* 22:179-86, 2011

- Mustacich DJ, et al, **Alpha-tocopherol modulates genes** involved in hepatic xenobiotic pathways in mice, *J Nutr Bioch*, 20:469-76, 2009

Mitochondrial Repair Is Crucial for Diabetes

Unfortunately many researchers in studies only use one or two nutrients. They actually treat nutrients as though they were a solo drug. They are oblivious to the orchestration of God's superior molecular biochemistry in the body. Also they usually do not assay the nutrients, much less balance them, which really skews the results. Just imagine the therapeutic power when medicine finally catches up with the 21st century.

Meanwhile the evidence is overwhelming. We know that the mitochondria cannot function without repair of their membranes nor without enough manganese in their exclusive antioxidant superoxide dismutase (SOD), and much more. We know how to assay the fatty acids and balance them. We know how to check the intracellular level of manganese, and we can even measure the CoQ10 levels to determine if the mitochondria are making sufficient electricity carriers, or enough ALC. Furthermore, we can measure whether the mitochondria have been damaged and just how much repair they need. This is all done in the **Cardio/ION**, an integral tool for healing diabetes, or any disease, for that matter.

Now before your eyes glaze over from this chemistry, remember that I wouldn't tell you about it unless it was pivotal in turning folks around, from death's doorstep to medication-free wellness. As one example, anyone repairing the mitochondria (shown by researchers to eventually be needed in all serious diseases) must check the RBC manganese (not to be confused with magnesium that you have learned about). For mitochondria were created with a special anti-oxidant in them called superoxide dismutase (SOD). It requires manganese. SOD acts like a sponge to sop up free radicals (naked destructive electrons) before they drill holes in the mitochondrial membranes. And these free radicals do more than just burn holes in mitochondrial membranes.

There are many ways SOD protects not only diabetics, but everyone. For example, one form of highly destructive free radical is called the superoxide anion (it is unavoidably produced when we make energy in the mitochondria). This **free radical stops insulin from working** (Gardner). But mitochondrial SOD provides **the first step in neutralizing** it to a peroxide. But this only happens if the mitochondrial SOD has enough of its **key mineral, manganese (in its SOD**; elsewhere in the body SOD depends on zinc and copper). For the next step in the body, another detox enzyme, glutathione peroxidase, finishes the detox job of detoxifying the formed peroxide. That enzyme is dependent on a molecule of selenium that you just learned about. Isn't the body miraculously designed? So a daily **Chelated Manganese** is essential, as well as a **Chelated Selenium**. If you don't know if you have a dinosaur doc or a dynamo doc, just ask him if he has checked your **intracellular manganese and selenium** yet. The response you get will tell you. And don't worry. We are going to map these out later. But because you are the first generation of man to have to learn how to heal yourselves, you need some more rudimentary background information.

Many other agents repair the mitochondria, but let's look at some simple things that you might do. Branched chain amino acids (leucine, isoleucine and valine) account for a fifth of all muscle proteins (Harper). And they improve sugar metabolism including hemoglobin A1C in poorly controlled diabetics as well as those who are losing muscle mass (Solerte). And when supplemented they can actually foster **making new mitochondria** (D'Antona). You can get branched chain amino acids as **Stress Guard**, with 500 mg of the 3 branched chain amino acids (leucine, isoleucine, valine). One a day should do it.

Clearly a cardiologist has slim chance of repairing a diabetic heart without attention to all the aspects of mitochondrial repair (Bugger, Shen, Wallace, Duncan, Finck, Rogers, Flarsheim). No wonder such garbage medical diagnostic terms have evolved such as "incurable diabetic cardiomyopathy", macular degeneration, motor neuron disease, fibromyalgia, polymyalgia rheumatica, NASH,

106

insulin resistance, restless legs syndrome, dry eye syndrome, PMS, polycystic ovary syndrome, etc. Anything and **everything is incurable if you don't look for the cause**. And diabetes, heart disease and cancer should head this list! I could go on with scores of papers proving that it should border on malpractice to fail to diagnose and repair mitochondrial dysfunction for every disease (Victor, Brooks, Stavrovskaya).

References:

• Nishikawa T, et al, **Normalizing mitochondrial superoxide production blocks three pathways of hyperglycemic damage**, *Nature* 404:787-90, 2000

• Green K, et al, **Prevention of mitochondrial oxidative damage as a therapeutic strategy in diabetes**, *Diabetes* 53:110-118, 2004

• Lowell BB, et al, **Mitochondrial dysfunction and type 2 diabetes**, *Sci* 307; 5708:384-87, 2005

• West IC, Radicals and oxidative stress in diabetes, *Diabetes Med* 17:171-80, 2000

• Gardner CD, et al, Hydrogen peroxide inhibits insulin signaling in vascular smooth muscle cells, *Exp Biol Med*, 228:836-42, 2003

• Murphy MP, Development of lipophilic cations as therapies for disorders due to mitochondrial dysfunction, *Expert Opin Biol Ther* 1:753-64, 2001

• Lortz S, et al, Importance of mitochondrial superoxide dismutase expression in insulin-producing cells for the toxicity of reactive oxygen species and pro-inflammatory cytokines, *Diabetologia* 48:1541-48, 2005

• Rosen P, et al, The role of oxidative stress in the onset and progression of diabetes and its of complications: a summary of a Congress Series sponsored by UNESCO-MCBN, *Diabetes Metab Res Rev* 17:189-212, 2001

• Bonnard C, et al, **Mitochondrial dysfunction results from oxidative stress** in the skeletal muscle of diet-induced insulin-resistant mice, *J Clin Investig* 118; 2:789-800, 2008

• Bugger H, et al, **Mitochondria in the diabetic heart**, *Cardiovasc Res* 88:229-40, 2010

• Shen X, et al, **Protection of cardiac mitochondria** by overexpression of **MnSOD reduces diabetic cardiomyopathy**, *Diabetes*, 55:798-805, 2006

• Wallace DC, **Mitochondrial** genetics: a paradigm for **aging and degenerative diseases**? *Science* 256:628-632, 1992

• Duncan JG, et al., **Insulin-resistant** heart exhibits a **mitochondrial** biogenic response driven by the **peroxisome** proliferator-activated receptor-a/PGC-1 alpha gene regulatory pathway, *Circulation,* 115:909-17, 2007

• Boudina S, et al, **Mitochondrial energetics in the heart in obesity-related diabetes**: direct evidence for increased uncoupled respiration and activation of uncoupling proteins, *Diabetes* 56:2457-66, 2007

- Finck BN, et al, A critical role for the **PPAR** alpha-mediated lipotoxicity in the pathogenesis of **diabetic cardiomyopathy**: modulation by dietary fat content, *Proc Natl Acad Sci USA* 100:1226-31, 2003

- Finck BN, et al, The cardiac phenotype induced by **PPAR** alpha overexpression **mimics** that caused by **diabetes** mellitus, *J Clin Investig*, 109:121-130, 2002

- Flarsheim CE, et al, **Mitochondrial dysfunction accompanies diastolic dysfunction in diabetic** rats heart, *Am J Physiol* 271: H192-202, 1996

- Shen X, et al, Cardiac **mitochondrial damage** and biogenesis **in a chronic model of type I diabetes**, *Am J Physiol Endocrinol Metab* 287: E896-905, 2004

- Murray AJ, et al, Plasma free fatty acids and peroxisome proliferator-activated receptor alpha in the control of myocardial uncoupling protein levels, *Diabetes* 54:3496-3502, 2005

- Nichols BJ, et al, Towards the molecular basis for the regulation of mitochondrial dehydrogenases by calcium ions, *Mol Cell Biochem*, 149-150:203-212, 1995

- Lehman JJ, et al, **Peroxisome** proliferator-activated receptor gamma coactivator-1 **promotes** cardiac **mitochondrial biogenesis**, *J Clin Investig,* 106:847-56, 2000

- Harper AS, Branched chain amino acids acid metabolism, *Ann Rev Nutr* 4:409-54, 1984

- D'Antona GM, et al, **Branched chain amino acids** supplementation **promotes survival** and supports cardiac and skeletal muscle **mitochondrial** biogenesis in middle aged mice, *Cell Metab* 12; 4:362-72, 2010

- Solerte SB, et al, Improvement of blood glucose control and insulin sensitivity during a long term (60 weeks) randomized study with amino acid dietary supplements in elderly subjects with type II diabetes mellitus, *Am J Cardiol* 101; 11A:82E-88E, 2008

- Victor VM, et al, Targeting antioxidants to mitochondria: a potential new therapeutic strategy for cardiovascular diseases, *Curr Pharmaceut Design* 13:845-63, 2007

- Brookes PS, et al, Calcium, ATP, and ROS: a mitochondrial love-hate triangle, *Am J Physiolog Physiol,* 287:817-33, 2004

- Stavrovskaya IG, et al, The powerhouse takes control of the cell: is the mitochondrial permeability transition a viable therapeutic target against neuronal dysfunction and death? *Free Rad Biol Med* 38:687-97, 2005

- Solerte SB, et al, Nutritional supplements with oral amino acid mixtures increases whole body lean mass and insulin sensitivity in elderly subjects with sarcopenia: *Am J Cardiol* 101; 11A:69E-77E, 2008

No Energy? Think Zinc

Zinc is also crucial in restoring mitochondrial function. It is part of the chemistry that creates the electricity or energy. Unfortunately, the unavoidable pollutants like plasticizers and many prescription medications like the statin cholesterol-lowering and blood pressure-lowering drugs, like calcium channel blockers and beta blockers, lower zinc. At least get 1 **Chelated Zinc** a day, remembering that as you take more you bottom out other minerals that are sort of on a teeter-totter with zinc, like molybdenum, manganese, chromium and other essentials. Balance is paramount.

And don't be hoodwinked by a "normal" level of zinc. Functional indicators on the **Cardio/ION** show if you need more zinc than you have on board, regardless of what your level is. Examples of clues: (1) if the beta-carotene is high normal and vitamin A is low normal, the enzyme that does this conversion is zinc-dependent. You need more. (2) If the neurotransmitters of happy mood are deficient, zinc is needed to convert vitamin B6 into its active form P5P to create happy moods. So even if your zinc is in the "normal" range, these show you need more, regardless.

Or (3) if your 8-OHdG is elevated (evidence of gene damage that could lead to cancer), zinc is needed in the enzyme RNA polymerase to restore the damaged gene to normal. Or (4) if you don't convert the omega-3 EPA to brain-saving DHA, zinc is crucial in the delta-6-desaturase enzyme that does this. (5) If you have recurrent infections, or brain fog from chemical exposures, zinc is crucial (Rogers, yes that's me). (6) If you have persistent inflammatory indicators like CRP or you are on a calcium channel blocker like Norvasc, these can be signs of a zinc deficiency (Shen, Gyulkhandanyan). And recall, zinc is needed in the enzyme pyridoxal kinase to convert B6 into P5P, needed not just for the brain's happy hormones, but to reduce glycation (A1C) and other overt predictors of the severity and progression of diabetes.

Don't worry, I won't give you all 300 zinc enzymes if you promise you've got the gist of how crucial zinc is and will take it forever. When you see the huge amount of years and money that hundreds of researchers have devoted to proving the necessity of zinc in not only preventing but curing diabetes, it boggles the mind why it's not standard to test for its adequacy (RBC zinc, not serum). Especially since zinc is actually part of (1) the pancreas and also (2) the actual insulin complex, and (3) most diabetics are low (Jansen).

References:

- Sensi SL, et al, **Modulation of mitochondrial function by endogenous Zn** 2+ pools, *Proc Nat Acad Sci, USA* 100:6157-62, 2003

- Rudolph E, et al, **Zinc induced apoptosis of** HEP-2 **cancer cells**: the role of oxidative stress and **mitochondria**, *BioFactors* 23:107-20, 2005

- Shen H, et al, **Zinc deficiency** induces vascular pro-inflammatory parameters associated with NF-kB and **PPAR signaling**, *J Am Coll Nutr* 27; 5:577-87, 2008

- Gyulkhandanyan AV, et al, The **Zn2+-transporting** pathways **in pancreatic beta cells**: a role for the L-type voltage-gated **Ca2+ channels**, *J Biolog Chem* 281:9361-72, 2006

- Rogers SA, Zinc deficiency as a model for developing chemical sensitivity, *Internatl Clin Nutr Rev,* 10;1:253-259, Jan 1990

- Jansen J, et al, **Zinc and diabetes** -- clinical links and molecular mechanisms, *J Nutr Biochem* 20:399-417, 2009

Did They Forget to Check Your Gamma Tocopherol?

Whether you're battling diabetes, a cancer, have just had a heart attack or are trying to stave off coronary artery disease or other inflammatory sequelae of diabetes, be sure your gamma tocopherol is checked. **Real vitamin E is really 8 entities, four tocopherols and four tocotrienols.** If just the alpha-tocopherol is checked and/or prescribed, you are being cheated. Why? Because one of the other parts of "vitamin E" is **gamma tocopherol. It has special anti-cancer and anti-chronic disease-fighting capacities that the other parts of vitamin E do not, and tests confirm most people are low in it.** Unfortunately when folks are unknowledgeable enough to only take **"vitamin E"** (which is usually synthetic alpha-tocopherol and does not work in the human body like natural alpha-tocopherol from foods), this actually **lowers the levels of gamma tocopherol**. This in turn leads to all sorts of complications from inability to heal diabetes, heart disease and cancers to the explosion into the myriad of inflammatory sequelae of diabetes. For example, the statin cholesterol-lowering Crestor® is promoted for **raising the HDL**, but **gamma tocopherol raises HDL twice as much and without the multitude of statin side effects, like increasing diabetes** as well as many other diseases, including Alzheimer's (as described in *The Cholesterol Hoax* and *TW).*

We have all heard the reports on TV and in the media of how vitamin E does not help in heart disease, or cancer. I would be utterly embarrassed to be affiliated with any of these studies. Whenever there is an article that says vitamin E doesn't help certain conditions, I scour the study to determine how they could come to such a ludicrous conclusion. And guess what I find! It's usually because they used only one of the 8 parts of real vitamin E, only alpha-tocopherol. That is as stupid as going to the car dealer and saying you can only afford to buy only one out of every eight parts of the car, but you expect it to work!

Also when you take only one of eight parts, this lowers other parts of vitamin E, like tocotrienols and **gamma tocopherol** (that you already learned is crucial in aspects of healing that alpha tocopherol lacks). All 8 parts of real vitamin E have unique healing qualities. For example, gamma tocopherol is **more potent for** healing various types of **cancers and heart disease** (evidence in past books and *TW*). More importantly, it **prevents full blown progression to diabetes from metabolic syndrome, improves insulin sensitivity** and even helps magnesium work better (which most folks as well as diabetics are low in) (Goepp).

Remember, a good sign of a lousy vitamin is if it just says on the label "vitamin E". They think you are too dumb to know the difference. Good daily protection for you is 1-2 **E-Gems Elite**, 1 **Gamma E-Gems** and 2 **Tocotrienols** to get super-healthy balanced levels of all crucial 8 forms of real Vitamin E. For even though **E Gems Elite** contains the 4 tocopherols and all 4 tocotrienols, it turns out that extra levels of **tocotrienols are particularly protective, not only for diabetes, but for cancers, the aging brain**, and so much more. So be sure to add one or two **Tocotrienols** twice daily to your regimen.

References:

• Paolisso G, et al, Pharmacologic doses of **vitamin E improve insulin action in** healthy subjects and non-insulin-dependent **diabetic patients,** *Am J Clin Nutr,* 57; 5:650-6, 1993

- Vucinic L, et al, **Gamma tocopherol supplementation prevents exercise-induced coagulation and platelet aggregation**, *Thromb Res* 125; 2:196-9, 2010

- Himmelfarb J, et al, **Gamma-tocopherol** and docosahexaenoic acid decrease inflammation in **dialysis patients**, *J Renal Nutr* 17; 5:296-304, 2007

- Gutierrez AD, et al, The response of gamma vitamin E to varying doses of a vitamin E plus vitamin C, *Metabolism* 58:469-78, 2009

- Goepp J, Combating the "Diabesity" epidemic, *Life Extension* (www.lef.org), 39-48 Aug 2010

- Osakada F, et al, **Tocotrienols prove the <u>most potent neuroprotective</u> among vitamin E** analogues on cultured striatal neurons, *Neuropharmacol* 47:904-15, 2004

- Sen CK, et al, Molecular basis of vitamin E action: <u>**tocotrienols potently inhibits**</u> **glutamate-**induced pp60c-Src kinase activation and <u>**death**</u> of HT4 <u>**neuronal cells**</u>, *J Biol Chem* 275:13049-55, 2000

- Ihara Y, et al, Antioxidant **alpha-tocopherol ameliorates glycemic control** in GK rats, a model of type II diabetes, *FEBS Lett* 473:24-6, 2000

Diabetics Do Not Have to Suffer Brain Deterioration

Diabetics are at more risk of early Alzheimer's and other brain abnormalities than the average person who doesn't have the free radical pathology of diabetes. Yet a combination of many of the nutrients that you will learn about here can literally stop brain deterioration in its tracks for either type. Alzheimer's brain deterioration is due to the deposition of amyloid, a special protein in the brain that literally glues down the nerves, then tangles them. But manganese (in the mitochondrial superoxide dismutase) can help reduce that (Dumont). **Vitamin E** is another example that helps prevent it (Yatin), but is **depleted by statins**. And fixing the mitochondria themselves is crucial (Arias), as is sopping up the free radicals like hydrogen peroxide to down-regulate Alzheimer's (Behl). But you have to have selenium in the enzyme glutathione peroxidase for it to work. Don't fret. I've mapped out the most commonly deficient nutrients for you in Chapter V.

Researchers have found that just having folks on the correct dose of **vitamin D** (whose deficiency is epidemic) can not only **protect the diabetic brain from deterioration**, but repair the calcium channels, reverse insulin resistance and/or diabetes (of course, all depending on the total deficiencies that the person has) (Kumar). The sad thing is this has been known for nearly 3 decades

(Nyomba). This is just one more reason why as soon as you get any symptom you had better find the cause and the cure. Otherwise you will soon be on the disease/drug roller coaster.

References:

• Yatin SM, et al, **Vitamin E prevents Alzheimer's amyloid** beta peptide (1-42)-induced neuronal protein oxidation and reactive oxygen species production, *J Alzheimer's Dis* 2; 2:123-31, 2000

• Behl C, et al, Hydrogen peroxide mediated amyloid beta protein toxicity, *Cell*, 77; 6:817-27, 1994

• Arias C, et al, Beta-amyloid neurotoxicity is exacerbated during glycolysis inhibition and mitochondrial impairment in the rat hippocampus in vivo and in isolated nerve terminals: implications for Alzheimer's disease, *Experiment Neurol* 176; 1:163-74, 2002

• Dumont AM, et al, **Reduction** of oxidative stress, **amyloid** deposition and **memory deficit by manganese** superoxide dismutase overexpression in a transgenic mouse model of Alzheimer's disease, *FASEB J* 23; 8:2459-66, 2009

• Kumar PT, et al, **Vitamin D3 restores** altered cholinergic and **insulin receptor** expression in cerebral cortex and muscarinic M3 receptor expression in pancreatic islets of streptozotocin-induced diabetic rats, *J Nutr Biochem* 22:418-425, 2011

• Brewer Al D., et al., **Vitamin D** hormone confers neuroprotection in parallel with the down regulation of L-type **calcium channel** expression in hippocampal neurons, *J Neurosci* 21:98-108, 2001

• Borissova AM, et al, The effect of **vitamin D3 on insulin secretion** and peripheral insulin sensitivity in type II diabetic patients, *Internat J Clin Pract* 57:258-61, 2003

• Nyomba BL, et al, Influence of **vitamin D status on insulin secretion** in glucose tolerance in the rabbit, *Endocrinology* 115:191-7, 1984

Key Nutrient Reverses Heart Failure, Even in Diabetics

In 2010 we heard about the failure of one pump that resulted in the worst pollution in the Gulf of Mexico in the history of the world (British Petroleum, August 2010). But in spite of staggering damages, the importance of that type of pump is miniscule. What's **the most important pump** in your life? It's the pump that began working when you were just a mass of unborn cells and has never stopped since. It works 24 x 7 and never gets a rest, your heart.

But like any good pump, it does need maintenance. Like any pump it requires (1) **an oil change** (for example, with something just as simple as cod liver oil and phosphatidylcholine and the 8 forms of vitamin E plus Acetyl-L-Carnitine, that you are beginning to memorize). As well, any plumber will tell you proper pump maintenance requires (2) **repair or replacement of worn-out parts** (like repair of vitamin A, R-lipoic acid, thiamine, niacin, DHA, magnesium, chromium, selenium and zinc deficiencies, as examples).

Besides changing the oil of any pump and repairing worn out parts, if you want it to last it also requires (3) **frequent cleaning**. And the heart is also no exception. That's why **getting the heavy metals out like lead, cadmium, arsenic, mercury, and aluminum, plus the plasticizers, pesticides, etc. are also crucial goals for keeping our hearts working properly**. I'll show you how (and for even further directions with more detail begin with *Detoxify Or Die*, followed by *The High Blood Pressure Hoax* and then *The Cholesterol Hoax*, regardless of the fact that you may not have the diseases in the titles. Some folks can be lucky and accomplish it with less detail as in *Is Your Cardiologist Killing You?*).

But when the heart fails, how does the specialist cardiologist take care of your precious pump? (1) He doesn't do any of the repairs such as an oil change, and (2) he doesn't replace worn-out parts or even clean it. In fact, (3) he goes one step further and purposely poisons the heart (that is already sick) in as many ways as possible. You find this hard to believe? Just look at the drugs prescribed by cardiologists to any person with serious heart failure. They usually include a **beta** <u>**blocker**</u> (like Toprol, Atenolol, Tenormin, Lopressor, Carvedilol, atenolol, metoprolol, Corgard, etc.) and an **ACE** <u>**inhibitor**</u> (like Lisinopril, Prinivil, Lotensin, Monopril, Capoten or Vasotec), a **calcium channel** <u>**blocker**</u> (like Norvasc, plus see names in *TW Dec.*/10) and/or an **angiotensin receptor** <u>**blocker**</u> (Atacand, Mycardis, Diovan, etc.). All these standard cardiology drugs block, inhibit and otherwise turn off or poison enzymes in the heart..... a heart that is already down and out. And by intentionally poisoning pathways, drugs also create a myriad of hidden deficiencies, leading to an avalanche of symptoms and (seemingly unrelated) new diseases.

In this common example, the "specialist" has attacked at least four enzymes that are crucial in the heart. He has intentionally poisoned them in attempt to "help" the heart not work so hard. Of course these medicines not only poison heart enzymes, but they **also create CoQ10 deficiencies, zinc deficiencies** and much more, all of which are crucial for actually healing heart failure, diabetes, cancer, or any disease. So now **your chances of recovery are dwindling by the day.**

Not only do the prescribed drugs create these nutrient deficiencies, but cardiologists do not routinely check to see if the patient needed them in the first place, much less check to see what nutrients the drugs have lowered. Meanwhile, the drugs are prescribed on the basis of your diagnostic label, according to the practice guidelines (the fixed recipes confabulated by "expert" physicians who are proven to be financially connected with the drug industry!). No wonder the median survival after heart failure (once it is diagnosed) is 5 years! That means it kills quicker than cancer, which has a median survival (all types lumped together) of 6 years. No one fixes what's broken.

And why do drugs get used instead of repairing the pump? As I've documented before from the *New England Journal of Medicine*, and other leading medical journals plus the *Wall Street Journal*, that **less than 11% of cardiovascular recommendations are based on scientific evidence. The rest are based on pharmaceutical influence. Also 87% of the "experts" who make the practice guidelines (the rules and recipes for treating every disease) have financial ties with the pharmaceutical industry.** You might say that the average physician who prefers to poison patients' pumps is merely a pimp or a puppet of the drug industry. You think this is harsh? You may change your tune once you see more evidence.

115

How does the average cardiologist fail the failing heart? It's been known for decades that the failing heart can no longer create energy. And by now you know where that occurs, inside the mitochondria. And you now know that when the mitochondria become poisoned through lack of the right nutrients and through toxins like the unavoidable plastics and heavy metals and pesticides, they can no longer efficiently create energy. **People experiencing this loss of energy think they are just getting old and tired. They have no idea that all they have to do is rejuvenate their pump,** starting with the mitochondria.

Remember, **heart failure is more dangerous than cancer** because the victim has a shorter median lifespan. Early signs of heart failure can just be shortness of breath, or the low number on your blood pressure (diastolic) climbs above 90, or your ankles swell. **Heart failure is totally curable in most folks. Yet this cure is not even sought by the average cardiologist** much less internal medicine or family practice physicians. Instead it is bludgeoned with often over half a dozen medications before the patient dies.

Let's use as our evidence example just one nutrient, ribose, a sugar I've introduced you to that is crucial in making ATP (the chemical that creates the energy we call "life") in the mitochondria. For starters, **folks with heart failure already have a minimum of 30% decrease in the amount of ATP** that they can make in a day compared with the normal person without heart failure. And this **mitochondrial poisoning which results in a decreased ATP (energy production) is a better predictor of early death than any of the standard tests used by doctors.** This includes a lot of nasty x-rays where you are injected with radioactive dyes.

In a nutshell, some folks with as little as one scoop (3000 mg) of **D-Ribose Powder** twice a day have **markedly improved their heart failure**. Of course, they are most likely low in many other things as well, for it takes a total package to bring each individual to the pedestal of wellness. Yet as you have learned like any good nutrient, D-Ribose has many other benefits in all spectra of folks, from sick to well. Recall **it shortens the recovery period from anything from a heart attack to over-doing with exercise, and if given right away when you have chest pain it makes the area of infarct (permanent heart damage) smaller. It improves folks with chronic fatigue and fibromyalgia,** and even angina and cardiomyopathy (which is erroneously considered by the clueless cardiologist as having "no known cause and no known cure").

Yet there's even a better use for **D-Ribose. It revives areas of the heart that were diagnosed as "dead" by heart scans.** So obviously when you have had a heart attack and they tell you that you have a certain amount of dead heart tissue, you want to **use D-ribose and other nutrients to resurrect this "dead" area.** The researchers who have discovered this then **labeled the resurrected heart as having been merely "hibernating"** all of this time. Yet even when I read papers by researchers from esteemed institutions like the Mayo or Cleveland Clinics or Johns Hopkins, they have totally missed the bottom line causes, the **heavy metal and phthalate toxicities that damaged the mitochondrial metabolism of ribose**. Their research focus appears to be to try to find a drug that will take the place of ribose, rather than using inexpensive and natural D-ribose. They are so close, yet so far away from the truth.

When you appreciate how simple cures can be and how utterly out of focus medicine is, there's no contest. **If you want to be independently healthy you must keep reading and take control, for medicine does not appear interested in cures. That is exactly why I have taken precious time to gather this information for you and to lovingly teach you this difficult state-of-the-art life-saving material. Medicine is caught in a seriously deceitful quagmire.**

As a **test**, just ask your physician how he is going to cure your heart failure. If you get a look or response that tells you are an idiot for even asking, for everyone knows there is no cure, you are in the wrong place. And when you find a practitioner who is interested in actually curing you, nurture him/her to your utmost. If any come to mind that you think would be interested in learning how to actually heal folks instead of merely drugging them, notify *orders@prestigepublishing.com* of their addresses and we will send a free sample copy of a newsletter.

References:

• Ingwall JS, et al, Is **the failing heart energy starved**? On using chemical energy to support cardiac function, *Circul Res* 95:135-45, 2004

• Omran H, et al, **D-Ribose improves diastolic function and quality of life in congestive heart failure patients**: a prospective feasibility study, *Eur J Heart Fail* 5:615-19, 2003

• Illie S, et al, **D-Ribose improves** myocardial function in **congestive heart failure**, *FASEB J*, 15; 5:A 1142, 2001

• Omran H, et al, **D-Ribose improves** myocardial function and quality of life in **congestive heart failure** patients, *J Mol Cell Cardiol*, 33;6: A173, 2001

• Gradus-Pizio I, et al, Effect of **D-ribose on the detection of the hibernating myocardium** during the low dose dobutamine stress echocardiography, *Circul* 100; 18:3394, 1999

Diabetics Need ALC for Neuropathy

Readers of our *Total Wellness* newsletter have asked some very good questions over its quarter century that you should know the answers to, as well.

Q. *My diabetes hasn't been under really good control and now I'm starting to lose sensation in my legs and get unusual needle-like pains as well. Of course, my libido is shot, too. I'm ready. Where do I start?*

A. You need to get very aggressive and quickly. The good news is it is reversible. First of all, **the very medications that most diabetologists, internists, and family doctors prescribe for diabetes actually raise your homocysteine and lower your folic acid and B12. These deficiencies alone can give bizarre pain, erectile dysfunction, numbness, loss of sensation, tingling, as well as depression, loss of memory, and promote faster aging**

118

and arteriosclerosis, as well as cancers. And this is only the tip of the iceberg. Furthermore, many other medications, for example, like those for the acid stomach like Prilosec, Nexium, Aciphex, etc. further reduce these nutrients making the symptoms cascade even quicker. As I evidenced a couple of years ago in *TW*, **vitamin D3 (a deficiency for which there is a hidden epidemic) works better than metformin**, the classic diabetes medication, and without the side effects.

As well, many other factors make sure the complications of diabetes remain rampant. For example, the plasticizers (the number one pollutant in the human body) damage the mitochondria where carnitine is made. **We not only need carnitine to keep us from heart disease and metastases in cancer, but also from muscle and nerve pain and loss of function. In fact, some diabetics have actually improved nerve function and gotten rid of the pain and loss of sensation of diabetic neuropathy with just ALC** (use **Acetyl L-Carnitine Powder** 1000 mg twice a day for starters).

Of course remember that no nutrient is to be used solo, as if it were a drug. Diabetics are usually also low in **Chromium, Vanadium, Molybdenum, Manganese, Magnesium**, as well as the components of **Cod Liver Oil** (EPA/DHA), **Phosphatidyl Choline**, the eight forms of vitamin E as in **E Gems Elite**, and much more. If you really value your health I would get the **Cardio/ION** and identify your deficiencies (I review them with select readers in over 10 countries on the phone), correct them, and then start getting the toxicities out. Many diabetics have even reduced or totally gotten rid of their medications. And remember **any neuropathy that cannot be reversed with some of the simpler methods above screams for heavy metal detoxification**.

There is a wealth of data proving that it should border on malpractice to fail to assay and prescribe ALC for diabetics. When nutrient deficiencies and environmental toxicities poison the mitochondria so they no longer make carnitine, the diabetic

119

cascade begins. But just **ALC has actually cured Syndrome X, repaired membrane function and enhanced regeneration of the pancreas, decreased insulin** and damaging lipoprotein(a), and even repaired damaged genes in the mitochondria, staved off kidney disease, anemia, made the size of the infarct or damaged area after a heart attack smaller, repaired the peroxisomes, raised HDL and albumin, lowered triglycerides and LDL, and, oh yes......**reversed diabetic neuropathy** (Molfino, Flanagan).

References:

• Sima AA, et al, Acetyl L-Carnitine Study Group, **Acetyl L-Carnitine improves pain, nerve regeneration, and vibratory perception in patients with chronic diabetic neuropathy**: an analysis of two randomized placebo-controlled trials, *Diabetes Care* 28; 1:89-94, Jan 2005

• Sahin M, et al, Effects of metformin or rosiglitazone on serum concentrations of homocysteine, folate, and B12 in patients with type II diabetes mellitus. *J Diabetes Complications* 21; 2:118-123, Mar-Apr 2007

• Molfino A, et al, Caloric restriction and l-**carnitine administration improves insulin sensitivity** in patients with impaired glucose metabolism, *J Parenteral Nutr*, 34:295-99, 2010

• Flanagan JL, et al, Role of carnitine in disease, *Nutr Metab* 7:30-44, 2010

What to Do When Nitroglycerin No Longer Works

Q. My husband was prescribed nitroglycerin under the tongue to dilate his coronary arteries for his attacks of angina. He needs this to protect him from having a heart attack, but now it no longer works. His doctor says he has developed a tolerance to nitroglycerin and that that's a common problem. They are offering angioplasty, stents and more drugs. What can we do?

A. Find a cardiologist who reads. As we showed in *The High Blood Pressure Hoax*, arginine is one of many nutrients that actually makes the body make its own nitroglycerin. In reality, nitroglycerin works by increasing the nitric oxide in the blood vessel lining, which then dilates the blood vessels allowing more oxygen and nutrients to the tissue (namely the heart when you're talking about coronary blood vessels). **Arginine is the rate-limiting amino acid for the body to make its own nitric oxide,**

which is nature's nitroglycerine. As well, you need sufficient levels of magnesium, and much more.

But there is much more dangerous ignorance on display here. For **when the heart is sick enough to require nitroglycerin in the first place, research clearly shows you must repair the mitochondria**. Once you've done that you may not even need the nitroglycerin. Sometimes the repair can be as simple as the membrane repair cited earlier, or require the detox cocktail, CoQ10, arginine, zinc, magnesium, manganese, selenium, molybdenum, or the many other nutrients that we have explained and referenced in *Is Your Cardiologist Killing You?,* plus in previous books and *TW* issues.

Where do you begin? If you are seriously committed to your husband's longevity, and seriously committed to becoming a "widow whacker", I would become an expert in the last six books and six years of *TW* newsletters. I don't know any place else where all this information is collated, explained and referenced for the most discerning folks, including physicians. If I did, I'd happily stop writing and improve my tennis game. I do know in looking back over 44 years of thousands of folks with a huge variety of ailments, that **those whose spouses became just as committed to learning as they were had the highest success rates. On the flipside, I could show you lots of unsuccessful cases where only one person was doing all the reading and work, while the other one was just along for the ride.** Remember, this is the first time in human history that lay people have had to learn how to cure, because medicine is instead focused on drugs. Team work!

Obviously you would want to get the **Cardio/ION** as soon as possible and an expert interpretation with both of you present.

References (and more in chapter 2):

• Esplugues JV, et al, Complex I dysfunction and tolerance to nitroglycerin. An approach based on mitochondrial-targeted antioxidants, *Circul Res* 99:1067-75, 2006

• McLennan PL, et al., Myocardial function, ischemia and n-3 polyunsaturated fatty acids: a membrane basis, *J Cardiovasc Med* (supple 1): S15-S18, 2007

• Parker JD, Nitrate tolerance, oxidative stress, and mitochondrial function: another worrisome chapter on the effects of organic nitrates, *J Clin Invest* 113:352-354, 2004

Nix on Norvasc

Q. *I've just been prescribed Norvasc for my blood pressure. What should I know about it? My doctor assures me it is the state-of-the-art treatment.*

A. Norvasc® is an example of one of many commonly prescribed drugs for high blood pressure, arrhythmias, angina, and more. It is from a classification of cardiology drugs called **calcium channel blockers**. You'll find other brand names in the 2010 *TW* and the book, *The High Blood Pressure Hoax*. Among the many bad things that calcium channel blockers do is **shrink the brain away from the skull, as proven by MRI** (Heckbert). **As well, testing of the person shows that their mental capabilities and IQ have dropped. In other words, folks get dumber on the drug, and the brain damage escalates the longer they take it.** It is usually prescribed for life, and the decline is chalked up to aging.

The measurable loss of brain size and I.Q. from calcium channel blockers happens within about five years of use. And even though it is usually prescribed for a lifetime, this is often without ever checking the induced nutrient deficiencies, much less the brain function and physical shrinkage. Users also have a higher risk for breast and other cancers and heart attacks (June 1998), since medications allow the doc to ignore fixing what's broken. If that were not bad enough, other categories of common drugs, like the cholesterol-fighters (statins) also damage the brain, so drugs that combine the two categories, like Caduet®, are doubly dangerous.

You must ask yourself: why did you need a drug to poison ("block") your calcium pores in the heart muscle and nerve linings? The **calcium channels can be repaired**. Sometimes it is as easy as doing the oil change. If you are new to this idea of actually curing rather than drugging, I would first read *Is Your Cardiologist Killing You?*, then go to *Detoxify Or Die* to begin to get the many chemicals out of the membranes that have accumulated over a lifetime. **Plasticizers, pesticides, auto exhaust fumes, fatty acid deficiencies, etc., all damage calcium channels**. Then read the vascular repair book, *The High Blood Pressure Hoax*, to get the heavy metals out. Your goal is to correct his blood pressure without drugs. With such a solid education don't be surprised if lots of other conditions clear up as you heal your husband, once and for all.

You may be among the lucky ones who have cured their blood pressure problems with just the following once a day: 1 tsp of **Super D Omega-3**, 1 heaping tsp of **HB-PC (Phosphatidyl Choline Powder)**, 2 **E Gems Elite**, and ½ tsp **Arginine Powder**. Also include 2 **Chelated Magnesium Glycinate** 400mg and 1 **Super 2 Daily**, each twice a day. **If poisoning your calcium channels with a drug that blocks the channels lowers blood pressure, then you can be sure the channels in your brain and elsewhere have become damaged and are deficient. They are screaming to be repaired**.

Besides the right fatty acids, Vitamin D, phosphatidyl choline and many nutrients are key in repairing the calcium channels such as zinc (Gyulkhandanyan), manganese, copper, silicon, selenium, and more. But this simple formula has cured many of hypertension by restoring nutrients and function to the membranes' calcium channels. And the beauty of it is that by fixing the membranes in his blood vessel lining, you have also repaired them everywhere else... as in his brain, penis (a major cure for erectile dysfunction), etc. **Nutrient repair is always a win-win situation.** The bottom line is only physicians ignorant of how to repair calcium channels would ever prescribe a calcium channel blocker that shrinks your brain and rots your intellect.

References:

• Gyulkhandanyan AV, et al, The Zn2+-transporting pathways and pancreatic beta cells: a role for the L-type voltage-gated Ca2+ channel, *J Biol Chem* 281:9361-72, 2006

• Huang JM, et al, Long-chain **fatty acids activate calcium channels** in ventricular myocytes, *Proc Nat Acad Sci USA* 89 (14): 6452-6, July15, 1992

• Das UN, Essential fatty acids and their metabolites could function as an endogenous HMG-CoA reductase and ACE enzyme inhibitors, and anti-arrhythmic, anti-hypertensive, anti-atherosclerotic, anti-inflammatory, cytoprotective and cardioprotective molecules, *Lipids Health Dis* 7:37-55, 2008

• Belke DD, et al, **Altered cardiac calcium handling in diabetes**, *Curr Hypertens Rep* 6:424-9, 2004

• Heckbert SR, etal, The association of antihypertensive agents with MRI white matter findings and with modified mini-mental state examination in older adults, *J Am Geriatric Soc* 45:1423-33, 1997

Don't Let a Dinosaur Lead You to Blindness

In chapter 1 you were exposed to just a few nutrient examples that dramatically protect against diabetic blindness, like DHA cutting the risk over 38%. No drug has that kind of power. But lest you think that is all there is to it, all the nutrients you will learn about are important for the health of the eye as well. One good daily insurance that you may not hear about is **Lutein with Kale** or **Lutein** (both containing hefty amounts of lutein plus zeaxanthin and more). Research we reported in *TW* 2011-12 shows that lutein is one of the nutrients the eye runs out of that triggers diabetic blindness as well as macular degeneration (the number one cause of blindness over age 50), glaucoma and cataracts, and even in non-diabetics.

References:

• Moustafa SA, **Zinc might protect oxidative changes in the retina and pancreas at the early stage of diabetic** rats, *Toxicol Appl Pharmacol*, 2001; 2:149-55, 2004

• Connor KM, et al., Increased dietary intake of **omega-3 polyunsaturated fatty acids reduces pathological retinal angiogenesis,** *Nat Med* 13; 7:868-73, 2007

• Jariyapongskul A, et al, Long-term effects of oral **vitamin C** supplementation on the endothelial dysfunction in the **iris micro vessels of diabetic** rats, *Microvasc Res* 74; 1:32-38, 2007

• Age Related Eye Disease Study Research Group, SanGiovanni JP, et al, The relationship of dietary carotenoids and vitamin A, E, and C intake with age-related macular degeneration and a case control study: AREDS Report#22, *Arch Ophthalmol* 125; 9:1225-32, 2007

• Cangemi FE, et al, TOZOL Study: an open case control study of an oral antioxidant and omega-3 supplement for dry AMD, *BMC Ophthamol* 7:3, Feb. 26, 2007

Beware of Nutrients That Cancel Each Other

As a quick example, you've learned that the zinc and chromium are indispensable in healing diabetics. Yet either one can unbalance molybdenum, manganese, copper and other minerals that are also absolutely necessary for healing. Likewise, vitamin B5 (pantothenic acid) and lipoic acid can unbalance biotin. Recall this is crucial for carbohydrate metabolism, improving pancreatic insulin, lowering the glycosylated hemoglobin, reversing insulin resistance, and much more. Sometimes a biotin deficiency can merely manifest itself as brittle nails. My point? Balance is key.

References:

• Liu J, et al, Memory loss in old rats is associated with brain mitochondrial decay and RNA/DNA oxidation: partial reversal by feeding acetyl-L-carnitine and/or R-a-lipoic acid, *Proc Natl Acad Sci USA* 99:2356-61, 2002

• Sethumadhavan S, et al, L-carnitine and a-lipoic acid improve age-associated decline in mitochondrial respiratory chain activity of rat heart muscle, *J Gerontol Biol Sci Med Sci* 61:650-9, 2006

• Kumaran S, et al, Age-associated deficit of mitochondrial oxidative phosphorylation in skeletal muscle: role of carnitine and alpha-lipoic acid, *Mol Cell Biochem* 280:83-89, 2005

• Albarracin CA, et al, Chromium picolinate and biotin combination improves glucose metabolism in treated, uncontrolled overweight to obese patients with type II diabetes, *Diabetes/Metab Res Rev* 24:41-51, 2008

• Koutsikos D, et al, Biotin for diabetic peripheral neuropathy, *Biomed Pharmacother* 44; 10:511-14, 1990

• Zempleni J, et al, Human peripheral blood mononuclear cells: inhibition of biotin transport by reversible competition with pantothenic acid is quantitatively minor, *J Nutr Biochem* 10; 7:427-32, 1999

• Hochman LG, et al, Brittle nails: response to daily biotin supplementation *Cutis* 51; 4:303-5, 1993

Balance is Key

I could fill volumes with the importance of every nutrient, many of which most folks have never even heard of, much less the more common nutrients. For they all have a role in healing. Take vitamin A, for example. Most diabetologists don't measure it so

125

they must not think it is crucial. But it has many roles in diabetes (Mukherjee). However, just giving it won't work if the receptor for vitamin A in the cell membrane is not repaired. Regardless of how much you give, it won't be able to turn on the cellular chemistry of healing. And as great as all the chemistry you have learned about for repair of membranes is, if folks are weighted down with environmental toxins (plasticizers, heavy metals, etc. that we all have and cannot escape), then nothing works until you get rid of them. I'll show you how.

Meanwhile "Why should someone be low in vitamin A to begin with?", you smartly ask. One of many reasons is because many medications and environmental toxins lower zinc, plus processed foods have had it yanked right out of them. As well, industrial and auto exhausts produce acid rain that depletes zinc from the soils and foods, etc. And if you do not have zinc, then you cannot convert beta-catotene (the vitamin A precursor found in lots of yellow and orange fruits and vegetables) into vitamin A. You may be starting to get the picture also that **the more that you can <u>assay all at once of all of your nutrients</u>, the better chance you have of repairing and balancing the whole package**. Piecemeal assays are counter-productive. But don't worry, I'm going to show you some shortcuts. I've done a lot of the work for you.

Reference:

• Mukherjee R, et al, Sensitization of diabetic and obese mice to insulin by retinoid X receptor agonists, *Nature* 386:407-10, 1997

Any Source of Nutrients Will Do? Not a Chance!

How wrong that is! Let's look at an example of one mineral, copper. Diabetes, unexplained depression, accelerated aging, anemia, fatigue, cardiac arrhythmias, nervous disorders, osteoporosis, recurrent infections, even gray hair and congestive heart failure and more can be signs of ignored copper deficiency. One problem is that **the American diet only supplies 50% of the RDA for copper (which itself is ridiculously low)**. Not only that but many types of medications, like anti-virals, can deplete it as well as can taking large amounts of zinc (as many men do for their prostates or others do for recurrent infections), as other examples.

On the flip side, many people are toxic with the wrong form of copper from copper water pipes at home or work. Industrial, landfill incinerators and vehicular exhausts are other sources. Unfortunately **one of the most deadly results of copper toxicity is Alzheimer's disease.** And **one of the chief causes of copper toxicity can be cheap multiple mineral supplements like those found in the grocery store**. In the *Journal of the American Medical Association* they showed one of the leading grocery store vitamins that you see continually advertised on television, Centrum®, produces no beneficial effects (2009 *TW*). And it shouldn't, because the abnormally low doses, unbalanced formulation, and cheap synthetic ingredients do not harmonize with the body's chemistry.

It turns out that **inorganic copper from cheap supplements by-passes the liver and can penetrate the blood/brain barrier.** My favorite forms of copper are **Zinc Balance** (15 mg of chelated zinc and 1 mg of copper, and very friendly to people's stomachs generally). For folks who need larger doses, use **Chelated Copper** (5 mg, but be sure to have it with a good-sized meal).

The bottom line? **Cheap nutrients can be toxic and accelerate brain disease**. I'm not connected with any companies that make or sell nutrients. In fact I don't design, manufacture, or sell my own nutrients, because I consider it unethical to be promoting my own when other companies may have come up with something better. I only sell knowledge. And once you have acquired it, it is yours forever. My mission is to find the best products I can for you and me. That is why you will find I have recommended certain nutrients in a book, for example, only to inform readers of a less expensive or better made one in subsequent *TW* newsletters. As the owners of nutrient companies age, they get bought out by folks with less discriminating ethics, etc. Things change. *It would* *be better to cut back on a more expensive nutrient that you trust and only have it twice a week than to take a cheaper one every day,* that harms you.

By the way, sometimes folks ask me if any old cod liver oil will do, but I don't know of another company that goes to such great lengths of immediately removing the cod livers and packing them in nitrogen right on the boat. Most manufacturers wait until enough fish have been caught, take the fish back to the dock and then ship them to the manufacturer's facility. This time lag produces a lot of free radicals that diminish the nutritional value. Another thing I detest are companies with no people's names attached to them, no photographs, not even an address sometimes. They are faceless corporations on the Internet. From cyber-space they send catalogs and merely sell wholesale nutrients, often stored in un-air-conditioned warehouses. Heat accelerates deterioration of nutrients. I have no idea about the people behind faceless nutrient manufacturers or their ethics. This is very disturbing to me and not someone I want to trust my nutrients to. That's just one more reason why most of the products I recommend are from people who have stood behind their quality, are proud of their names, and have been upfront about their commitment to my patients and readers, answering my questions, and substantiating their claims with research.

And why is quality so important? Did you know there is a continual dance going on inside your body? A powerful microscopic look at our fatty acids in the cell membranes is nearly incomprehensible. **Molecules are not sitting there motionless. There is a continual high frequency dance of all of our molecules.** And this miraculous movement is enormously bogged down by not only trans fatty acids from french fries, GMO canola oil and commercial salad dressings, but heavy metals as from our "silver" dental fillings, the plasticizers that we can no longer avoid, and much more.

That is the very reason why I try to find the best quality nutrients for you, since they have to maintain **this "dance of life" that determines health**. If you have inferior quality cut-rate cheap, improperly stored cod liver oil, for example, just how easily will it enable the molecules in your cell membrane to gyrate to the tune of life? To oscillate to the frequency of health? This **"flip-flop" flexibility of nutrient molecules is literally the dance of life. This cadence is the backbone of health**.

References:

• Kamp F, et al, pH Gradients across phospholipid membranes caused by fast **flip-flop** of un-ionized fatty acids, *Proc Natl Acad Sci*, 89:11367-70, Dec 1992

• Kamp F, et al, Fatty acid **flip-flop** in phospholipid bilayers is extremely fast, *Biochem* 34:11928-37, 1995

• McLennan PL, et al., Myocardial function, ischemia and n-3 polyunsaturated fatty acids: a membrane basis, *J Cardiovasc Med* (supple 1): S15-S18, 2007

• Brewer GJ The risks of **copper toxicity contributing to cognitive decline** in the aging population **and to Alzheimer's disease**, *J Am Coll Nutr* 28; 3:238-42, 2009

"How Would I Ever Figure Out What is Needed?"

You have witnessed just a smidgen of the overwhelming evidence that **diabetes and in fact all diseases have only two causes**. Over a lifetime (1) nutrient deficiencies and (2) toxicities have accrued. That's why we and others have been so successful in reversing diseases that are still taught in medical schools to have no known cause and no known treatment. *We no longer care what the label or title of a disease is. All we care about is finding the cause and cure.* The motto? First find what's broken and fix it. But medical schools, physicians, insurance companies, medical boards and others are pharmacy-focused, with surgical, laser, and other forms of destruction as a last resort. Sure, we have gene manipulation on the horizon and increasingly more new body parts and devices available as well, but again these do not cure the whole body.

So where do you start? With the best test that I have seen in over 44 years of being a medical physician, the **Cardio/ION**. It is 13 pages of your vitamins, minerals, fatty acids, amino acids, organic acids and other important indicators such as hsCRP (indicating hidden inflammation or infection), fibrinogen (indicating abnormal coagulation and imminent clots), 8-OHdG (indicating damage to genes that can lead to diabetes, cancers, neuropathies, and other chronic conditions), and much more.

And more important than actual levels of nutrients are the "functional assays" which show if *you* as an individual need more of particular nutrients than the average person. Again, we don't care where "normal" range lies for everybody else. We only care where *yours* should be.

Besides that, you should recall that "normal" is an erroneous government-mandated concept. It is merely defined by looking at hundreds of blood samples to determine where 95% of the values fall. These are samples from people who know nothing about health, are foolish enough to have regular diets of **damaging trans fats in processed white breads, french fries, donuts, or diabetes-producing trans fats disguised as canola oil,** as examples. In other words, these levels are not what you and I would want. They are not optimal. But by fabricated definition they are the "norm". As a simple warning, if your doctor looks at the test and merely decides what you need by seeing if things fall in the "normal" range you have been exorbitantly cheated.

Who can order it? Your family doctor, internist, diabetologist, chiropractor, naturopath, etc. And the *Wall Street Journal* gave a website where folks can get lab tests ordered if their doctors are unknowledgeable about them, directlabs.com, which is legal. And when you think about it why shouldn't every person be able to get their own lab tests that they pay for? It's their health, their lives. Why should your results be the secret possession of someone who is clueless about the molecular biochemistry of healing? Furthermore, a website, anylabtestnow.com, tells you where to find a lab to draw and process the test if your local lab refuses.

If your physician is new to the idea of cause and cure, share this book, with him. Or if you think he is particularly resistant, give him an even quicker read and yet highly referenced and convincing book *Is Your Cardiologist Killing You?* If he doesn't have time to read a book less than 200 pages that would take him maximum 10 minutes a day for two weeks in spite of his hugely busy schedule, then scratch him off your list. He is closed to learning. What you see is what you get, and he is most likely not going to be growing any further.

Once you get the prescription that says "Cardio/ION", call the 800 number for MetaMetrix Laboratory, have them send you the kit, then carefully read the directions. Schedule your blood collection at a local lab or office. After collecting and freezing the morning urine, take it and the kit as described in *TW* 2012 (being sure to fill out tube I.D. and paperwork beforehand) to the lab. In that way you are less likely to overwhelm them and be rejected. Also gently remind them you don't want your blood to lay around the lab all day going bad. They need to return it in its Fed-Ex® mailer promptly, and keep it refrigerated after it has been processed.

And do not be afraid to test any physician who is going to interpret your 13-page assay. That's why I have given you many simple tests scattered throughout here that you can use to surreptitiously test a perspective physician. Many physicians who label themselves as holistic, alternative, integrative, environmental, or functional medical "specialists" are totally unprepared to spend an hour gratis reviewing your last three years of laboratory and specialists' reports and then spend another hour with you personally interpreting your Cardio/ION. Frankly, they just do not have the cumulative knowledge, which is very quick and easy for you to prove one way or the other. Don't forget your life depends on it.

Looking at 2 Inches of the Elephant

Watch out for the lab or physician who thinks they have a better test. I have consulted on hundreds of our readers in over a dozen countries and have seen just about every lab test going. I have seen nothing to equal this. But I have seen many people waste a huge amount of money with their doctors piece-mealing a few minerals and fatty acids from other labs. **The more information you have all at once about your total package as a human being leads to a more clinically useful and cohesive strategy**, especially when it is collated with your medical, environmental, dental, surgical, and other histories as well as a review of your last few years of physician visits and laboratory and x-ray data, as I do with our readers who qualify on the phone.

Just imagine if someone gives you a tiny peep hole in a wall to look through to diagnose what is on the other side. Each time that you are stumped the hole gets a little larger. But when it's 1 inch, 1 foot, or even 3 feet wide you still may not be able to identify what is on the other side of the hole. By the time the hole is finally big enough, you realize why all of your guesses before never made the mark. It was an elephant behind the wall. Just as mineral levels are useless without fatty acids, and vitamins are useless without organic acids, mitochondrial poisoning cannot be repaired without all of this. **We need the largest possible and most complete picture of your molecular biochemistry all at once** to adequately diagnose what's broken, because each parameter interacts with dozens of others on other pages.

Furthermore, reviewing all of your records from all of the physicians from the previous 2-3 years makes the interpretation even better. Likewise, **the more of the books and past newsletters folks have read, the higher the level of interpretation and implementation we can soar to together**. Folks who have only read two or three books and a year of newsletters cannot hope to soar to as high a level of wellness in the hour consultation as someone who has read much more. It forces me to remain at what I term a "kindergarten" level of interpretation, because their lack of reading leaves them asking questions that unnecessarily deplete the time and were covered in books and newsletters. Remember, I never leave anyone out, regardless of what a book title might suggest. The more you read (and re-read) the smarter you get.

Watch Out for the Doc Who Orders the Wrong Tests

Many physicians very easily flaunt their ignorance about nutritional medicine. A simple test is if they order a serum magnesium which will usually just say "magnesium" on the lab report. It has been known for over two decades that **the serum magnesium is extremely inferior and in fact, so useless that it could look totally normal but you could walk out of the office and die from a sudden heart attack caused by low magnesium.** To quote from just one of dozens of papers, "*Serum magnesium can be normal in the presence of intracellular magnesium depletion*, and the occurrence of the low serum level usually indicates significant magnesium deficiency." (Al-Ghandi). Unfortunately this researcher stopped short and is not aware of the fact (evidence given earlier) that as an intracellular magnesium gets further depleted this can make the serum magnesium actually *look too high*. This gives a super dangerously false sense of security to the physician and assures he will *never* discover your true magnesium deficiency. There are many other useless tests described in the books and newsletters.

Because people progressively eat more processed foods, the world is more chemically polluted, and nutrient levels are declining faster (partly because of more prescription medication use), **norms have been "dumbed down" over the last decade**. For example, in some labs the norm for magnesium was 40-80 ng/dL. But after a few years it dropped in some labs to 15-40. This allows folks to have serious deficiencies but be labeled "normal". Vitamin D is a good example, since most labs (referenced earlier) have a cut-off of 30-40, but research clearly shows we need to be over 60 ng/dL. Likewise, the norm for toxins like mercury and lead have quadrupled, allowing folks to have higher amounts and still be called "normal". As folks are more toxic the government has foolishly raised the "norm". Lead is a good example that I have referenced voluminously where the current "safe" "norm" of 10 mcg/dL has been shown to cause a measurable drop in I.Q. and intelligence (Canfield, *TW*).

And there's even an appalling lack of knowledge among researchers. For example, they will show that there's a double amount of osteoporosis in diabetics and then they don't even assay intracellular minerals or essential fatty acids to find the cause and cure of the bone loss. So it should not be a surprise that their conclusion is that it's a "mystery" why diabetics have more osteoporosis (Masse). Anyway, you know why.

References:

• Masse PG, et al, **Bone metabolic abnormalities associated with well-controlled type I diabetes** (IDDM) in young adult women: **a disease complication often ignored or neglected**, *J Am Coll Nutr* 29; 4:419-29, 2010

• Al-Ghandi SM, et al, Magnesium deficiency: pathophysiologic and clinical overview, *Am J Kidney Dis* 24; 5:737-52, 1994

• Canfield RL, et al, **Intellectual impairment in children with blood lead concentrations below 10** mcg per deciliter, *New Engl J Med* 348; 16:1517-26, 2003

Beware of Erroneous Interpretations

Another common mistake is folks will be advised to just take the nutrients that are listed on the report, the computer-generated "cheat-sheet". This only gives you at best 50% of what you need. Another dinosaur clue is when a physician takes 5 or 10 minutes to read the report. There's much more information than that and it usually takes an hour minimum.

In terms of heavy metals for example, many physicians have told folks not to worry because their levels were all in the "normal" range. This just shows they have no concept of the provocation needed to diagnose heavy metal toxicity. Remember from *The High Blood Pressure Hoax* that the only way you know what heavy metals the body is screaming to get rid of is with a provocation test (that is all explained in there).

134

For that reason MetaMetrix Laboratory divides the government-mandated "normal" ranges on the Cardio/ION into quintiles or five parts. This is a pivotal contribution, because for many nutrients you want to be in the top or 5th quintile or higher, whereas for many toxins you want to be in the first or even lower. As an example, if you are **in the fifth quintile** for lead, the doctor who knows nothing about this tells his patient that he is okay and looks normal. But that **translates to 200 ppb of lead which is equal to 20 mcg/dL. This is enough to seriously destroy your brain**, kidneys, cause high blood pressure, promote coronary artery plaque, cancers, diabetes, and much more. And even the next lower quintile, the fourth quintile, is equivalent to 100 ppb which is 10 mcg/dL. As I show below in Canfield's research right from the *New England Journal of Medicine,* there is definite brain damage in children who have less than 100 parts per million (ppm) which is equivalent to 10 mcg/dL (micrograms per deciliter) of lead in the blood. But the government still dangerously registers that as a "normal" level in spite of years of research, even from their own government medical journals like *Environmental Health Perspectives.* In fact, real researchers have shown **there's no safe level of lead.**

The government's double standards in medicine continually amaze me. A commonly used lab, Quest Diagnostics, one of the leading conventional laboratories for patient medical data in the United States, used by Kaiser Permanente and lots of other high-profile organizations, lists the normal for blood lead as less than 10 mcg/dL. This is in spite of the fact that even the *New England Journal of Medicine* showed over seven years ago that serious brain damage occurs in children with levels below this. And I've given the references in past *TWs* by many other scientists proving that the blood lead level is an inferior test.

Clearly anyone who has read all of the evidence in *The High Blood Pressure Hoax* would understand that **the provocation test is much more diagnostic of the levels of heavy metals that the**

135

body is screaming to get rid of. The bottom line is many children are unnecessarily having lower IQ and brain damage because the powers that be severely lack knowledge in their very own fields as well as intellectual honesty and concern for the public. No one will ever know how smart these kids could have been. And then in terms of the adults, as they get duller and less intelligent with age, everyone just chalks it up to mere "normal" aging.

Even Harvard research published in the government's leading environmental journal last year doesn't seem to make any impact. They clearly showed that the **decline in brain function as folks age is related to the rising level of lead that slowly accumulates throughout life, with no occupational exposure, but just "normal' living in the U.S.** Remember, it's not old age, it's heavy metal build-up (as from hair dye) that results in memory loss, brain destruction, and diseases like diabetes.

Even worse are the double standards of some of the states. For example, New York State allows this lab to perform blood tests on their residents, but they penalize their residents by disallowing more important assays. They are the only state that I have seen in consultations from nearly every other state that does not allow measurements of, for example, gamma tocopherol, 8-OHdG, D-arabinitol, and many other highly referenced and extremely pertinent indicators of serious problems that need correcting.

Plus my reader consultations in Canada have to come across the border to have the number one adrenal hormone drawn, DHEA (dehydroepiandrosterone), because their government will not allow it. Go figure! It's enough to confuse any layperson who is just trying to get the best health for himself in this distorted medical era which features drugs over cures.

Meanwhile, because the evidence of our ever-escalating levels of heavy metals is so overwhelming, I see no need to even provoke, anymore. Just get rid of them, and you will learn how in ensuing chapters. And that is a lifetime job. After you have corrected your nutrient deficiencies for several months (usually 2-6 depending on the person) then you're ready to start the detoxification of toxins beginning with *Detoxify Or Die* and then progressing to *The High Blood Pressure Hoax* and another detox protocol in 2010 *TW* and here. Meanwhile, if you need proof (above and beyond the Cardio/ION) that you have **Phthalate** toxicities, **Pesticides** and other toxins like **Volatile Solvents**, those tests are also available through MetaMetrix as well. More on these later.

References:

• Canfield RL, et al, **Intellectual impairment** in children with **blood lead concentrations below 10** mcg per deciliter, *New England Journal Medicine* 348:1517-26, 2003

• Lanphear BP, et al, **Low-level and environmental lead exposure** and children's intellectual function: an international pooled analysis, *Environl Health Persp* 113; 7:894-99, 2005

• Weuve J, et al, Cumulative exposure to lead in relation to cognitive function in older women, *Environmental Health Perspectives* 117; 4:574-80, 2009

"What if I Can't Afford the Test?"

"Couldn't I just start with some nutrients?" Absolutely. The old 80/20 rule shows us that 80% of people will be better with only 20% of what we have to offer. To look at it another way, if you look at the Cardio/IONs of the last hundred people with diabetes and other associated maladies like high blood pressure, obesity, syndrome X, early macular degeneration or cataracts, elevated cholesterol or triglycerides or low HDL or inability to lose weight, kidney or liver failure, heart disease, arrhythmias, arthritis, or neurologic problems, many folks share the same deficiencies and toxicities.

So I'll map out the most commonly deficient nutrients in subsequent chapters, then you and your doctor can decide how to integrate some or all of it into your plan, depending upon what you think you might need. But remember the functional assays in the Cardio/ION can be indispensable. What does that mean? As an example, if you are among the third of folks who don't metabolize their folic acid as well as others, then taking of normal doses will not stop you from fatal diabetic kidney disease, arteriosclerosis, etc. But the functional assays (as an elevated organic acid formiminoglutamate) shows if you need more folic acid than the average person. In that case I often recommend the best form of folic acid, Folinic acid as in sublingual **Folixor.** That's also why I consider genomic testing rather useless without this test first. Then usually this test negates the need for any genomics. Who cares what your genes show. Food and nutrients talk to genes and control them. We just need to know exactly what *you* need. Likewise, if the **methylmalonate** is elevated then your diabetes medication is probably stripping you of B12 which leads to numbness, tingling, painful neuropathies, impotence, loss of memory and brain function, poor vision, and much more.

At the risk of sounding self-serving, the more books and newsletters (all at prestigepublishing.com) you read, the higher the level of wellness you can attain. Also, **re-reading is very important**. As the sole researcher, writer and editor of all of them, even *I* still re-read them. There is much too much for all of us to assimilate at once and remember. Also that is why I repeat things for you to try to make learning easier. In my semi-retirement, I'm fulfilling a life-long dream, learning to play cocktail piano of the old romantic tunes of the 30s and 40s. I find that even here I must re-read jazz theory books that I finished months ago. And the cool thing that I find is that when I re-read a book, because I am at a different level of understanding compared with where I was when I first read it, I get more out of it that completely went over my head the first time. The same goes for this form of medicine. Unfortunately for you, you have to learn the molecular biochemistry of healing because the majority of medicine frankly is not interested.

References:

• Hasegawa G, et al, The association between end-stage diabetic neuropathy and methylene tetrahydrofolate reductase genotype with microangiopathy in type II diabetes mellitus, *Exp Clin Endocrinol Diab* 111:132-8, 2003

138

- Ames BN, et al, High-dose vitamin therapy stimulates a variant enzymes with decreased enzyme binding affinity (increased Km): relevance to genetic disease and polymorphisms, *Am J Clin Nutr* 75; 4:616-58, 2002

"How Can I Test My Physician?"

Another simple test of the Cardio/ION interpreter would be to ask "I'm taking extra lipoic acid to stave off the nasty side effects of diabetes. What organic acid will show if I need extra biotin to compensate for this extra lipoic acid?". (The answer is **beta hydroxy iso-valerate**). If he doesn't know right off the top of his head, most likely the rest of the 13 pages of your complex molecular biochemistry will also be a mystery to him.

Likewise, you recall how important chromium and vanadium are for healing diabetes. You might just ask him, "Are you going to check my beta hydroxybutyrate?" For this is a functional assay of not only whether you need more of these minerals, but also if you are approaching metabolic acidosis, have unrepaired mitochondrial damage, or are even in the cachectic starvation stage of end-stage cancer that screams for repairs. Or as you learned earlier, carnitine is absolutely crucial for nerve regeneration, especially when you have developed any type of paresthesias, painful neuropathies, erectile dysfunction, loss of memory, etc. from diabetes or from the medications. So how will your physician know if you need more? Tests like **adipate, suberate**, and **ethylmalonate** show if you need additional carnitine. These are just a smattering, but will serve you well. Also metametrix.com has a range of books and courses to help in interpretation. As soon as you see a new physician you want to ask him up front if he plans on doing any of these tests. If not, he doesn't plan on curing you.

Reference:

- Lord RS, Bralley JA, eds, *Laboratory Evaluations for Integrative and Functional Medicine, 2nd Edition*, 2008, metametrix.com

Getting Your Cardio/ION Covered by Insurance

Did you know that in the *Archives of Internal Medicine* researchers decided that a procedure could be considered cost-effective if it resulted in a better quality of life and cost less than $50,000 a year. If you look at it that way, the **Cardio/ION** is an absolute bargain. In fact, you could have one monthly, buy a far infrared sauna plus all your nutrients and detox protocols for the year, and even buy dozens of books and newsletter subscriptions for your friends, relatives, and physicians and still have enough money left over for a car! So check with your insurance company, or even try to educate them, too. In addition, *TW* documents FDA approval and insurance coverage for chemotherapies that cost over $100,000/year and often only buy a few months of extra life. So if you can cure your diabetes, that is infinitely more cost effective than for example, $93,000 for four months of extended life as with a common prostate cancer treatment, Provenge®. But don't forget if they refuse, their primary focus is not your health, but their business of making money.

Reference:

- Yao L, Knee replacements are determined to be cost-effective, *Wall Street Journal,* D2, June 23, 2009
- Burton TM, Medicare to cover drug for prostate cancer, *Wall Street Journal*, B4, July 1, 2011

I kept my promise and did not even give you 1,000th of the evidence for the necessity of nutrients to bring about total healing of diabetes. I'm sure your eyes glazed over as you read some of this chemistry. But in your 2nd time through you will amaze yourself at how you have a handle on the *joy of rejuvenation*. But before we put your nutrient program together let's look at another important item, your gut.

Chapter IV

Dinosaur Diabetes Docs Deny Dysbiosis

The Road to Health is Paved With Good Intestines

Is there something else to be considered before starting your nutrient program? Indeed. Like, are you going to be able to absorb and assimilate all your nutrients? You see, many folks will never heal their diabetes, much less any other disease, merely because their guts are too sick. Never forget that **the gut houses (1) half the immune system** (and diabetes is an auto-immune disease) and **(2) half the detoxification system** (and recall diabetes gets rapidly worse when you don't detoxify all of your everyday chemicals) for the entire body. That is why when a doctor neglects to check the health of the gut, it becomes a stumbling block for any hope of healing. Let me make this absolutely clear: **Unidentified intestinal dysbiosis (or bad bugs) in the gut can keep folks from healing any disease indefinitely.** And you don't have to have any gut symptoms as a clue!

For starters, you have to have a healthy gut in order to absorb your nutrients. But two out of three people have a bacterial infection (*H. pylori* or *Helicobacter pylori*) in the stomach, for example that can be silent, or cause heartburn, or mimic GERD (gastroesophageal reflux disease). Worse, the bug can migrate to the heart arteries and form plaque in the coronary arteries, or destroy the lining of the stomach. This silent destruction of the acid secreting cells of the stomach is called **atrophic gastritis** which then stops you from absorbing nutrients, regardless of how wonderful they are. Also if you have been on acid inhibitors like Prilosec, Nexium, Acifex, etc. these also **can cause atrophic gastritis** (as well as interfere with absorption of B12, magnesium and other minerals, trigger pneumonia, and much more). Furthermore, by killing your stomach acid, these drugs actually act as fertilizer for this bug, H. pylori. Yet the FDA has ruled has that these drugs magically became safe enough to no longer require a prescription once their money-making patents expired. Go figure!

But there are other hidden sources of gut toxicity. A vast number of diabetics have overgrowth of a yeast in the gut called *Candida albicans*. It thrives on sugars, especially elevated diabetic blood sugars. Furthermore, antibiotics act like fertilizer, plus steroids and other hormones can trigger it mercilessly. When this yeast (fungus) grows in abnormal amounts in the gut, the symptoms can masquerade as irritable bowel syndrome, colitis, chronic fatigue, GERD, indigestion, heartburn, MCS, interstitial cystitis, prostatitis, recurrent infections, fibromyalgia, and much more. It can also reside around the pancreatic ducts and interfere with other pancreatic enzymes needed for digestion of the fats (necessary to heal the cell membrane where insulin receptors reside and to heal the mitochondria where energy is made). An elevated **D-arabinitol** on the **Cardio/ION** is one indicator of Candida overgrowth. And an elevated **indican** suggests the bugs may be higher up in the intestines interfering with pancreatic secretions. If you have gas and bloating after meals you might consider taking some pancreatic enzymes with bile to promote absorption of your fat soluble nutrients as a temporizing measure. Use 1-3 **Digestive Aid #34** with meals.

If you have any indication that your gut is not 100% normal, then you must get it cured before you can cure anything else. Why? Because the gut is not only responsible for absorption of our nutrients and housing half the immune system and half the detoxification system for the entire body. **The gut makes 95% of the happy hormones like serotonin.** That is one reason why some will never cure their depression or motivate themselves to heal, because no one checked the gut.

Anti-depressants like Prozac work by increasing your serotonin, one of our "happy hormones" in the brain (by poisoning its breakdown so it lasts a longer). The problem is any self-respecting psychiatrist *knows* that 95% of the body's serotonin is not made in the brain. It is made in the gut! Often depression is at a standstill until the doctor thinks of healing the gut where the neurotransmitters of happy mood are made. Meanwhile the patient can suffer the agony and expense of a continual trial of medications, most of which have suicide as a side effect. You might also say **the road to mental health is paved with good intestines** (*Depression Cured At Last!* covers the multitude of curable causes of depression. Further healing of the gut is in *No More Heartburn*. Also check *Wellness Against All Odds* on celiac, a common yet frequently undiagnosed form of allergy that comes on at any age, that impairs nutrient absorption and silently destroys the brain). You need to be happy to work at healing.

Clearly, to put someone on Prozac, Celebra, etc., without looking at the gut much less the other minerals and vitamins that could heal the brain (as described in *Depression Cured At Last!*) is not what I would call intelligent medical practice. Furthermore, Prozac contains three molecules of toxic fluoride which are actually damaging to the brain enzymes and other chemistries of the body. This in part explains why suicide is a common side effect of taking these drugs. The prescriber has failed to look for the cause and cure, which must include the gut. Furthermore, studies from researchers at my own medical school have shown that prescribing **anti-depressants at normal doses acts like fertilizer for any cancers** (reference in June 1998 *TW*).

When in doubt about your gut, get a stool study that shows which unwanted bugs are living there, and does a job far superior to any hospital lab tests that I have ever seen. The test you want is called **Comprehensive Stool with Purged Parasites X3** from Doctors Data Lab (doctorsdata.com). Even if you do not suspect parasites, I would suggest that part, since it is often the only place to find Candida. Besides that, we no longer have to leave the country to get "foreign" diseases, since the rest of the world has come here. And when folks have limited education, job and language skills, they can always get a job in a restaurant kitchen preparing your food. If the gut is still a problem, and you did not find your answers, a more sophisticated test looks at the genetics of the intestinal bugs as well as other parameters and is called **G.I. Effects** by MetaMetrix (metametrix.com). Folks with severely damaged guts or long-standing problems need both tests as well as the Cardio/ION. I must admit that combination has been a massive disease-breaker in the most recalcitrant of cases.

Nix on Nexium

While we are on the subject of the gut, let me give you a couple of other signs of a clueless dinosaur physician. One is if he prescribes Nexium. Don't take my word for it. Let me back you up so you can decide for yourself. Prilosec was the first "blockbuster drug" in the history of the world, and in fact that's where the term originated from. When its patent ran out, the pharmaceutical company merely attached a sidearm onto it in order to create a "new" (and now again patentable and expensive drug) and called it Nexium®.

The problem is when you take Nexium, your body must first metabolize this side arm off. The work of doing this uses up nutrients that should have been used for healing. Now with the side arm off, you have the original Prilosec, which is now over-the-counter, needing no prescription and far cheaper (generic omeprazole). Nexium is about $4 a capsule, while Prilosec is about $0.32. So I ask you, what doctor in his right mind would prescribe something that is (1) over 10 times more expensive and (2) causes more metabolic work for your already over-worked and sick body? Only one who has no idea of what he is prescribing.

Meanwhile, the gut drugs **Nexium, Prilosec, Acifex**, etc. are what we call **proton pump inhibitors**. They poison the stomach cells that produce acid needed to digest food, promote nutrient absorption and kill unwanted bugs. And these drugs act as fertilizer for everyday bugs that then go on to raise havoc. **When prescribed for hospitalized patients, they increase pneumonia**

30% (*TW*). This is **what lots of folks die from once they end up in the hospital**. And these acid-axers lower magnesium, zinc, and B12, creating bone loss, Alzheimer's, bizarre neurological problems that no one figures out, and more (references page 115 *Is Your Cardiologist Killing You?*). Yet recall, once their patents expired they magically become safe enough for OTC (over-the-counter or non-prescription) designation by the government agency meant to protect us from drugs, the FDA.

I repeat: **Nexium or Prilosec increase the chance of getting pneumonia in the hospital 30% (and it's a common cause of death) by inhibiting the absorption of priceless nutrients**. Worse, acid inhibitors counteract medications like **Plavix** (clopidogrel) which are prescribed to decrease unwanted clotting (Ho, Dunn, Gilard). So physicians are unknowingly propelling the patient toward a heart attack, even though the FDA quietly warned about acid inhibitors canceling out the effects of Plavix years ago.

References:

• Ho PM, et al, **Risk of adverse outcomes** associated with concomitant use of **clopidogrel and proton pump inhibitors** following acute coronary syndrome, *J Am Med Assoc* 301:937-44, 2009

• Sibbing D, et al, Effect of **proton pump inhibitors on the antiplatelet effects** of clopidogrel,*Thromb Haemost* 101:714-9, 2009

• Dunn SP, et al, Baseline **proton pump inhibitor use is associated with increased cardiovascular events** with and without the use of clopidogrel in the CRDEO trial, *Circulation* 118: S815, abst, 2008

• Gilard M, et al, Influence of **omeprazole on the antiplatelet action of clopidogrel** associated with aspirin: the randomized, double-blind OCLA (Omeprazole CLopidogrel Aspirin) study, *J Am Coll Cardiol* 51:256-60, 2008

• U.S. Food and Drug Administration. Information for Healthcare Professionals: Update to the labeling of Clopidogrel Bisulfate (marketed as **Plavix) to alert health care professionals about a drug interaction with omeprazole (marketed as Prilosec and Prilosec OTC)**. Available at: HTT:\\www.FDA.gov/Drugs/DrugsSafety/PostmarketDrugSafety

• InformationforPatientsandProviders/Drug SafetyInformationforHealthcareProfessionals/UNC 190787. htm

Caution: Antibiotics Can Start Your Downhill Demise

There's nothing like the pain of an abscessed root canal to give you a vast appreciation for the power of antibiotics. But as much as antibiotics have rescued us, they can also be the beginning of the end. So let's make sure you understand enough so this does not happen to you.

Many folks are getting dental implants for example, which necessitate weeks and sometimes months of antibiotics along with cadaver bone graphs. As wonderful as antibiotics are, they do not make a beeline to the place we are trying to treat, but go to every nook and cranny of the body. In fact, if you're not taking enzymes to help the antibiotics beat their way into the inflamed sore, abscessed area, the antibiotics will actually end up in higher levels every place else in the body and at lower levels where you actually need them. So refer back to your previous *TW* issues which give you a choice of half a dozen different types of **enzymes** (and their double night-time doses) that **promote getting the antibiotics at a higher level into the tissues that actually need them the most**. Also 2011-12 *TW* has several issues on the importance of destroying **biofilms, a protective barrier that bugs secrete making them immune to antibiotics**. Enzymes do this.

Meanwhile, once you have been on antibiotics, there's an inevitable overgrowth of yeasts like *Candida albicans* (as just one example of hundreds). And this yeast is even more common in diabetics, since it thrives on sugar. Unfortunately, it has been the beginning of the end for many people. For example, once you have Candida growing silently in the gut, the body can make antibodies against it, which also are similar to our thyroid tissue. So now you start attacking your own thyroid and "out of the blue" get Hashimoto's auto-immune **thyroiditis or hypothyroidism** or other thyroid maladies. Yeasts also produce acetaldehyde, a metabolite that creates "mysterious" **brain fog or depression** for seemingly no reason. Or they produce **thiaminase**, an enzyme that **destroys vitamin B1** before it even has a chance to get absorbed. So no mater how much you take, you **cannot heal the diabetic kidney or failing heart** even if this deficiency is the cause (*No More Heartburn*).

Or the Candida organisms can inflame the gut lining creating leaky gut (intestinal hyper-permeability), which then can go on to create new **auto-immune disorders** like rheumatoid arthritis, multiple sclerosis, lupus, etc., and ....yes, **diabetes.** Recall the articles from the *New England Journal of Medicine* on **juvenile diabetics** that showed these kids **had high antibodies against milk antigens that attacked their pancreases.** Then there are folks on record for whom clinicians gave diabetics an equal amount of calories. But if they gave them in the form of a food to which the diabetics were unknowingly allergic, it made their blood sugars go twice as high. In essence **the pancreas can become an allergic target organ.** And anyone develops food allergies at any time.

To drive home the point of how widespread the damage from one undiagnosed yeast in the gut can produce, let me repeat and expand on two common examples. **Candida can make an enzyme called thiaminase that destroys the B1 vitamin** before it gets a chance to be absorbed. This silent B1 deficiency can lead to not only heart failure (usually fatal within 5 years), but poor energy, poor recovery from exercise, and **worsening of diabetes** (with mysterious inability to bring down the hgb A1C). But far worse, B1 deficiency can create **albumin loss in the kidneys leading to** kidney destruction and the need for $60,000 of **dialysis** a year for the rest of the person's life. This in turn creates aluminum , phthalate and cyclohexanone toxicities that trigger Alzheimer's (see chapter 1)..... and all because the doctor failed to check the gut for Candida. Remember, one good indicator of Candida in the gut is an elevated organic acid, D-arabinitol, which is also on the Cardio/ION.

And the problems do not end here. For example **the yeast can make acetaldehyde which mimics <u>brain fog, unexplained depression, inability to concentrate and bizarre dizziness.</u>** Or it can leak toxins through the inflamed and damaged gut which then mimic the migrating muscle and joint pains of **fibromyalgia or polymyalgia rheumatica or the deadly exhaustion** of **chronic**

fatigue or **mysterious irritable bowel syndrome**. Yet how many "specialists who treat these diseases do a complete analysis of the gut? And hospital based gut tests are not as complete.

The problem is most physicians and dentists prescribing antibiotics have never read *No More Heartburn* and don't know how to protect folks against getting Candida and its sequelae. The other problem is they often do not see the patient for months. By then their new symptoms seem unrelated to anything they could have done to the patient, especially since the new symptoms may now propel the patient to seek treatment from a different type of specialist. For example, if months after an antibiotic for your tooth you insidiously develop hypothyroidism, heart failure, chronic fatigue or fibromyalgia, who is going to suspect it came from the antibiotic-induced overgrowth of a yeast?   And for many practitioners Candida basically doesn't even exist in their thought processes. That's why I want to be sure that you can direct your physicians/dentists to give you the best care.

After you have had any antibiotic treatment for 10 or more days, **it's best to get rid of the Candida as quickly as possible so that there's less of it to deal with, making it easier and faster to heal.** The longer it persists, the more recalcitrant it becomes. You need to tell the practitioner that he needs to prescribe two items for you. First is **generic Nizoral called ketoconazole**. You want **200 mg of Ketoconazole**, one a day for anywhere from 5 to 15 days depending on how long you had antibiotics. It is a systemic anti-fungal, meaning it goes into the bloodstream and **reaches cells from the inside of the body**. If he writes the prescription for Nizoral instead of its generic twin, the capsules are about $7 each versus $1.

At the same time you have to be also killing the yeast from the "outside" (which is actually the inside of the gut lumen or canal) with **Nystatin Pure Powder (USP)**. Many physicians will not write it because they don't know how, so you can instruct them that you want 50 million units per gram in a 10 gm bottle with several refills, and that you will be taking 1/8 to 1/2 teaspoon 2-3 times a day as tolerated. Since the dose varies from lot to lot, 1/4 teaspoon is average 1,000,000 units (use NDC#00574040405). Follow the directions on how to hold it in the mouth, do the diet, follow up with a probiotic, etc., after the two prescriptions are done (the directions are in *No More Heartburn,* and for physicians the scientific backup is in that book). More in Chapter V.

If you cannot afford that, many folks are lucky in that just a 3 week slamming of the bugs with a proprietary herbal combo like **ParaGard** (3-4 capsules) and **Kyolic Liquid** (2 swigs) each three times a day can knock out unwanted bugs. ParaGard proprietary herbs include goldenseal (Hydrastis), grapefruit seed extract and more, resulting in a wide spectrum of antibacterial/anti-fungal activity. And I've given you a huge amount of references on Kyolic Liquid in the past (including Budoff's study that showed it even markedly retarded coronary plaque formation). Follow this with 2 weeks of a probiotic (to restore the good bugs that will help heal the gut and inhibit yeasts) like **ABX Support** 2-3 twice a day. It contains the three top most needed probiotics, Lactobacillus, Bifidus, and Saccharomyces (see *TW*).

And while we're briefly looking at antibiotic substitutes don't forget things like **Argentyn 23** (*TW*) that is a non-colloidal homeopathic silver that you can use with the dropper applicator in the nose for sinus infections, in the mouth for gum infections and cold sores, or take it internally for Candida. Unlike colloidal silver, it does not cause heavy metal toxicity.

References:

• Booth AA, et al, **Thiamine pyrophosphate and pyridoxamine inhibit** the formation of antigenic advanced **glycation** end-products: comparison with aminoguanidine, *Biochem Biophys Res Commun*, 220:113-19, 1996

• Scazzocchio F, et al, Antibacterial activity of *Hydrastis canadensis* extract and its major isolated alkaloids, *Planta Med* 67:561-64, 2001

• Cvetnic Z, **Antibacterial activity of grapefruit seed**, *Acta Pharm* 54:243-50, 2004

- Reagor L, et al, The effectiveness of processed **grapefruit seed extract as an antibacterial agent**, I. An in vitro agar assay, *J Altern Compl Med* 8:3 325-32, 2002

- Heggers JP, et al, The effectiveness of processed **grapefruit seed extract as an antibacterial agent**, II. Mechanism of action and in vitro toxicity, *J Altern Compl Med* 8:3 333-40, 2002

Common Mistakes Made by Physicians Treating Candida:

Over three decades, since my departed adorable colleague, Dr. Billie Crook, and Dr. Orion Truss discovered Candida's dangers, I have seen many of the same mistakes occur regarding Candida treatment. So let's be sure you are experts in this.

(1) Docs who haven't studied it don't treat it soon enough, i.e. right after they have prescribed the antibiotic. Unfortunately many times folks wait 2-3 years as symptoms slowly and insidiously emerge. By that time, the Candida is so well entrenched that it takes a long time and much more aggressive therapy to get rid of it. Plus the long-standing inflammation of the gut has impaired their nutrient levels. This makes them even more vulnerable for the chronicity, as undiagnosed nutrient deficiencies make it even more difficult to heal. So **the easier path is to aggressively get rid of it in just a few days as soon as the antibiotic is finished**, as opposed to needing months of treatment. And please! **Never treat yeast while on an antibiotic**. It merely fosters the growth of resistant yeast forms.

(2) You do not want the brand name Nizoral® since it is seven times more expensive than the generic Ketoconazole. This goes into the bloodstream and in between cells in the lining of the gut. Caution: many diabetes medications interfere with the liver's detoxification of Ketoconazole, so the physician needs to monitor liver function tests even more carefully.

(3) Unknowledgeable physicians prescribe only Nizoral or the generic Ketoconazole but without the Nystatin Pure Powder. They do not understand that **Candida puts out little fingers called mycelia** that interdigitate or tightly grab in between the cells of the intestinal wall. Because of this **you have to treat it from the**

inside of the blood vessels (as with Ketoconazole which goes into the bloodstream), as well as from the inside of the gut lumen, as with Nystatin powder. **Nystatin is not absorbed, but it kills by contact from the inside of the gut.** That's also a good reason why you want to do a colon cleanse such as in *Wellness Against All Odds* beforehand to reduce the amount of stool that has to be treated. This can also increase the topical killing power of the nystatin. Think about it. If you have reduced the amount of stool to be treated and cleansed the gut wall thereby exposing more Candida, you have decreased the treatment time as you increase the efficacy of the treatment.

(4) If he wants to prescribe Nystatin **capsules** instead of the powder **do not accept them.** This shows he does not understand that Candida often grows in the mouth, the esophagus and the stomach as well as the small intestines and the large intestine. A capsule does not open up until it has gotten into the stomach or small intestine. As a consequence, since it only kills by contact and is not absorbed, you never kill the Candida in the mouth or the esophagus or upper stomach. So it keeps coming back after treatment (it keeps seeding itself from the untreated upper gut), and **the person mysteriously never gets well.** Meanwhile, the fungus becomes even more deeply entrenched in the victim and the doctor cannot understand why the patient never gets well. Be sure to use the oral powder protocol in *No More Heartburn* to kill Candida all the way from mouth to stomach.

So there you have it. Refer back *No More Heartburn* for the necessary other details, as these are the main *faux pas* we have seen in over three decades of treating Candida. In there you will learn about many other heart-destroying bugs to get rid of (also more in *Is Your Cardiologist Killing You?*). Meanwhile, there's no reason in this era to suffer the consequences of undiagnosed Candida.

Do You Need a Battery Boost?

If your computer mouse stops working, two-to-one it needs a new battery. If your car suddenly won't start, it could merely need a new battery. Coenzyme Q10 is like a battery. It shuttles the electrons through the mitochondria to make the electricity we call "life". But environmental chemicals poison the ability of the mitochondria to make CoQ10. As well, some prescription drugs, especially the cholesterol-lowering statins, like Lipitor, diabetes, blood pressure, and anti-depressant drugs seriously poison the chemistry for CoQ10 synthesis. There is a wealth of data of how supplementing CoQ10 has improved many of the complications of diabetes from hypertension to cardiomyopathies. Since it so effective, yet simple and harmless to supplement, why not?

Until you repair your mitochondria (and many folks' mitochondria are rapidly aging) and learn how to shed drugs after symptoms have been cured, taking exogenous C0Q10 can give an extra boost to healing. So why did I bring this up again in the gut section? Since we don't know how good your gut is yet in terms of absorption, taking a sublingual (absorbed under the tongue like a nitroglycerine is) form of CoQ10 makes more sense. In this way you avoid one more capsule (that may not get broken down if you lack enough digestive enzyme capacity yet). For that reason, I suggest 2-3 **Q-ODT** once or twice a day dissolved under the tongue (ODT stands for "oral dissolving tablet").

Foods to Use and Foods to Lose

Food is not just for nourishment. **Food talks to genes, while drugs poison them**. Not only does food supply nutrients and biochemical balance, but food also controls whether a gene becomes dedicated to diabetes, cancer, heart disease, or health. The good news is even if you have a bad family history, **you can override bad genes with the right foods.**

A simple but effective start is just to make sure you have whole grains and fresh lightly steamed vegetables every day, which can cut your diabetes risk minimum 16-36% (Hobson). Many patients have completely cleared not only diabetes (McCulley), but reversed heart diseases (Ornish, *TW* 2012), and even end-stage wildly metastatic cancers where folks were given 48-hours to live and medicine had nothing else to offer (Rogers-1). Whether you're a carnivore and need your meats or are a dedicated vegan, *Macro Mellow* provides recipes and instructions for whole foods cooking.

If you have really serious disease and have decided to go on the macrobiotic program, start with *You Are What You Ate* and then progress to *The Cure Is In the Kitchen* (Rogers-2). If any of your friends are diagnosed with cancer, just have them ask for a free sample issue of the *TW* newsletter on cancer (Dec. 2006), and they can learn first-hand how potent the diet is in a thoroughly documented case. In this case, a 46 year old non-smoking nurse with inoperable and wildly metastatic lung cancer, reduced to 72 pounds, bed-ridden, unable to use chemo or radiation, was given 48 hours to live. I introduced her on a cruise lecture 5 years ago and she was perfectly well then, 13 years later, all with the diet.

References:

- Yamaoka S, et al, **Mitochondrial function** in rats **is affected by modification of membrane phospholipids with dietary sardine oil**, *J Nutr* 118:290-96, 1988

- Storlien LH, et al**, Fish oil prevents insulin resistance** induced by high-fat feeding in rats, *Sci* 237; 4817:885-88, 1987

- Carpentier YA et al, **n-3 fatty acids and the metabolic syndrome**, *Am J Clin Nutr*, 83 (6 supple): 1499S-1504S, 2006

- Hobson K, **Brown rice to lower diabetes risk**, *Wall Street Journal*, D4, June 15, 2010

- Lawlor DA, et al, **Avoiding milk is associated with a reduced risk of insulin resistance** and the metabolic syndrome: findings from the British Women's Heart and Health Study, *Diab Med* 22; 6:808-11, 2005

- McCulley D, *Death To Diabetes*, Death To Diabetes.com

- Ornish, references in 2012 *TW* and *The Cholesterol Hoax*, available from prestigepublishing.com or 1-800-846-6687

- Rogers-1, described in *Total Wellness* 2006, available from prestigepublishing.com or 1-800-846-6687

- Rogers-2, *Macro Mellow, You Are What You Ate,* and *The Cure Is In the Kitchen* compose the *Macro Trilogy* available from prestigepublishing.com or 1-800-846-6687

No Diet is Perfect for Everyone

In spite of the fact that the macrobiotic diet has the best proven track record for literally curing cancers of any other diet that I have investigated in over 40 years of medical practice, it's not for everyone. And internist Dr. Dean Ornish successfully reduced and reversed coronary plaque with a modified macrobiotic diet, but he used a lot of processed foods and arthritis-provoking nightshades that I wouldn't recommend because of arthritis (Ornish). Then there are folks who never eat grains or folks who juice most of their fruits and vegetables, or the folks who eat mainly raw foods with soaked or sprouted grains and beans. And it is not unusual for folks' dietary needs can change over a lifetime.

A great macrobiotic cookbook is by a young lady who could not afford surgery for ovarian cancer in 1993, so cured herself with macrobiotics. Then in 2001 she had a life-threatening auto accident from which she was not expected to survive, much less ever walk again. Not able to afford the hospital stay, she was bedridden at home for over a year before she was even able to get in a wheelchair for another year. The bottom line? She is very well and has written a recipe book with the most beautiful photography I've ever seen in a cookbook, all done by her loving husband and fellow cook and healer. Even if you don't go macro, you will **learn how to start making smarter food choices that have enormous life-promoting power** in *Love, Sanae. My healing journey*, by Sanae Suzuki (www.LoveEricInc.com or 1-310-450-6383).

I've seen people heal chronic conditions with the macrobiotic diet and then go back to being carnivores. Many people need meat and even more so in this era to balance the body chemistries poisoned by the unprecedented level of toxins that we all bear. In fact, in

154

one study in the American Heart Association's journal, *Circulation,* researchers showed that **red meat is not associated with a heightened risk of coronary heart disease, strokes or diabetes**. But it is the **processed meats** with all the chemicals (also known as delicatessen or luncheon meats like bologna and salami, that contain nitrates and other additives) **that *are* associated with a 42% greater risk of having a heart disease and 19% risk of having diabetes** (Micha). The key is always to be as close to nature as possible with as few as chemicals as possible.

Some diabetics thrive with more meat. During this global economic meltdown one of the least expensive and most nutritious meals could be sardines (don't buy the boneless, skinless, but the whole fish), which can be seasoned with low-sodium soy sauce or tamari, Ponzu, pear-infused vinegar, etc., on whole grain toast. They will give you not only protein but the omega-3 oils you need to repair the mitochondrial membranes. And eggs for breakfast supply phosphatidyl choline for starting your "oil change".

Don't confuse carnitine (ALC) with carnosine which is an amino acid found primarily in red meat. A typical red meat meal may provide 250 mg of carnosine. Carnosine lowers blood glucose, enhances insulin sensitivity and helps prevent type II diabetes from emerging. It is a natural antioxidant and anti-glycation substance found in normal human tissues predominantly the brain and the heart. No diet is for everyone, nor is it forever.

References:

- Ornish D, Intensive lifestyle changes for reversal of coronary heart disease, *J Am Med Assoc*, 28; 23:2001-2007, 1998

- Nagai K, et al, Possible role of L-**carnosine in the regulation of blood glucose** through controlling autonomic nerves, *Exper Biol Med* (Maywood), 228; 10:1138-45, 2003

- Sauerhofer S, et al, L-carnosine, a substrate of carnosinase-1, influences glucose metabolism, *Diabetes* 56; 10:2425-32, 2007

- Micha R, et al, Red and **processed meat** consumption and **risk of** incident coronary heart disease, stroke, and **diabetes**. A systematic review and meta-analysis, *Circulation* 121:2271-83, 2010

The Spices of Life

I have told you how the mineral **vanadium acts like insulin** and helps diabetics improve, lower their insulin, and thwart the damaging effects of diabetes, plus help weight control. It turns out that the spice from tree bark, **cinnamon, also is an insulin mimic**. Think of as many ways as you can to add fresh organic herbs like this containing polyphenols to your cooking. You will be surprised how well it adds zip to meats, enhances salad dressings, soups, desserts and more.

Curcumin or turmeric is yet an even more potent root. It has huge fat burning activity as well as lowers oxidative stress in the kidney and liver. Furthermore, it improves insulin resistance as well as has improved NASH, diabetic nephropathy and encephalopathy, lessens mitochondrial damage and brain peroxidation, delays the onset of cataracts, inhibits platelet aggregation (dampens unwanted clot formation), lowers glycosylation, lessons obesity, and much more (Goepp). And more importantly, it activates the peroxisomes (one of the mechanisms of diabetes medications is also to activate peroxisomes or their receptors, PPAR), but does so more safely than via drugs. **Curcumin** has other properties such as decreasing the chance of a diabetic getting cancers and other complications, as well as helping to **improve mitochondrial function**, decreasing free radicals, and more (Yun).

An interesting old-time remedy of organic vinegar (preferably with the "mother") can lower glucose as well as help with dieting and satiety (feeling full and content) (White, Mettler). **Artemesia also known as Russian tarragon** (a perennial herb that has marked ability to lower glucose) improves insulin levels (Wang). Its phytonutrients can **lower aldose reductase** levels, a chemical diabetics make that leads to eye damage like **cataracts**.

These are just some quick examples of the anti-oxidant power of fresh herbs and spices. Be creative. There is an overwhelming amount of data for their protection and healing properties. In fact, think twice before you throw any of nature's foods away. For example, you made Caesar dressing with membrane-building anchovies and are discarding the lemon rind? Why not grate it? **Lemon zest** adds punch to a variety of dishes from soups, rice dishes, or fish to a fruit compote with maple syrup, while it supplies priceless phytonutrients. You might say it adds zest to your life in multiple ways! And why not **plant an herb garden**, even in pots or on your windowsill or porch? Fresh herbs like tarragon and spices like ginger are natural diabetes fighters. **Natural Lifestyle** is the most complete place I know of to fill all your culinary needs regardless of diet type and where you live (1-800-752-2775, Naturallifestylemarket.com).

References:

- Wang ZQ, et al, An extract of *Artemesia dracunculus L.* enhances insulin receptor signaling and modulates gene expression in skeletal muscle in KK-Ay mice, *J Nutr Biochem* 22:71-8, 2011

- Jarvill-Taylor KJ, et al, A hydroxychalcone derived from **cinnamon functions as a mimetic for insulin in** 3T3-L1 **adipocytes**, *J Am Coll Nutr*, 30:327-36, 2001

- Khan A, et al, **Cinnamon improves glucose and lipids of people with type 2 diabetes**, *Diabetes Care* 26; 12:3215-8, 2003

- Anderson RA, et al, Isolation and characterization of polyphenol polymers from **cinnamon with insulin-like biological activity**, *J Agric Food Chem* 52:65-70, 2004

- Kirkham S, et al, The potential of **cinnamon to reduce blood glucose levels in patients with type II diabetes and insulin resistance**, *Diab Obes Metabol* 11; 12:1100-13, 2009

- Qin B, et al, **Cinnamon extract prevents the insulin resistance** induced by a high-fructose diet, *Horm Metab Res* 36; 2:119-25, 2004

- Anderson RA, Chromium and polyphenols from **cinnamon improves insulin sensitivity**, *Proc Nutr Soc* 67; 1:48-53, Feb 2008

- Yun JM, et al, Epigenetic regulation of high glucose-induced pro-inflammatory cytokine production in monocytes by curcumin, *J Nutr Biochem* 22:450-58, 2011

- Rastogi M, et al, **Curcuminoids modulate** oxidative damage and **mitochondrial dysfunction** in diabetic rat brain, *Free Rad Res* 42; 11-12, 999-1005, 2008

- Sharma S, et al, **Curcumin**, the active principle of **turmeric** (Curcuma lomga), **ameliorates diabetic nephropathy** in rats, *Clin Exper Pharmacol Physiol* 33; 10:940-5, 2006

- Goepp J, Combating the "Diabesity" epidemic, *Life Extension* (www.lef.org), 39-48 Aug 2010

- White AM, et al, **Vinegar** in digestion **at bedtime moderates waking glucose** concentrations in adults with well-controlled type II diabetes, *Diab Care* 30; 11:2814-15, 2007

- Mettler S, et al, Additive postprandial blood glucose-attenuating and **satiety-enhancing effect of cinnamon and acetic acid,** *Nutr Res* 29; 10:723-7, 2009

- Al-Amin ZM, et al, **Antidiabetic** and hyperlipidemic **properties of ginger** (*Zingiber officinale*) in streptozotocin-induced diabetic rats, *Brit J Nutr* 96; 4:660-66, 2006

- Su HC, et al, Resveratrol, a red wine antioxidant, possesses an insulin like effect in streptozotocin-induced diabetic rat, *Am J, Physiol Endocrinol Metab,* 290; 6:E 1339-46, 2006

The Canola Con...It's Worse Than the Soy Ploy

Just as important as what you eat is what you don't eat. Often folks who believe they are knowledgeable about the best things to put in their bodies are proud to tell you that they use canola oil for cooking. Furthermore, they choose mayonnaise, salad dressings, baked goods, and other processed foods containing canola oil. They'll tell you it has omega-3 oils (the helpful ones in cod liver oil) as well as monosaturated oleic (the oil that predominates in olive oil) and many other benefits. As well, the major fast food chains brag that they no longer have trans fats, but have switched to canola oil. They use it for their french fries, burgers, salad dressings and baked goods, exchanging it for trans fatty acid-laden genetically engineered soybean oil. Would I eat it? No.

Knowing that **canola oil is a genetically engineered product** (not a seed oil that was created by God), I was very suspicious there was something wrong. Besides, there is no canola plant! The thing that really motivated me to check it out however, was finding progressively **more damaging** trans fatty acids in the **Cardio/ION** panels when I reviewed them with you readers. The kicker was that you folks were not eating any sources of trans fatty acids, at least not knowingly. So my research began.

The bottom line for you folks who don't really want a lot of molecular biochemistry is that **canola oil actually has a higher level of trans fatty acids than the soybean and vegetable oils that it replaced**. Once again the public has been duped! You see, in the interim the definitions changed that allowed this ruse. Clearly the politics of the food industry are so potent that this information will not come out for at least another couple of decades. Why? Because unknowledgeable regulatory agencies (not having done their research) have been deceived into believing that canola is the next best oil. Now they have vested their legislative careers in the oil change, so there's no way it's going to be turned around quickly. Remember it took literally decades before the dangers of trans fats were finally exposed.

And in spite of the enormous proof of the dangers of trans fats (some of which were reported by Harvard researchers decades ago), the FDA (whose goal I naively thought was to protect consumers) has caved to the clout of food manufacturers. In this decade **the FDA actually legalized lying to consumers**. As of 2006, the Federal Register has allowed food manufacturers to put the words **'NO TRANS FATS"** to be plastered on any label if there are less than **500 mg of trans fats per puny ½ cup** serving. This of course assumes that the FDA is also clairvoyant and knows exactly what foods you eat and how much of them, so that you don't exceed your daily allotment. Of course **Harvard researchers showed ages ago that there is <u>no</u> safe level of trans fats,** since trans fats have grossly changed the fundamental chemistry of our cell membranes (recall evidence in chapter 3).

So why are **there more trans fatty acids in canola oil than in the soybean oil** that it replaced? Because **canola oil has a higher level of omega-3 oils**. So in order to make that bottle last on a shelf, plus be able to withstand high heat cooking, you need over a dozen chemical stages to process canola into an oil that will not go rancid. These processes include not only **hydrogenation but deodorization** of the omega-3. This process **can form as much as 40% trans fatty acids in canola, even more than soybean oil.**

Behind all this is the need to create high profit fast foods. It's one more example of how the arrogance of man makes him think he can one-up God and create a more healthful seed oil by changing the genetics of the rapeseed to make canola. Eating out now, although it is a pleasurable social pastime, becomes increasingly more dangerous to our health. I know it's going to be difficult to get canola out of our diets, since I've only found one commercial mayonnaise without GMO canola oil or nightshades (www.followyourheart.com or 1-888-394-3949). And we can always make our own mayo (the recipe is in *Macro Mellow*) and it is much more nutritious and tastes better, plus it's fresher.

Meanwhile, **the canola con (CON-ola?) is even greater than the soy ploy I warned about decades ago**. And it will most likely persist even longer. It's one more reason why people all around us mysteriously deteriorate into chronic degenerative diseases. They have literally changed their body chemistries. Meanwhile, regulatory "authorities" have managed to ignore even the warnings of the **Harvard School of Public Health that stated decades ago that there is no safe level of trans fats.**

For you folks who are new to the idea of trans fatty acids and have never had a Cardio/ION that can measure your trans fats (along with your vitamins, minerals, fatty acids, organic acids, etc.), start with the oil change in *Detoxify Or Die*. You can't hope to be well without knowing all of the hidden sources of trans fatty acids in our foods. For just like plasticizers and other pollutants, they damage the very fundamental chemistry of the body creating not only diabetes, but stubborn obesity, cardiovascular diseases, cancer, etc. Remember, once you have repaired your cell membranes (the computer keyboard and hormone docking site of the body), there is an artful balance of all fatty acids needed in order to orchestrate and perpetuate perfect health. And yes, we can benefit from butter, meats, cheeses, etc. How much depends on your individual environmental toxic burden, genetics, health of your gut, and the results of your fatty acid assays (see *TW* 2012).

Clearly, as we showed in *The Cholesterol Hoax*, cholesterol is not the bad guy. It is merely the messenger, the band-aid. We need healthful levels of cholesterol for daily cellular repair and longevity. Unfortunately unknowledgeable folks who are trying to eat a low cholesterol diet, taking the dangerous statin drugs and using canola are on a fast track for developing further diseases, with diabetes leading the list. **The brain is particularly vulnerable to early degenerative changes.** But now you no longer have any excuse for being among these unknowledgeable folks with dwindling intellects.

There's even more to the canola con. First of all, **canola depletes vitamin E.** But you recall the media did such a good hatchet job in slandering vitamin E that many people stopped taking it. Of course, the researchers only used one of the eight parts of E and then it was synthetic, so it doesn't adequately fit into God's molecular biochemistry of the body. Furthermore, Lipitor for cholesterol and many other drugs deplete vitamin E. Consequently, we are going to be paying for more chronic diseases like heart, cancer, Alzheimer's, and diabetes than ever before in history. And progressively younger people are getting these diseases, partly because folks are being fed more canola oil than ever before in the history of the planet. In *TW* you saw the reference where over **95% of wealthy kids under 5 were already deficient in vitamin E.** This alone can foster unending medical maladies.

Of course there are no human studies on canola; who's going to support them? There's no money in showing people how to be healthier. In animal studies however, **canola has increased the rigidity of membranes** (which is a major aging factor and trigger for degenerative diseases like diabetes). It actually damages hearts creating fibrosis (depending on animal genetics), impairs the action of vitamin E (crucial in inflammation), and changes the size of cells. Plus **canola retards growth so well that the FDA has outlawed it in infant formulas (Federal Register,** 1985)! Fancy that. They knew a quarter of a century ago that it was not good for babies, but now it's suddenly okay for everyone else. Go figure. Studies in other countries that involved humans showed there was an increase in lung cancers as well as heart damage.

But let's look at some of the animal studies that have been done on canola. In some it **shortens the lifespan of the animals** and in others it **lowers the platelet count and increases the size of the platelet cells**. Platelets you remember are crucial in blood clotting, inflammation, arteriosclerosis, blood vessel repair, cancer and much more. And since canola oil increases the bleeding time by damaging platelets, it means that **surgeons who tell you to go off vitamin E before surgery had better start telling you to go off canola oil.** And another thing it does **is raise the nervonic acid** level on your Cardio/ION, and no one quite knows the ultimate effect of that.

And researchers find canola oil contains traces of some "unique sulfur compounds" that nobody knows anything about, and of course it contains small amounts of erucic acid which is known to be very damaging to the heart and toxic to other tissues. In fact, this is why they genetically modified rapeseed (which was 20% erucic), to make canola oil in the first place. And canola is still not totally devoid of toxic erucic acid (contains about 1.2%). In fact this is precisely why **canola oil is outlawed for baby formula**: (1) there are no human studies, and (2) the accumulation of **erucic acid is toxic and damaging to the body**, including the **brain**.

In another study daily **canola oil raised the triglycerides a staggering 47%** (Calabrese). The sad thing is many people think they are safe and knowledgeable in choosing canola oil, because they have fallen for the hype without finding out the facts for themselves. The bottom line is you **don't want to ingest any food containing GMO canola oil or hydrogenated vegetable oils**. Butter, grape seed oil, olive oil (preferably cold-pressed, unfiltered, extra virgin) are great for cooking. And of course olive, grape seed, flax seed, hemp seed, walnut and macadamia nut oils are great for salad dressings. Even organic unrefined coconut oil is good for once a week low temperature cooking and especially good for folks who are fat-starved for saturated oils. There are so many nut and vegetable oils that are organic and expeller-pressed or cold pressed (not hydrogenated). It goes without saying any **oil in dark glass is preferred** over plastic as well.

There is overwhelming evidence that trans fatty acids (endorsed by the American Institute of Nutrition) promote genetic damage, chronic diseases, metabolic syndrome, high cholesterol, high blood pressure, obesity as well as diabetes. And simple cod liver oil (as in your oil change) can fix all of that as well as repair much of the damage done by bad fats and plasticizers (Duque-Guimaraes).

References:

• Calabrese C., et al, A cross-over study of the effect of a single oral feeding of medium chain triglyceride oil vs. canola oil on post-indigestion plasma triglyceride levels in healthy men, *Altern Med Rev* 4; 1:23-28, 1999

• Enig M, *Know Your Fats* (Bethesda Press, 2000), *The Oiling of America*, also website: westonaprice.org/know your fats/canola

• Kramer JKG, et al, Hematological and lipid changes in newborn piglets with milk-replacer diets containing erucic acid, *Lipids,* 33; 1:1-10, 1998

• Innis SM, et al, Dietary canola oil alters hematological indices and blood lipids in neonatal piglets fed formula, *J Nutr* 129:1261-68, 1999

• Sauer FD, et al, Additional vitamin E required in milk replacer diets that contain canola oil, *Nutr Res* 17; 2:259-69, 1997

• Kwon JS, et al, Effects of diets high in saturated fatty acids, canola oil, or safflower oil on platelet function, thromboxane B2 formation and fatty acid composition of platelet phospholipids, *Am J Clin Nutr*, 54:351-58, 1991

• MacDonald BE, et al, Comparison of the effects of canola oil and sunflower oil on plasma lipids and lipoproteins and on *in vivo* thromboxane A2 and prostacyclin production in healthy young men, *Am J Clin Nutr* 50:382-88, 1989

• Kramer JKG, et al, Myocardial changes in newborn piglets fed sow milk or milk replacer diets containing different levels of erucic acid*, Lipids* 25:729-37, 1990

• Duque-Guimaraes DE, et al, Early and prolonged intake of **partially hydrogenated fat alters the expression of genes** in rat adipose tissue, *Nutr*: 782-9, 2009

Dying for a Diet Coke

After workouts and sports I commonly see folks dive into a pitcher of diet coke. You should avoid that like the plague. I don't think there is a restaurant table in the U.S. that doesn't have little packets of aspartame (**NutraSweet®, Equal®**) on them, plus choices of other fake sugars. As far back as 1996, the TV show "60 Minutes" did an exposé on it, and a senior FDA toxicologist testified before Congress that **beyond a shadow of a doubt aspartame caused brain tumors (Congressional Record SID 835:131, August 1,**

163

1985). And even in Searle's (subsequently bought by Monsanto) own inter-office reports they admitted there was "complete conversion to DKP (diketopiperazine, a brain tumor agent). And the original studies by Searle confirmed this in animals. Later when a U.S. attorney was assigned to re-investigate aspartame, he conveniently stalled until the statute of limitations had expired and coincidentally then went to work for Monsanto (with a much larger salary). You have to be an ass to use as-partame.

In past issues of *TW* I have dealt with this plus the noted neurosurgeon Russell Blaylock, M.D. and Dr. H. J. Roberts both wrote books on it (*Excitotoxins-The Taste Kills, Aspartame Disease: An Ignored Epidemic*) and Dr. Betty Martini has an extensive website documenting this, and more.

In short, aspartame is metabolized to phenylalanine, aspartic acid and **methanol which then is metabolized into formaldehyde**. Methanol you recall from articles on proving how well the **Lumen** gets rid of joint pain (*TW* 2005, 2011) is the chemical they **used to cause blindness** in experimental animals. And clearly **formaldehyde, used to embalm corpses,** is damaging to nerve/brain/cardiac/genetic, etc. tissues as well. Furthermore, in some folks formaldehyde is **addicting and lowers dopamine and serotonin** as part of its brain-damaging and **depressive** effects.

There are reports of sudden death, seizures, atrial fibrillation, low platelet counts, arthritis, brain tumors, and much more with over 92 reported side effects. Unfortunately unknowledgeable producers of chewable vitamins will include it, and of course everywhere you look you see folks clutching a soda as part of their daily quest to apparently destroy their brains.

And it goes without saying that the high fructose corn syrup that is also in most sodas is not a healthful alternative since that contributes to pre-diabetic metabolic syndrome, high cholesterol, triglycerides, and obesity (Stanhope). In fact if you have looked closely at the titles of many reports here, this type of **fructose is**

used to create diabetes in experimental animals (Song, Rajasekar, Qin). Yes, you read that correctly. The FDA condones high fructose corn syrup in a multitude of foods and drinks even though it is known to contribute to the diabetes/obesity/metabolic syndrome/etc. epidemics . Furthermore, when researchers want to show how important zinc deficiency is, they use prescription drugs like the cholesterol-lowering statins and tranquilizers like chlorpromazine to create zinc deficiency in the experimental animals. It so much easier and less expensive that way. Who needs to use phthalates to create a zinc deficiency when prescription medications and grocery store foods will do it?! (Mouat). Or if they want to **create insulin resistance and poison biotin they will use calcium channel blockers** like nifedipine, Norvasc, etc. (Vilches-Flores). Meanwhile, high fructose corn syrup and fake sugars are environmental toxins that you don't need. When I choose my poisons these are not among them.

References:

• Vilches-Flores A, et al, Biotin increases glucokinase expression via soluble guanylate cyclase/protein kinase G, adenosine triphosphate production and autocrine action of insulin in pancreatic rat islets, *J Nutr Biochem* 21:606-12, 2010

• Stanhope KL, et al, Consuming **fructose-sweetened, not glucose-sweetened, beverages increases visceral adiposity and lipids and decreases insulin sensitivity** in overweight/obese humans, *J Clin Investig* 119:1322-34, 2009

• Song D, et al, Chronic N-acetyl cysteine prevents **fructose-induced insulin resistance and hypertension** in rats, *Europ J Pharmacol* 508; 1-3:205-10, 2005

• Rajasekar P, et al, Renoprotective action of l-carnitine in **fructose-induced metabolic syndrome**, *Diab Obesity Metab* 10; 2:171-80, 2008

• Qin B, et al, Cinnamon extract prevents the **insulin resistance induced by a high-fructose diet**, *Horm Metab Res* 36; 2:119-25, 2004

• Mouat MF, et al, **Zinc uptake** into MCF-10A cells is **inhibited by cholesterol depletion**, *J Nutr Biochem,* 14:74-80, 2003

The Pancreas as an Allergic Target Organ

Did you know the pancreas can be an allergic target organ just like the nose, chest or skin? In fact, type I diabetes is recognized as an auto-immune disease…one where the body becomes allergic to its own tissues and attacks them. And in keeping with that is the fact that the *New England Journal of Medicine* years ago published how juvenile diabetics had higher levels of food antibodies directed toward (or cross-reacting with) the pancreas (Karajalainen). Having specialized in allergy and immunology for over 30 years, treating folks from a dozen countries, I can vouch for the fact that **the number one and two most common food allergies are wheat and dairy products**.

What most folks don't appreciate is **you can develop an allergy to anything at any point in time. But if you were never allergic to this food before, it's the last thing you think of. Yet once you do develop a food allergy, it can attack any area of the body and produce any symptom.** Food allergy can be the perfect disease-mimic, yet rarely does any specialist check it.

If it produces immediate skin rashes anybody can diagnose it. If it produces asthma or chronic sinusitis or migraine headaches or irritable bowel, often a food allergy is not even thought of. And if it produces something like diabetes, should you suggest an allergy, most physicians would think it was bordering on quackery and readily dismiss the notion. This is in spite of the fact that for over two decades **milk allergy is just one example of a food allergy associated with juvenile diabetes**, even in the *New England Journal of Medicine*. It's a complicated issue and the book on environmental illness, *The E.I. Syndrome,* shows you how to diagnose your own food, mold and other environmental allergens as a curable cause of symptoms, at home without tests. For remember **food allergies have a dozen different mechanisms**. When you do a blood test for food allergies, you are only looking at one of those mechanisms. Therefore it's a lot less expensive to learn how to diagnose food allergies at home by manipulating your own diet.

But remember phthalates can trigger allergies, just as can trans fats. Both permeate the standard American diet, which many countries are foolishly emulating. Phthalates are plasticizers in food packaging, whereas trans fats are chemically changed natural fats to make them last on the shelf and not go bad. **Both food allergy triggers are hidden in processed foods**. And another common cause of evolving food allergies is **leaky gut** from antibiotic-induced Candida yeast overgrowth.

Rarely is a natural food bad, but the more that's done to it in a factory the more damaging it can be in the body. Just putting spring water in plastic bottles gives enough phthalate level to the unknowledgeable mother for her to program her unborn fetus for not only food allergies, but prostate and breast cancers, and, oh yes, diabetes. As a simple example, **folks who had whole milk products** as opposed to dairy fats fractionated in a factory (and called reduced fat, dietetic, low fat, etc. where more processing has been done) were **61% less likely to develop diabetes** (Mozaffarian). The more food processors try to one-up nature, the more diabetes they can induce.

And don't always think that every reaction is a food allergy. Stuffy nose or brain fog from red wine can often be cured by fixing the molybdenum deficiency (since it runs the enzyme sulfite oxidase, see *Tired Or Toxic?*). Irritable bowel can be from an unsuspected lactase deficiency where avoidance of milk products heels the gut. Or reactions to MSG (Chinese restaurant syndrome) can be overcome by fixing a B12 deficiency, as tiny examples. It all depends on your specific deficiencies. And food allergies, like any other type, are not cast in stone. I got rid of over 85 food allergies while also getting rid of debilitating chemical sensitivities.

Remember health is a process. It doesn't appear over night. It is a result of your cumulative knowledge, which is why I never leave anyone out when I write a book, regardless of title. The more I can teach you, and the more I can release you from the restrictions of current medical thinking, the higher you can soar.

References:

- Mozaffarian D, et al, **Trans fatty acids and cardiovascular disease**, *New England Journal of Medicine* 354:1601-13, 2006

- Karajalainen J, et al, A bovine albumin peptide as a possible trigger of insulin dependent diabetes mellitus, *New Engl J Med* 327:302-307, 1992

- Gerstein H., **Cow's milk exposure and type I diabetes mellitus**. Preliminary studies have found that early introduction of cows' milk formula feeding increases the risk of developing type I diabetes, *Diabetes Care* 17:13-9, 1994

- Elliott RB, et al, Type I (insulin-dependent) **diabetes mellitus and cow's milk**: casein variant consumption, *Diabetologia* 42:292-6, 1999

- Eisenbarth KGS, Type I diabetes **mellitus: a chronic autoimmune disease**, *New Engl J Med* 314:1360-8, 1986

- Dahl-Jorgensen K, et al, Relationship between **cows' milk consumption and incidence of IDDM** in childhood, *Diabetes Care* 14:1081-83, 1991

- Mozaffarrian D, et al, Trans palmitoleic acid, metabolic risk factors and new onset diabetes in U.S. adults, *Annals Internal Medicine* 153:790-99, 2010

- Vally H, et al, Role of sulfite additives in wine-induced asthma: single dose and cumulative dose studies, *Thorax* 56:763-9, 2001

Pancreatic Enzyme Deficiencies Also Promote Cancer

Even worse than diabetes, is cancer. And it is well-known that cancer is much more common in diabetics. Why? Because you already have to have nutrient deficiencies in order to get either one, so that propels you faster toward the other. That's why I want to take this time give you a brief highly simplified primer on cancer. **You will have a tough time killing a cancer without sufficient pancreatic enzymes**. Don't be surprised if you find most oncologists do not know this. Did you ever wonder how the immune system can fight off virulent bacteria and viruses, but cannot fight off a cancer cell? It is because cancer cells are smarter and secrete a suit of armor around themselves (a sialoglycoprotein) that basically makes them invisible to the immune system. The antigenic recognition sites on the surface of cancer cells are covered by a slimy protein. So when the immune cells come looking for cancers to destroy they don't even see them. This "coating" makes them "invisible".

But the pancreas doesn't just make insulin. It also makes pancreatic enzymes. And one of their most crucial roles is to **dissolve the**

"suit of armor" off from cancer cells so that they can now be recognized and gobbled up by the immune system (see *Wellness Against All Odds* and modifications in subsequent *TW* for details on how to do it). Lowered pancreatic function can be the beginning of the end for many who shrug off indigestion as inconsequential, and merely mask it with drugs. Big mistake.

An elevated **indican** on the Cardio/ION and elastase on the **GI Effects** test can indicate unwanted bacteria are in the upper bowel that are **damaging pancreatic function**. And an elevated indican can be too low once the pancreas has burned out. An important sign of dwindling pancreatic function can be stools that actually float (too much undigested fat). Taking pancreatic enzymes like **Digestive Aid #34** (contains pancreas and bile) can correct this, and of course getting the best *live* stool study, **Comprehensive Stool Study**, to identify which bugs are actually growing in the gut and what to use to get rid of them is important. Caution: using the fake sugar artificial sweetener **saccharin can elevate indican**. Clearly you want to identify the bad bugs first. Remember **pancreatic enzymes** are not only important for digestion of fats plus all the fatty acids in the membranes, but fat-soluble vitamins A, D, E, K, CQ10, and beta-carotene, as well as proteins. And they are essential if you plan on killing cancer.

For over a decade and a half now I've presented the evidence in numerous *TW* articles confirming the importance of pancreatic enzymes in digesting off the suit of armor from cancer cells so that the immune system can now recognize them and gobble them up. Yet I still never see oncologists who are recommending this simple inexpensive yet life-saving procedure to folks. In one study **pancreatic enzymes doubled the survival time of experimental animals with pancreatic cancer,** and the tumors that did occur were much smaller. Even though this was supported in part by the American Cancer Society, they never recommend it. And of course the original work was done over a century ago by Dr. John Beard in **1903**, so there's really no excuse for your oncologist not having heard of it. And there is so much more.

Then even in the last decade it was shown that folks again with one of the worst cancers, **pancreatic cancer, more than had tripled survival at one year using pancreatic enzymes.** Furthermore, folks who had had all that medicine could offer, **quadrupled survival** at two years **using pancreatic enzymes.** And at three years they still had 36% survival for folks using enzymes and supplements, but **there were <u>no survivors at three years</u> in those having all that conventional care could offer <u>with no enzymes or supplements</u>.** The enzyme/supplement users even had **regressions where the tumors melted in size.** Even though there are no side effects from enzymes, I never hear of them being recommended. This is a travesty since pancreatic cancer is one that has such a dismal track record that many people are dead in just six months.

If you have any cancer whatsoever, past or present (and diabetics have a higher rate than others), please devour *Wellness Against All Odds*. It's an inexpensive, easy read (infinitely easier than this book!) and has saved lives. You could use **Digestive Aid #34,** which contains pancreatic enzymes that protect against stomach acid degradation and as well contains bile acids needed for detoxification. Many other enzymes do not possess these important qualities. But remember once you have killed off a lot of those dead cells, you must do the detox enema to remove those toxins or you can die from the toxic overload of dead cancer cells. The details are all in the book. Like many other answers in medicine, if it doesn't make a huge amount of money for the drug industry, you'll never hear about it.

This is seriously important if you have cancer and even if you do not. For **all of us have cancer cells already growing in us every day.** Our bodies are busy fighting them off and destroying them before they develop their suit of armor. When our nutrient deficiencies and toxicities finally reach a critical level, we lose the battle. Many cancers won't show up for 10 years. You may want to keep up with *TW*, for we have tests coming up to diagnose them 10 years earlier. The beauty of knowing this is that you have plenty of time to make slow adjustments and catch up on your reading. And just as important, you have time to **dissolve off that protective suit of armor that surrounds those cancer cells so that your immune system can destroy them** *now*.

References:

• Miloszewski K, et al, Increase in urinary indican excretion and pancreatic steatorrhea following replacement therapy, *Scand J Gastroent* 10; 5:481-85, 1975

• Lawrie CA, et al, The urinary excretion of bacterial amino acid metabolites by rats fed saccharin in the diet, *Food Chem Toxicol* 23; 4-5:445-50, 1985

• Surac M, et al, **Pancreatic enzyme extract improves survival** in murine pancreatic cancer, *Pancreas* 28:41-12, 2004

• Gonzalez NJ, et al, Evaluation of pancreatic proteolytic **enzyme treatment of adenocarcinoma of the pancreas**, with nutrition and detoxification support, *Nutr Cancer* 33:117-24, 1999

• Shively FL, *Multiple Proteolytic Enzyme Therapy of Cancer*, Dayton: Johnson-Watson, 1969

• Sakalova A, et al, Retrospective cohort study of an additive therapy with an oral enzyme preparation in patients with multiple myeloma, *Cancer Chemotherap Pharmacol* 47 (suppl): S. 38-44, 2001

The Celery Solution

Sounds silly? You already learned in *The High Blood Pressure Hoax* how **a mere 4 stalks of celery has lowered (and in some cases completely cured) high blood pressure** so well that medications were no longer needed. It turns out that **luteolin (tetra-hydroxyflavone) from celery has the potential to heal or repair the peroxisomes** (structures in our cells that are commonly damaged by environmental plasticizers and that help bring on diabetes).

Luteolin has performed so well that insulin resistance, diabetes, hypoglycemia, high triglycerides, cholesterol, weight gain that just will not budge, and other symptoms have also improved or melted away. Of course, how much of an effect a solitary item has on one's improvement depends on the total load that each person

171

brings to the table. For some folks still have too much of a load of heavy metals for anything to make a difference until they get rid of them (I'll show you how). Heavy metals are a huge roadblock for any type of healing (the protocol for getting rid of these is in *The High Blood Pressure Hoax* and 2010 *TW*, yes, even if you do not have high blood pressure).

Meanwhile, because of its 4 hydroxyl groups, luteolin is a potent anti-inflammatory agent, but there are many other mechanisms that I won't bore you with. It also contains an aromatic compound, androstenone, that gives celery its flavor. Because we all have different genetics, half of all people cannot smell it, 15% think it smells woody or floral, and the rest think it smells like stale urine.

Meanwhile, why not find as many ways to eat raw celery each day and see what happens. As an example, you can serve celery as a crudity and make bean dips or hummus, etc. (*Macro Mellow* has recipes). Since the studies were not done with cooked celery, I would suggest raw, and of course, organic (which most groceries carry now). In addition, the fiber is excellent for the gut. If nothing else, just the fiber and bulk could make you feel fuller and enable weight loss. So celery yourself silly!

References:

• Ding L, et al, **Luteolin enhances insulin sensitivity via activation of PPARgamma** transcriptional activity in adipocytes, *J Nutr Biochem* 10;21:941-7, 2010

• Musso G, et al, **Lipoprotein metabolism mediates** the association of MTP polymorphism with **B-cell dysfunction** in healthy subjects and in nondiabetic normolipemic patients with **nonalcoholic steatohepatitis**, *J Nutr Biochem* 10;21:834-40, 2010

• Shi RX, et al, **Luteolin sensitizes tumor necrosis factor**-alpha-induced apoptosis in human tumor cells, *Oncogene* 23:7712-21, 2004

• Lin Y, et al, **Luteolin, a flavonoid** with potential **for cancer prevention and therapy**, *Curr Cancer Drug Targets* 8:634-46, 2008
• Chen CY, et al, **Luteolin suppresses inflammation**-associated gene expression by blocking NF-kappa aB and AP-1 activation pathway in mouse alveolar macrophages, *Life Sci* 81:1602-14, 2007

• Weir K, 20 things you don't know about taste, *Discover*, 80, Dec 2010

Tea Time

Do you want something else that is incredibly simple that can have a bearing on healing? Green tea has a long history of sopping up free radicals, and the greener it is, the stronger the antioxidant power. In fact, we can fill whole books with just the improvement in prevention and treatment of diabetes plus ameliorating its legions of complications (Romeo). Yet its benefits extend far beyond, including strong anti-cancer properties. How simple yet effective can it be to be sipping on green organic tea? I get organic green tea from two trusted sources, **Naturallifestylemarket.com** (1-800-752-2775) and **indigo-tea.com**.

References:

• Sabu MC, et al, **Anti-diabetic activity of green tea polyphenols** and their role in reducing oxidative stress in experimental diabetes, *J Ethnopharmacol* 83:109-116, 2002

• Romeo L, et al, The major green tea polyphenol **ECGC, induces heme oxygenase** in rat neurons and acts as an effective neuroprotective agent against oxidative stress, *J Am Coll Nutr* 28; 4:492-99, 2009

• Tsuneki H, et al, Effects of green tea on blood glucose levels and serum proteoglycans patterns in diabetic (db/db) mice" and glucose metabolism in healthy humans, *BMC Pharmacol* 4:18-27, 2004

• Bose M, et al, The major **green tea** polyphenol, (-)-epigallocatechun-3-gallate, **inhibits obesity, metabolic syndrome**, and fatty liver disease in high-fat fed mice, *J Nutr* 138:1677-83, 2008

• Cao H, et al, **Green tea** polyphenol extract **regulates the expression of genes involved in glucose uptake and insulin** signaling in rats fed a high fructose diet, *J Agric Food Chem* 55:6372-8, 2007

• Kuriyama S, et a Green tea consumption and mortality due to cardiovascular disease, cancer, and all causes in Japan, *J Am Med Assoc* 296; 10:1255-65, 2006

• Hininger-Favier I, et al, **Green tea** extract decreases oxidative stress and **improves insulin** sensitivity in an animal model of insulin resistance, the fructose-fed rat, *J Am Coll Nutr* 28; 4:355-61, 2009

Drink Your Way to Health

"Hey, now you're talking!" Actually we're exploring a special type of water that has an over 40 year history for improving diabetes. Think about it. What causes all diabetes and in fact all disease? If you drop down to the microscopic chemical/electrical level, it is destructive free radicals (naked electrons). These electrons create disease by burning holes in cell membranes, thereby making cells spill their guts and die. That is why *anti-oxidant* vitamins, as an example, are able to heal so much in the body. They are sponges for free radials (these naked destructive electrons or free radicals are also called reactive oxygen species or ROS). Well, wouldn't it be great if our water contained some free radical sponges as well? It can.

For over 4 decades scientists have **electrolyzed water to increase the number of hydrogen atoms that sop up or neutralize harmful free radicals**. As well, we know an acidic pH is present in disease, whereas an optimally alkaline pH (as you get from a diet high in fruits, vegetables and whole grains and beans) promotes healing. On the flip side, dead processed foods from factories make the body more acidic. Remember when a diabetic goes into fatal coma it is preceded by diabetic keto-*acidosis*. Also when folks show up in the emergency room from a serious accident or with a near fatal infection, they are in acidosis.

Clearly this water should also have a slightly alkaline pH. Now the proof of the pudding comes in seeing if it can not only prevent diabetes, but improve it once it has appeared. And study after study confirms decades of use in Japan and elsewhere of **electrolyzed water, high in free radical-scavenging hydrogen ions in protecting against diabetes**. And once diabetes has appeared, alkaline water has reduced blood sugars, insulin, free radicals, improved pancreatic function, reduced diabetic complications, improved glucose tolerance, and many other measured parameters in animals as well as in humans. And it has been important for folks with end-stage renal disease on dialysis.

You can make this water at home and drink it daily. The **Akai Spring Alkaline Water** machine has been faithfully available to our readers for over a decade now, from High Tech Health. Never forget **the number one detoxifier is water**. It dilutes then flushes out toxins. And now if it is an anti-oxidant and alkaline as this is, (as the old song says) "Who could ask for anything more?"

References:

- Jin D, **Anti-diabetic effect of alkaline-reduced water** on OLETF rats, *Biosci Biotechnol Biochem*, 70; 1:31-37, 2006

- Kajiyama S, et al, Supplementation of **hydrogen-rich water improves lipid and glucose** metabolism **in patients with type II diabetes** or impaired glucose tolerance, *Nutri Res* 28:137-43, 2008

- Kim MJ, et al, **Anti-diabetic effects of electrolyzed reduced water** in streptozotocin-induced and genetic diabetic mice, *Life Sci*, 79:2288-92, 2006

- Huang K, et al, **Reduced** hemodialysis-induced oxidative stress in **end-stage renal disease** patients **by electrolyzed reduced water**, *Kidney Internat* 64:704-14, 2003

- Kim MJ, et al, **Preservative effect of electrolyzed reduced water on pancreatic** B-cell mass in diabetic db/db mice, *Biol Pharm Bull,* 30; 2:234-36, 2007

- Li Y, et al, **Protective mechanism of reduced water against** alloxan-induced **pancreatic B-cell damage**: Scavenging effect against reactive oxygen species, *Cytotechnology* 40:139-49, 2002

- Li Y, et al, Suppressive effects of **electrolyzed reduced water** on alloxan-induced apoptosis and **type I diabetes mellitus**, *Cytotechnology*, 2010

- Lenzen S, et al, Low anti-oxidant enzyme gene expression in pancreatic islets compared with various other mouse tissues, *Free Rad Biol Med* 20:463-66, 1996

- Ohsawa I, et al, **Hydrogen acts as a therapeutic antioxidant** by selectively reducing cytotoxic oxygen radicals, *Nature Med* 13:688-94, 2006

- Pennathur S, et al, Mechanisms for **oxidative stress in diabetic** cardiovascular disease, *Antiox Redox Signal* 9:955-69, 2007

- Minich DM, Bland JS, Acid-alkaline balance: role in chronic disease and detoxification, *Alternative Therapies* 13; 4:62-5, Jul/Aug 2007

The Detox Cocktail to the Rescue

What simpler way to rev up detoxification of both the blood and gut all at once than with the 3 basic ingredients of the detox cocktail (which I first created for *Detoxify Or Die* if you need further references)? Since detoxification involves 2 phases, I chose a major detoxifier for each one and added another anti-oxidant to recycle them to get even more mileage.

In brief, (1) it is whatever dose you best tolerate of vitamin C for phase I, remembering the body must have it since we do not make it. Let too lose a stool be your limiting factor, and the dose often

175

varies from ½ -1 heaping tsp of **Vitamin C Powder** (2-6 gm). By now you are an expert in knowing that free radicals create inflammation, and inflammation creates not only diabetes and other diseases, but accelerates its complications. One dangerous indicator, for example, that your disease is on the fast track is an elevated **hsCRP (high sensitivity C-reactive protein). This marker of inflammation is so serious that once it climbs above 3 mg/L you are in serious risk of early heart attack, stroke, cancer, senility**, and more.

On the flipside it could mean that you have a smoldering tooth infection or intestinal abscess that you're not aware of.   A dentist, Douglas L. Cook, DDS gives the explanations and evidence for how an unhealthy tooth, root canal, implant, or even empty cavitation site (from an old tooth extraction) can affect organs "downwind" that are sharing the same acupuncture meridians. **There are many folks who will never get well until a specific diseased tooth is dealt with**. And you know what a reference-junkie I am, so you know that he provides plenty of evidence in this book as well. You will learn what a good biological dentist should know in *Rescued By My Dentist. New Solutions To a Health Crisis* (1-920-842-2083, or www.dentistryhealth.com, or 1-888-232-4444 or www.traford.com). In *Pain Free In 6 Weeks*, I've given you the dental map of which teeth affect which organs. Sometimes repairing a tooth in the acupuncture meridian (electrical pathway) of the pancreas can correct diabetes.

Meanwhile prescription drugs like Crestor® are recommended by dinosaurs because it lowers the CRP by about 33%. Sounds like a good idea? But as we referenced in *TW* gamma tocopherol (one of the 8 forms of natural vitamin E) does double that.   The Cardio/ION measures this non-damaging part of vitamin E that lowers CRP 66%. It comes as **Gamma E Gems** or **Natural Gamma E**, usually one or two a day is all that is needed. Furthermore, vitamin C (and only 1000 mg a day) can do as much as some statin drugs (Block).

The next ingredient (2) is the best referenced form of glutathione, the major detoxifier of the body, and we do make this, but not nearly in the quantity that is needed to detoxify our 21st century daily onslaught of toxins. That is why in every disease, there is a deficiency of it. **Recancostat** is a special reduced GSH (glutathione) because it contains an anthocyanidin to recycle it, improving its lifespan. I've referenced articles in *TW* where they used this specific brand for children near Chernobyl to protect them from the hypothyroidism, cancer, and other effects of the excessive radiation.

(3) Last is 300 mg **R-Lipoic Acid** (remember you already learned how indispensible this antioxidant is in diabetes in guarding against its lethal side effects, in restoring memory and vitality, etc. in Chapter 3). We make this in mitochondria, but not in the amounts needed in this century of unprecedented pollutants, and especially in the face of the demands of diabetes. It recycles vitamins C, E, CoQ10 and other anti-oxidants, extending their therapeutic lives, plus it chelates heavy metals. Most importantly it down-regulates the multitude of side effects of diabetes. It's so potent it is even used in emergency treatment for poison mushrooms, for which there is no other (recognized) treatment. Avoid products that just say "lipoic acid" or "alpha-lipoic acid", since 50% is unusable by the body (and it is another indicator of an inferior nutrient or prescriber).

NAC is the poor man's glutathione, since the body uses this rate-limiting amino acid to make glutathione. It is another important adjunct in reversing insulin resistance (Song). And you will notice once again from the references that one way researchers create diabetes for their studies is with high fructose corn syrup, something that laces American fast-foods, processed-foods, convenience-foods, diet and soft drinks, and is even added to fruit juices that are hyped as healthful (Qin).

And for folks who are not ready to make their own detox cocktail, or want it sweetened with natural stevia, or need it in handy single dose packets for travel, or all the above, one company makes **Happy Bodies' Detox Cocktail** (but add 2 **R-Lipoic Acid** 100 mg capsules to it).

Some folks **lower their biotin with lipoic acid** so you need to have your doctor check your beta hydroxy iso-valerate, the functional test for biotin deficiency (it's on your Cardio/ION). For recall that **biotin must be repaired in order to prevent as well as treat diabetes**, and it inhibits many side effects. Lipoic acid and Biotin are both crucial for diabetes control, but the former can lower the later. Biotin is also lowered by medications for seizures, and other diseases (Monograph).

References (*TW* and our books contain so many more references proving it should be considered malpractice to neglect giving lipoic acid to diabetics, that they have not been duplicated here. As well, remember any reference not included here is in previous books or *TW*s):

- Block G, et al, **Vitamin C treatment reduces elevated C-reactive protein**, *Free Rad Biol Med* 46; 1:70-77, 2009

- Monograph, Biotin, *Altern Med Rev* 12; 1:73-78, 2007

- Song D, et al, Chronic **N-acetyl cysteine prevents fructose-induced insulin resistance** and hypertension in rats, *Eur J Pharmacol* 508; 1-3:205-10, 2005

- Qin B, et al, Cinnamon extract prevents the **insulin resistance induced by a high-fructose diet**, *Horm Metab Res* 36; 2:119-25, 2004

- McLennon SV, et al, Changes in hepatic glutathione metabolism in diabetes, *Diabetes* 40, 344-48, 1991

- Jennings PE, et al, Vitamin C metabolites and microangiopathy in diabetes mellitus, *Diabetes Res* 6:151-4, 1987

- Sreemantula S, et al, Influence of antioxidant (L-ascorbic acid) on tolbutamide-induced hypoglycemia/anti-hyperglycaemia in normal and diabetic rats, *BMC Endocr Disord*, 5:2, 2005

- Young IS, et al, The effect of ascorbate supplementation on oxidative stress in streptozotocin-induced diabetic rats, *Free Rad Biol Med* 12:41-6, 1992

- Paolisso G, et al, Plasma **GSH/GSSG affects glucose homeostasis** in healthy subjects and non-insulin-dependent **diabetics**, *Am J Physiol* 263 (pt 1): E435-40, 1992

- Paolisso G, et al, Metabolic benefits deriving from chronic vitamin C supplementation in non-aged non-insulin-dependent diabetics, *J Am Coll Nutr* 14:387-92, 1995

- Shih PH, et al, Anthocyanins induced the activation of phase 2 enzymes through the antioxidant responsive element pathway against oxidative stress-induced apoptosis, *J Agri Food Chem* 55:9427-35, 2007l,

- Packer L, et al, Molecular aspects of **lipoic acid in the prevention of diabetes complications,** *Nutr* 17; 10:888-895, **2001**

- Jacob AS, et al, Oral administration of our RAC-a-**lipoic acid modulates insulin sensitivity** in patients with type II diabetes mellitus: a placebo-controlled pilot trial, *Free Rad Biol Med* 27; 3-4:309-14, 1999

- Estrada D, et al, Stimulation of glucose uptake by the natural coenzyme a-lipoic acid/thioctic acid: participation of elements of the insulin signaling pathway, *Diabetes* 45; 12:1798-1804, 1996

- Anonymous, Alpha lipoic acid, *Altern Med Rev* 11; 3:232-7, 2006

- Lord RS, Bralley JA Eds, 2nd Ed, *Laboratory Evaluations for Integrated and Functional Medicine*, metametrix.com (1-800-221-4640, also check on many other newer books on interpretation), 2008

Where is the Diet?

If you are diabetic you have already seen many books and magazines and internet sites loaded with diets and recipes. I'm here to tell you that the American Diabetes Association and the American Heart Association's recommended diet is 30% fat. This diet has never and I repeat, NEVER, been proven to reverse any disease. However, another diet has not only reversed diabetes, but end-stage heart diseases in folks for whom no more medications or surgeries were available, and everything medicine had to offer prior had failed. As well it has even improved cancers. The diet is outlined and referenced in 10 issues of *Total Wellness* 2012-2013.

The reason I have not repeated it here is in trying to keep this book small enough to entice people who are scared off by large volumes. The second reason is I would rather see you absorb for yourself forever an enormous amount of information that you cannot get in any other single place, so that your daily decisions about your health are more firmly based in scientific evidence. I'm a strong believer that we should show people how to fish, not give them a fish. If I just say "take these nutrients and eat this diet", I consider myself a failure. My goal is to provide you with so much solid thought-provoking information that you start to make your own decisions much better than anyone else could, especially one who has never examined you nor assayed your nutrients and toxicities. I want to see you get too smart to fail.

If you remember nothing else from your first go round with this chapter, bear in mind 3 facts. (1) The higher sugar levels of diabetes fosters Candida growth. (2) Candida can destroy any organ including the pancreas. (3) Candida can also create new food allergies that you never had before that can also create and perpetuate diabetes.

Clearly the road to health is paved with good intestines, whereas the road to disease is paved with ill-informed intentions and misinformation. O.K., I'll bet you are ready for a nutrient program to be mapped out for you.

Chapter V

Dinosaur Diabetes Docs Don't Deliver Doses for Cure

Fixing What's Broken

"Can't we just make it simple?" "I can't deal with a lot." "How about just giving me the top nutrient categories?" you ask. That's a bigger task than you may realize. The evidence is overwhelming that **diabetics have starving cell membranes**, they are **deficient in minerals**, and the **mitochondria** where energy is made **are poisoned**. Clearly each person carries his own personal load of deficiencies and toxicities. Having said that, let's see what a focused practical repair can do for you. But remember, without all the information that preceded this chapter, you limit your chance of success incredibly. Your goal is *not* to just try to take everything here (which would be impossible), but to learn how to sort through and make a more intelligent decision on what is best for *you*. There is enormously more information in past and future *TW* and books. For *real health is a continually evolving growth process*. Most of all: Remember, I don't want to just throw you a fish. I want to teach you how to catch your own for a lifetime. I want to help you *get too smart to fail* in your health goals.

How Do You Cure Diabetes? Start With the 7-M Focus

It's very straightforward and the evidence for each aspect is overwhelming. But don't worry. I will guide you through it, section by section. For more information about each individual item, you can find it in the previous books and *TW* newsletters, which are a *must*. **Health is a growth process**. One book cannot answer all your needs. Furthermore, everyone starts with a different base of knowledge (and lack thereof). But remember **the average person does not need all of these things.** Yet since I have never examined you, nor taken your history, nor seen your lab results, **I don't know which things you can skip**. The following (and what you have learned in the preceding chapters) represent the most common deficiencies and repair needs I've seen to reverse recalcitrant disease in over 40 years.

For the **7-M focus**, you need to repair

(1) the cell **membrane**, then
(2) the **minerals**, then
(3) the **mitochondria**, then
(4) your **meals**, next
(5) **miscellaneous** gut and hormone issues, then if you're still not better
(6) the heavy **metals** and other **meridian** pollutants must be gotten rid of. But never forget:
(7) the **mind, motivation, and mood**

(1) Membrane Healing

If you look at the last hundred **Cardio/IONs** from diabetics as well as other "incurable" or recalcitrant diseases, they have what I call **starving cell membranes**. It doesn't matter if it is atrial fibrillation, an undiagnosable motor neuron nerve disease or end-stage cancer. Most disease starts here. So let's repair the damage to cell membranes which also hold the insulin receptors, for it takes 120 days to make a new red cell. In the last hundred people who cured or dramatically improved their diabetes, these would be the statistically most often deficient nutrients plus the average corrective doses and the best sources I could find. I can't check every company (and they continually change formulations and suppliers, owners retire or sell, etc.), but have seen many products I would not take. I have not given you the volumes of evidence for the indications for every single nutrient because they are described and referenced in the other books and 24 years of *TW* newsletters. For if I repeated all of this evidence this book would be so big no one would ever with want to tackle it, and you'd need a wheelbarrow to carry it to the beach.

Cod Liver Oil, Lemon Flavored a tablespoon every other day
                             carlsonlabs.com 1-800-323-4141
GLA   one a day
                             carlsonlabs.com 1-800-323-4141
Phosphatidyl Choline Powder a heaping teaspoonful daily or
                             one tablespoon every other day
                             happybodies.com 1-800-427-7926
E-Gems Elite   two a day
                             carlsonlabs.com 1-800-323-4141
Gamma E-Gems   one a day
                             carlsonlabs.com 1-800-323-4141
Tocotrienols   two a day
                             carlsonlabs.com 1-800-323-4141
Solar D Gems, 4000 mg   one a day
                             carlsonlabs.com 1-800-323-4141
Vitamin K2   one a day
                             carlsonlabs.com 1-800-323-4141
PS-100   1-2 twice a day
                             carlsonlabs.com 1-800-323-4141
Magnesium Chloride Solution 200 mg/cc
(Rx written by your doctor as follows:
Disp. 18 oz   Sig. ½ tsp b.i.d., ref 20),
then call the Windham Pharmacy (Windham, NY) to get it
properly filled (518-734-3033).
If you cannot get a prescription, at least use 1-2 heaping teaspoons
of Natural Calm (NEEDS.com, 1-800-634-1380) a day or **Happy
Bodies' Mag** (happybodies.com, 1-800-happybo).

(2) Minerals

Because there are limited mineral transporter proteins to carry
minerals across the gut wall and into the bloodstream, we have
found that *they are not all absorbed if you to take a handful at
once* or a "multiple mineral". But they are absorbed well if you
space them out with just a few minerals (maximum 3-5 minerals
at a time) in the morning and then a few more several hours later,

and a few more several hours after that. It helps to have a tad of food in your stomach, even if it's just 3 soaked almonds or a handful of blueberries or a bite of an organic banana. It doesn't have to be much food, just something to buffer your stomach and trigger digestive enzymes. You will notice other crucial minerals have been relegated to other categories. Having said that, most of the remaining mineral deficiencies can be rectified with one a day (or every other day) of each of the following:

Zinc Balance	jarrow.com	1-800-726-0886
Iodoral	optimox.com	
	use needs.com	1-800-634-1380
Silboron	intensivenutrition.com	1-800-333-7414
SeaSel	"	
IntraMin	druckerlabs.com	1-888-881-2345
Moly B	carlsonlabs.com	1-800-323-4141
Chelated Vanadium	"	
Chelated Chromium	"	
ACES with Zinc	"	
BioSil	happybodies.com	1-800-427-7926

(3) Mitochondrial Repair

Since mitochondria (the organelles inside of cells where energy is created) are a mass of membranes, **the preceding membrane and mineral repairs are likewise paramount for the repair of damaged mitochondria**, which are all too common in this era. In fact dozens of scientific reports of the highest caliber now prove that **disease and death hinge on mitochondrial health** or lack thereof. The most commonly deficient nutrients (in addition to the ones you just learned) include the following:

Acetyl L-Carnitine Powder	1000 mg/ once or twice a day
	carlsonlabs.com 1-800-323-4141
Arginine Powder	same dose and supplier

Chelated Manganese	one a day	
	carlsonlabs.com	1-800-323-4141
Nutra Support Joint	two/day	"
Q-ODT	3 dissolved under the tongue twice a day	
	intensivenutrition.com	1-800-333-7414
D-Ribose Powder	3000 mg/day	
	carlsonlabs.com	1-800-323-4141
B Compleet-100	one a day	
	carlsonlabs.com	1-800-323-4141
Niacin Time	1 twice a day	
	carlsonlabs.com	1-800-323-4141
P-5-P	1-2 a day (before three o'clock)	"
Vitamin B1	one a day	"
Glycine Powder	1000mg/ day	"
Super Milk Thistle X	one twice a day	
	integrativeinc.com	1-800-931-1709
Detox Cocktail	once or twice a day	
	happybodies.com	1-800-427-7926
R-Lipoic Acid	2 twice a day	
	intensivenutrition.com	1-800-333-7414

It sounds like a lot? Sure! Why do you think you have diabetes or any other disease? These are the most common deficiencies that we have identified in hundreds of 13-page assays of folks' vitamins, minerals, fatty acids, amino acids, organic acids and other crucial laboratory parameters. But do not despair. It took you a lifetime to get sick. It is a lot quicker to repair. And you don't have to take it all in one day. In fact it is preferable not to, but, rather in the beginning to **spread one day's worth of nutrients out over 2-3 days**. Anything is better than what you're doing now. I repeat: if you can't manage (or afford) all your nutrients in one day then spread a day's worth out over a few days, especially if you have any abnormal kidney function such as an elevated BUN (blood urea nitrogen) or low albumin (albuminuria is a protein lost in the urine, a sign of diseased diabetic kidneys). If you have to take the slow boat to China, so be it. At least you are on a focused path to improve your nutritional status, to fix what's broken, to heal. That's better than the path you were on.

(4) Meals

(1) Basically you want to avoid the trans fatty acids which include canola and other foods with the legalized lying labels that say "NO TRANS FATS". Because it is so important, I repeat: According to the Federal Register the FDA now allows food manufacturers to say this if a food contains less than 500 mg of damaging trans fatty acids per puny half cup serving. As we've referenced in the past from Harvard and other prestigious centers **there is no safe level of trans fats.**

(2) You want to avoid the phthalates as much as possible which means not drinking out of plastic water bottles whenever possible (and disregard "No BPA", just as you would "No trans fats" (refer to *TW* 2012 and the next chapter). Try to buy foods that are unpackaged, organic, and locally fresh. Avoid those shipped from far away, since even if the food starts out organic, it will not stay that way after the ship hold is invariably sprayed (fumigated) for the rest of the non-organic produce. Bugs can delay perishables at customs.

(3) Avoid any foods with Olestra (they often say they are guilt-free or fat-free). It inhibits absorption of fat-soluble life-saving vitamins like A, D, E, K, CoQ10, beta-carotene, the fatty acids, all essential for curing diabetes.

(4) Avoid any fake sugars or sugar substitutes including high fructose corn syrup. Don't forget it is used to create diabetic animals in the laboratory so that researchers can experiment on them with drugs. With all the decades of evidence against high fructose corn syrup (see references below), it boggles the mind how that can still permeate the processed foods and drink industry while the FDA

vigorously attacks repair nutrients and detoxification supplements.

(5) The maximally low fat diet has effortlessly allowed weight loss of pounds that have evaded all types of diets over decades. More importantly it has reversed some of the most recalcitrant diabetes and cardiovascular diseases that have resisted all that medicine has to offer. This oil-free modification of the Ornish plan has even melted away coronary plaque (details in *TW* 2012-13).

(6) The **macrobiotic diet** has literally cured people with end-stage cancers who were given just hours to live (ask for your free sample *Total Wellness* December 2006 newsletter that describes one such case who is still enjoying vibrant health over 17 years after her 'death sentence'). It also has enabled folks to get rid of their diabetes. You start with *You Are What You Ate* then proceed to *The Cure Is In the Kitchen*. The recipe book is *Macro Mellow* (the composite of all 3 books is called *The Macro Trilogy*). Another option is the whole foods diet, having about 70% raw foods to which can be added cooked whole grains, beans, and meats, fish, poultry. Even if you don't go macro, you will learn how to start making smarter and more expanded food choices that have enormous life-promoting power with *Love, Sanae. My healing journey*, by Sanae Suzuki (www.LoveEricInc.com or 1-310-450-6383).

References:

- Gaby AR, Adverse effects of dietary fructose, *Altern Med Rev* 10; 4:294-306, 2005

- Tokita Y, et al, **Fructose ingestion enhances atherosclerosis** and deposition of advanced glycated end-products in cholesterol-fed rabbits, *J Atheroscler Thromb* 12; 5:260-7, 2005

- Beck-Nielsen H, et al, **Impaired** cellular insulin binding and **insulin sensitivity induced by high-fructose feeding in normal subjects**, *Am J Clin Nutr* 33; 2:273-8, 1980

- McPherson JD, et al, Role of **fructose in glycation** and cross-linking of proteins, *Biochemistry* 27; 6:1901-7, 1988

- Moeller SM, et al, Consult on Science and Public Health, American Medical Association. Effects of high fructose syrup, *J Am Coll Nutr* 28; 6:619-26, 2009

- Angelopoulos TJ, et al, The effect of **high fructose corn syrup consumption on triglycerides and uric acid**, *J Nutr* 139; 6:1242S-1245S, 2009

- Stanhope KL, et al, Endocrine and metabolic effects of consuming beverages sweetened with fructose, glucose, sucrose, or high fructose corn syrup, *Am J Clin Nutr* 88;6:1733S-7S, 2008

- Forshee RA, et al, A critical examination of the **evidence relating high fructose corn syrup and weight gain**, *Crit Rev Food Sci Nutr* 47;6: 561-82, 2007

- Ouyang X, et al, **Fructose consumption is a risk factor for non-alcoholic fatty liver disease**, *J Hepatology* 48;6: 993-9, 2008

- Hallfrisch J, et al, Effects of dietary fructose on plasma glucose and hormone responses in normal and hyperinsulinemia men, *J Nutr* 113; 9:1819-26, 1983

(6) Miscellaneous: **Gut, Hormones**

As you learned in the previous chapter, **the gut houses half the immune system and half the detox system for the entire body. All healing of many diseases is stalled until the gut is repaired**. And you have already learned a bit about how pivotal the detox nutrients are as a sponge for free radicals. These are generated by the harmful 21st century toxins like plasticizers and pesticides, statin-resistant Teflon-types and flame retardants impregnating myriads of products, auto and industrial gases, and more. Clearly, free radicals are often the ultimate destroyers of the pancreas and insulin receptors on the cell surfaces. And you know that diabetes is an auto-immune disease, meaning the body's bug-fighters are mistakenly attacking its own tissues, namely the pancreas. Most auto-immune disease begins in the gut when its walls become "leaky".

Yet the gut is also the home of many hormones, like serotonin, one of your brain's "happy hormones" that anti-depressants like Prozac increase. Actually they poison its breakdown so that it lasts longer in the brain, hence, making you feel happier. But a knowledgeable doc is aware that 95% of the body's serotonin is not made in the brain. It is made in the gut. So if the gut is not healthy, you can't be happy. And poisoning the brain with anti-depressants? They act like fertilizer for cancer patients, while Prozac also contains three molecules of fluoride which are toxic for brain enzymes and neurotransmitters (see *TW* and chapter IV for more).

The chief gut problem for diabetics is an overgrowth of yeast in the intestines called *Candida albicans*. When it grows excessively (it thrives on sugar), it does may bad things.

(1) It causes **heartburn**, GERD, gastritis, irritable bowel syndrome, colitis, indigestion, and more.

(2) It creates **new food allergies** that you never had before, like nightshades being a totally curable cause of all sorts of arthritis and even mimicking ruptured discs, sciatica, ganglion cysts, tendonitis, fibromyalgia, solo painful joints or multiple joints as in rheumatoid arthritis, and much more (see *Pain Free In 6 Weeks* for details of cause and cure). Candida creates new food allergies by first creating the "leaky gut" (the causes and cures of which are described in *No More Heartburn*).

(3) Candida in the gut also releases acetaldehyde which can cause depression, mimic fibromyalgia and bizarre muscle and joint disease, depression, *brain fog*, and more.

(4) Candida also fosters the development of **thyroid auto-antibodies** that attack and destroy your thyroid. That is right! No disease occurs out of the blue and for no reason. Phthalates, Candida, nutrient deficiencies and heavy metals are just some of the causes for a pancreas, thyroid or any gland or organ to suddenly stop working. But if no one is checking for Candida overgrowth or thyroid auto-antibodies, then you continue to have weight gain, depression, hair and tooth loss, constipation, and exhaustion, all chalked up to old age! (5) And Candida makes an enzyme, thiaminase that kills your B1 vitamin, silently leading to fatal heart failure, depression, exhaustion and, oh yes, "incurable" diabetic nephropathy. Did I repeat these things? You bet! It's one of the easiest ways for you to learn new and difficult facts pertinent to your future health.

TW 2011 goes into the most commonly made mistakes by doctors attempting to treat Candida. And as an addendum to that article you will have to teach your doctor that probably the only way he can now order **Nystatin Pure Powder** for you is through a manufacturer's (Paddock, 1-800-328-5113) distributor like McKesson-Robbins which sends it directly to your local pharmacy. When he calls the pharmacy or writes the Rx, he must **use the NDC # 00574040405**. This will provide a 50 million unit bottle, which taken as ½ tsp t.i.d. will last about 3 weeks (since potency varies lot-to-lot). Most docs need this instruction to order it.

I wish that were all that this silent gut-killer does, but there is much more. The bottom line is that if you do not have a healthy gut, get a stool study to diagnose the bad bugs, like Candida. It thrives in diabetics. After over 40 years of seeing lab results from famous clinics and hospitals, I can unequivocally say the two best stool tests are the **Comprehensive Stool Study with Purged Parasites X3** (by Doctor's Data) and the **GI Effects** (by MetaMetrix). Why two? Because one cultures the live bugs and the other identifies them by their genetics. And both tests also include other unique assays critical for gut health. The combination of the two tests gives the most superior results that no hospital lab has duplicated. Now you see why many folks will never heal because the gut was never checked and healed. To cure the gut read *No More Heartburn*, <u>**for the road to health is paved with good intestines!**</u> Other bugs in the gut produce an organic acid that chelates out your magnesium (tricarballyate), while others raise your indican level, signifying the pancreas is in real trouble. All these hidden warning parameters and much more are on the **Cardio/ION** blood/urine test.

In terms of hormones, it would take volumes to cover them all. But you have seen how *unsuspected Candida can destroy the thyroid*. More importantly, the *vast majority of environmental toxins* from our air, food and water, regardless of what chemical category they are in, are **EEDs or environmental endocrine disruptors**.

Whether they are pesticides, plasticizers, heavy metals, volatile organic hydrocarbons or anything else, the EEDs target glands and destroy them. A commonly destroyed or worse yet, silently hypo-functioning gland is the adrenal or stress gland. When that's not working up to par you can just feel vaguely low in energy. The best test is the **Adrenal Stress Panel** (metametrix.com). It is easy to do since you merely saturate cotton wads with saliva and send them back in the pre-paid FedEx(® mailer. It assays over a 24-hour period your adrenal hormone functions and deficiencies.

A commonly low adrenal hormone is DHEA (dehydroepiandrosterone), the #1 one adrenal hormone. In fact it gets lower in most people as we age, especially after the age of 50. If that were not enough, it's usually lower in people with any type of chronic disease, especially diabetes. We don't know what comes first the chicken or the egg. Probably the same deficiencies and toxicities that create the diabetes add to the demise of the adrenals. Clearly chronic disease also limits the protection of the adrenal glands against developing deficiencies and toxicities. Fortunately, sometimes something as simple as a trial of one to two **25 mg DHEA** daily can restore energy and help you balance your body's diabetic response. Also DHEA metabolizes into testosterone, another hormone that is severely impacted by environmental chemicals leading to impotence. Having low DHEA also promotes not only diabetes but arteriosclerosis and accelerated aging. Because DHEA can metabolize into other hormones including testosterone and progesterone in the human body, women usually need a lower dose or they may develop unwanted facial hair.

Of course as always my goal is *not* to have you take hormones. My goal is to teach you how to **repair the gland** that produces the hormones by restoring the depleted nutrients and getting rid of the toxins that created the dysfunction. Now the gland can make sufficient hormone again all by itself. For remember, when you take a hormone for an extended period of time, the *"feedback inhibition" can turn off any further production of hormone* by your gland. You don't want that. You want to heal it. So the shorter the hormone "rescue", the better. And if repairing the gland fails, remember you also often have to **fix the hormone receptors on the surface of the cell membrane** with your membrane repair and "oil change". The site on the cell surface that is like a lock and key must be healthy enough to allow the hormone to turn on cellular function. Otherwise, if the receptor is not repaired, you can take hormones forever, but they "don't work". If you need, there's more about this in *Total Wellness*.

References:

• Boudou P, et al, **Hyperglycemia acutely decreases circulating dehydroepiandrosterone** levels in healthy men, *Clinl Endocrinol* (Oxford) 64; 1:46-52, 2006

• Dhatariya K, et al, **Effect of dehydroepiandrosterone replacement on insulin sensitivity** and lipids in hypoadrenal women, *Diabetes* 54; 3:765-9, 2005

• Villareal DT, et al, **Effect** of **DHEA on abdominal fat** and insulin action in elderly women and men: a randomized controlled trial, *J Am Med Assoc* 292; 18:2243-8, 2004

• Diamond P, et al, Metabolic effects of 12-month percutaneous dehydroepiandrosterone replacement therapy in postmenopausal women, *J Endocrinol* 150 suppl: S43-50, 1996

• Yamashita R, et al, Effects of dehydroepiandrosterone on gluconeogenesis enzymes and glucose uptake in human hepatoma cell line, HepG2, *Endocrinol J,* 52; 6,727-33, 2005

• Kapoor D, et al, Androgens, insulin resistance and vascular disease in men, *Clin Endocrinol* (Oxford) 63;3:239-50, 2005

• Kupelian V, et al, Low sex hormone-binding globulin, total testosterone, and symptomatic **androgen deficiency are associated with development of the metabolic syndrome** in non-obese men, *J Clin Endocrinol Metab* 91; 3:843-50, 2006

• Bain J, The many faces of testosterone, *Clin Interv Aging* 2;4:567-76, 2007

• Traish AM, et al, **The dark side of testosterone deficiency II. Type 2 diabetes and insulin resistance**, *J Androl* 30; 1:23-32, 2009

(6) Metals and Other Meridian **Pollutants**

By just correcting the nutrient deficiencies in the membranes, minerals and mitochondria sections, many will be cured. For others, they need to go further. **Heavy metals are one of the most stubborn causes of all chronic diseases**, for they are unavoidable. How do they destroy body chemistry? They sit in enzymes, kicking out the minerals that make them work. Hence that particular chemistry comes to a screeching halt or performs unpredictably abnormally. For example, in the pancreas or in the membrane insulin receptors, when the zinc is replaced by mercury or lead, cadmium, arsenic or aluminum, you have diabetes.

We cannot escape heavy metals in this era. We all have mercury (from coal-fired power plants, dental amalgam fillings, seafood, etc.), cadmium, arsenic, lead, aluminum, and more from industrial/manufacturing exhausts, pesticides, and more in our air, food and water. Heavy metal detoxification is not taught in medical schools primarily because the majority of funding comes from the pharmaceutical companies. That is why all diseases merely look like a deficiency of the latest drug. The three primary protocols for removing heavy metals can take from one to several years depending on the person. But it has been the basis for many people, myself included, for curing multiple "impossible to heal" medical conditions. And compared with IV chelation (that increases dangerous cardio-toxic plasticizers and cyclohexanone in the body from IVs) the protocol for getting rid of heavy metals described in *The High Blood Pressure Hoax* is 5 times safer and more economical than IV chelation, and does not require a prescription (like I say, every book has essential information for everyone including this, even though you may not have the title's high blood pressure).

I feel after having reversed over 20 "incurable " maladies in myself, and having seen others do the same and even more spectacular accomplishments, that **we have to detoxify forever**. Follow the protocols very carefully for the DMSA (Captomer) and EDTA (Detoxamin or prescribed compounded suppositories), for the uninformed have gotten themselves into serious trouble. I have consulted on physicians who thought they could plow ahead with less reading. They released toxins, but didn't prepare for the removal of them from the body. Hence toxins tanked up in joints, leaving some in wheelchairs. *And all because they tried to skimp on reading.* As one example of how to avoid toxin overload as you mobilize them, you must use the absence of the sulfur smell in your urine to determine your next dose of DMSA. For it can vary from 1-2 capsules 1 to 3 times a day, depending on the individual. And you must take no minerals the days you are on it. More on toxins and their removal in chapter VI.

Likewise the EDTA dose can vary from 1-3 suppositories, and you must take all the minerals before 2 p.m. when you are on this. Recently the FDA has forced the non-prescription version off the market even though it has been an FDA-approved food additive for over 50 years. But your doctor can prescribe it through compounding pharmacies. *The High Blood Pressure Hoax,* subsequent *TW* and books will guide you with even more detoxifiers and updates. Much depends on the severity of your poisoning. In the next chapter I'll give you a gentler detoxification protocol to start with.

Recall that Dr. Douglas L. Cook, DDS gives the explanations and evidence for how an unhealthy tooth, root canal, implant, or even empty cavitation site (from an old tooth extraction) can affect organs "downwind" that are **sharing the same acupuncture meridians** (*Rescued By My Dentist. New Solutions To a Health Crisis).* Sometimes a person can relate the appearance of a diseased organ, like the pancreas, to shortly after a particular dental procedure like a mercury amalgam filling or implant, or a hidden infection developing in an old root canal. Many folks who will never get well until a specific diseased tooth is dealt with.

Beyond what I could deal with here, in *TW* we'll be showing how an electrical system of the body disguised as the web of myo-fascial tissue and trigger points masquerades as every painful malady from a bad hip or knee to crippling arthritis. But I'll give you one pertinent example later of how it mimics a hip that needs joint replacement before we close this chapter. The bottom line? Heavy metals and other toxins (next chapter) choke normal function, but it's all blamed on aging.

And it goes without saying that detoxifying the body with a daily **far infrared sauna** (High Tech Health or Sauna Ray) and an **alkaline spring water machine** (High Tech Health) as detailed in *Detoxify Or Die* should precede the heavy metals protocol. For these are so fundamental to health that they should be begun in childhood. Don't forget that diabetes is even more rampant in children than ever before, as much as one in eight. And by the time U.S. children are 6 years of age, most children have toxin levels that it used to take us from a different generation until age 40 to accumulate. They are on a path of accelerated disease and aging, one reason the *New England Journal of Medicine* had an article showing many children will now not outlive their parents.

(7) Mind, Mood, and Motivation

If I hadn't seen it in my own physician colleagues who had some of the most "incurable" diseases, it might never have gotten my attention. But when I asked them what turned around the course of their diseases, they said it was learning how to forgive. If you have any doubt about the power of negative thoughts over your body's function, the best and most comprehensive proof that I have ever found is in a book by Dr. Art Mathias, Ph.D., *In His Own Image* (907-563-9033 or www.akwellspring.com). *In His Own Image* is the best, most concise, readable and highly referenced exposé on **how harmful emotions can unmercifully trigger diseases in our bodies**. Then I would suggest the sequel, *Biblical Foundations Of Freedom* which takes the reader even further, since as Dr. Mathias teaches, **if a memory hurts, it's unresolved, not forgiven, and can negatively impact the health of the body** (1-907-563-9033 or www.akwellspring.com). Regardless of your spiritual persuasion or lack thereof, this provides an integral awakening of the need to **detoxify your emotional trash**, convincing you to **free yourself from the mental toxins that we all carry**.

If you don't feel you are worth it, I readily recommend reading *Inner Journey: Finding Happiness Within* (1-585-872-0688 or www.gockley.com/gockleyinstitute@gockley.com, or 1-877-buy-book or www.buybooksontheweb.com). In fact I challenge you to be able to come away from reading it totally unchanged and unimproved. There's enough negativity in the world and not nearly enough positivity. Dr. Gockley and his wife show how we can unburden our minds to improve our mental health by changing ourselves, mentally and emotionally. Too often we wallow in how we would change the world, but rarely consider changing ourselves. And yet in reality *the only person you can change is you*. This mind-challenging, mind-opening, refreshing and thought-provoking book shows we all come equipped with our own individual emotional baggage and how to clean it out.

In over 40 years in medicine, I have seen highly educated attorneys, physicians, engineers, etc., not choose to heal themselves. Then a truck driver or farmer or a high school drop-out grabs the bull by the horns and they heal themselves from maladies that stumped the most highly-educated specialists. I'm thoroughly convinced that **education level has no bearing, nor does socioeconomic level. There is some inner ability to take control, to take responsibility for one's destiny** that some folks have and others simply do not. Or do they just *choose* not to have control? I don't know. But clearly *original sin began with abrogation of personal responsibility.* Didn't Adam, when asked by God what he had done, try to first blame it on that woman that God had given him? When that failed to hold water, then he blamed the only other person left in his universe, the Creator Himself, as he reminded God that it was *He* who had given her to him. **Do you also have an unending litany of excuses why you will never have the time to make your health a priority?**

Reference:

•   *The Student Bible, New International Version,* Zondervan Publishing House, Grand Rapids MI, 1986 (the best beginners' *Bible* I have seen with very helpful explanations as you read along)

So there you have an outline of my plan for you. But before we close this chapter on nutrients, there are some more life-saving concepts for you.

How About an Easier Start?

There are many natural herbs that also improve diabetes and I'll just give you an example of a few products and the logistics for their combination of ingredients. One herb is *a fruit from the cucumber family called* momordica. Its common name is *bitter melon*. It has reversed diabetes and repaired the pancreas and lowered the hemoglobin A1C, lowered triglycerides and LDL cholesterol, and increased insulin (Fernandes). I don't know of any prescription medication they can do all of that.

Now if you were to combine this with some *chromium* which you know enhances insulin sensitivity (Anderson, Bahijiri, Althius), and *magnesium* which has an indispensable role in improving insulin secretion (Paolisso), and some of the *B vitamins* that are known to enhance insulin secretion and protect against insulin resistance, plus help maintain normal blood glucose levels (Polo, Kolb, Inubushi, Romero-Navarro, Sun), this could certainly work synergistically to improve the many damaged areas of diabetes metabolism. While don't forget the average Rx diabetes medicine actually lowers your B vitamin levels!

But wait! We could add more things to our cocktail like *lipoic acid* which decreases glycation and lipid oxidation, plus increases insulin sensitivity and secretion, as well as glucose transport across cell membranes (Henriksen, Jacob, Konrad, Evans). And we have only just begun. What about the long time herb *Gymnema silvestre*, known to stimulate the regeneration of the pancreas and to help maintain healthy sugar and insulin levels (Shanmugasundarum, Persaud, Kanetkar)? And let's not forget other bioactive compounds that are not only in the bitter melon, but the novel *Bababa leaf* (containing corosolic acid) called *lagerstroemin* (Liu, Kakuda, Judy, Fukushima). And wait. We haven't even talked about things like *green tea* which are also able to improve insulin sensitivity (Wu).

Fortunately, one company has put all of these diabetic regulators and more into a single product, called **Glucose Optimizer** (Jarrow.com). And I have by no means given you back-up for all the ingredients nor as many references as I could for each one. But you get the gist of it. Why not try 1-3 with meals (2-3 times a day)? You may be lucky and not have to do anything further.

References:

• Fernandes NPC, et al, An experimental evaluation of the antidiabetic and anti-lipidemic properties of a standardized *Momordica charantia* fruit extract, *BMC Compl Altern Med*, 7:29, 2007

• Anderson RA, et al, Elevated intakes of supplemental **chromium improve glucose and insulin** variables in individuals with type II diabetes, *Diabetes* 46:1786-91, 1997

• Bahijiri SM, et al, The effects of inorganic chromium and Brewers yeast supplementation on glucose tolerance, serum lipids and drug dosage in individuals with type II diabetes, *Saudi Med J*, 21:831-7, 2000

• Althuis MD, et al, Glucose and insulin responses to dietary chromium supplements: a meta-analysis, *Am J Clin Nutr* 76:148-55, 2002

• Paolisso G, et al, **Improved insulin response** and action **by chronic magnesium** administration in aged NIDDM subjects, *Diabetes Care* 12:265-9, 1989

• Polo S, et al, Improve insulin secretion and metabolic control in the leading type II diabetic patients with secondary failure to sulfonylureas, *Acta Diabetol* 35; 1:61-64, 1998

• Kolb H, et al, Nicotinamide in type II diabetes. Mechanism of action revisited. *Diabetes Care* 22; 2:B16-20, 1999

• Inubushi T, et al, Effects of vitamin B6 on glucose utilization and serum insulin level in mice, *Vitamins* 76; 9:403-11, 2002

• Romero-Navarro G, et al, **Biotin regulation of pancreatic** glucokinase and insulin in primary cultured rat islets and in biotin-deficient rats, *Endocrinology* 140; 10:4595-4600, 1999

• Henriksen, EJ, Oxidative stress and antioxidant treatment: effects on muscle glucose transport in animal models of type I and type II diabetes. In: Packer L, et al eds., *Antioxidants in Diabetes Management*, 1st Ed, New York, Marcel Dekker, 2000, pages 303-17

• Jacob S, et al, Oral administration of RAC-a-**lipoic acid modulates insulin sensitivity** in patients with type II diabetes mellitus: a placebo-controlled pilot trial, *Free Rad Biol Med* 27:309-14, 1999

• Konrad T, et al, **Lipoic acid treatment decreases serum lactate and pyruvate** concentrations and improves glucose effectiveness **in lean and obese patients with type II diabetes**, *Diabetes Care* 22:280-7 1999

• Evans JL, et al, **a-Lipoic acid**: a multi-functional antioxidant that **improves insulin sensitivity** in patients with type II diabetes, *Diabetes Technol Therap* 2:401-13, 2000

- Shanmugasundarum ERB, et al, Use of *Gymnema sylvestre* leaf extract in the control of blood glucose and insulin-dependent diabetes mellitus, *J Ethnopharmacol* 30:281-94, 1990

- Persaud SJ, et al, **Gymnema sylvestre stimulates insulin release** in vitro by increasing membrane permeability, *J Endocrinol* 163:207-12, 1999

- Liu F, et al, An extract of Lagerstroemia speciosa L. has insulin-like glucose uptake-stimulatory and adipocyte differentiation-inhibitory activities in 3T3-L1 cells, *J Nutr* 131; 9:2242-7, 2001

- Kakuda T, et al, Hypoglycemic effects of extracts from Lagerstroemia speciosa L. leaves in genetically diabetic KK-AY mice, *Biosci Biotechnol Biochem* 60; 2:204-8, 1996

- Judy WV, et al, Antidiabetic activity of a standardized extract (Glucosl) from Lagerstroemia speciosa leaves in type II diabetes. A dose dependence study, *J Ethnopharmacol* 87; 1:115-7, 2003

- Sun Y, et al, **Effectiveness of vitamin B12 on diabetic neuropathy**: systematic review of clinical controlled trials, *Acta Neurol Taiwan*, 14; 2:48-54, 2005

- Anonymous, Mormordica charantia (bitter melon), Monograph, *Altern Med Rev* 12; 4:360-63, 2007

- Fukushima M, et al, Effect of corosolic acid on post challenge plasma glucose levels, *Diab Res Clin Pract* 73; 2:174-77, 2006

- Kanetkar P, et al, Gymnema Silvestre: A memoir, *J Clin Biochem Nutr* 41; 2:77-81, 2007

Is it Really a Bad Hip?

Do you have pain in your hip? Do you get pain with certain motions such as getting out of the chair or taking a step forward or climbing stairs? Can you no longer cross your legs when sitting or have painful feet when you get up in the night? Or is it pain or weakness that migrates to knees, shins or feet and then back to the hip or back? This package of migrating disability and pain anywhere from low back to feet is a common beginning for the downhill course that makes folks abandon sports and eventually fall for joint replacements or other surgeries after medications fail. And the reason this is here? Because this devastating **pain limits enthusiasm for learning** anything else regarding healing of the body. So let's take a quick look at some common causes.

It may just be that you can totally heal this by yourself with some simple things. Hopefully you've already read *Pain Free In 6 Weeks* and ruled out a major hidden cause of any type of joint pain, namely hidden nightshade sensitivity. It is more than white potatoes, tomatoes, vodka, tobacco, and bell peppers, as you will learn. And don't forget that **modified food starch and modified food protein are some of the most disguised forms, since they are derived from potato starch.** They are often injected into poultry like turkeys and chickens to plump up the weight, as well as in deli meats and processed foods and substitutes for gluten–free foods. Plus the open-ended term "spices" on any label usually includes one of the deadly forms such as paprika, cayenne, pepper flakes, chili, curry, etc.

Hip pain is becoming another epidemic, as are joint replacements occurring in younger folks. For a crash course in its anatomy, you can find the top of the hip bone (greater trochanter) by going straight from your pubic bone across the groin to the outside of your hip. The bone that sticks out is the greater trochanter or the head or top of the femur (the long thigh bone). Underneath this is the ball and socket joint which can become painful or arthritic for a multitude of reasons, like unsuspected newly developed food, chemical or mold allergies (see *Depression Cured At Last!*). The causes may seem staggering, so let's break them down into more workable common categories.

The silent development of (1) nightshade allergies is the easiest to prove (see *Pain Free In 6 Weeks)*, followed by (2) leaky gut, often the underlying cause of other newly created food allergies (see *No More Heartburn*). (3) Then nutrient deficiencies triggering osteoarthritis, degenerative arthritis, rheumatoid arthritis, and other forms of arthritis (see *The Cholesterol Hoax, TW* and *ICKY*, my abbreviation for *Is Your Cardiologist Killing You?*). Just a **magnesium or vitamin D deficiency** (both of which are epidemic) **can mimic** anything from a ruptured disc to chronic hip pain. Another common cause that accelerates these deficiencies would be medications themselves such as **pain relievers** like nonsteroidal anti-inflammatory drugs (Celebrex, Naprosyn, Aleve, Motrin, ibuprofen, etc.), because they **actually deplete nutrients while they deteriorate the chemistry of cartilage renewal.** This is a big factor leading to our epidemic of joint replacements.

Then (4) the most hidden and difficult causes are the toxicities, like phthalates (see *Detoxify Or Die*) and heavy metals (see *The High Blood Pressure Hoax*). You'll learn more about these in the next chapter. Now you also appreciate why most folks will never get themselves well. They would not have the initiative to read so much to empower themselves to find the causes and the cures. So be it. But let's be sure chronic pain doesn't dampen your quest.

There is yet another hidden cause of hip pain. Over that greater trochanter there lies a bursa which can become inflamed producing *trochanteric bursitis*. However, there's (5) another condition that's even more common called *pseudo*-trochanter bursitis. Why is it called pseudo - or fake? Because it really is **referred pain from the tensor fasciae latae** (we'll just call it the TFL!). You see the TFL is a *web of fascia* (membrane gristle-like film encasing muscles, you see it when you cut chicken or streak) that runs throughout the body from low back to feet. The pain can be just in the hip or anywhere along that pathway. These hip pain victims with toxic and inflexible TFL have all sorts of symptoms like an intolerance for prolonged sitting, extremely painful soles of the feet or shins in the night, plus the pain prevents them from walking rapidly or running, or even crossing their legs while sitting. Plus when they get up from sitting there in much more pain for a while. And they usually have to use their arms to hoist themselves because their muscles are so weak as well as painful.

So where do you start? All along that entire leg there may be **tender trigger points which are actually areas of poor circulation with trapped toxins**. You can learn to **massage them out** with the references I give. But for now, a simple diagnostic and treatment maneuver will work for a number of people. Merely stand midway in the doorway and hang onto the moldings with your arms out to the side at shoulder level while you press your hip to the door frame and then try to move it forward beyond the door frame. Do this gently 2-6 times, then work the opposite hip in like manner. As you persist, you should over the weeks gain progressively more range of motion and could shortly be painless.

This not only gently stretches the muscle, but the "gristle" or fascia (TFL) that covers all muscles. Why is this important? Because these **tissues (fascia, tendons, ligaments and muscles) stockpile the nasty toxins that create pain and limit motion**. They overload our bodies every day, creating minute areas of inflammation as the body attempts to get rid of toxins or at least wall them off. If we don't mobilize them or turn them loose into the circulation so they can be gotten rid of, they torture us indefinitely, beginning with pain and resulting in scar tissue with progressively more restricted motion or loss of flexibility. Multiple modalities can release these toxins, from deep tissue massage or trigger point therapy to myo-fascial release, specific yoga, isolated stretching and strengthening, cranial-sacral or activation chiropractic, neuromuscular chiropractic, or all and more. Tantamount to success however, is all that you have learned here, especially correction of detox deficiencies and then the ultimate depuration (dumping) of toxins.

And now you can begin to appreciate the tie-in with all that you have learned here. **Old age and disease begin with damaged mitochondria**, the organelles that make energy. Their **membranes also become stiff and inflexible** as they lose the correct fatty acids/phosphatidyl choline and other nutrients. This inflexibility also translates to the cell membrane and rest of the cell. These are the micro-works for building any tissue. On the macro-works level, no wonder the body likewise becomes less flexible and more stiff all over as we age, since it's microscopic parts began the journey long before we had any symptoms. **Clearly our lifetime accumulation of deficiencies and toxicities have created the micro inflammations that lead to serious restrictions or loss of flexibility that we associate with the bent and painful body of old age.**

In the early stages of TFL pain, this maneuver (what I call the "door-jam maneuver") may actually duplicate your pain. But if you gently persist in stretching out the hip and massaging the trigger points it may become therapeutic and one more tool to help you open up the hip joints that become so contracted with age. And an easy adjunct to this would be to stand a foot or more back from the counter when you are preparing food, putting on make-up, or shaving. Lean your hips forward to stretch the TFL, resting your hips on the counter. Think of the many ways you can get those lower hips forward and stretch them in everyday postures, as opposed to being hunched over like an old geezer.

Going further and *properly* learning stretch and properly learning gentle yoga is enormously beneficial (if not held too long to exhaust and damage the stretched area). Done in moderation, it has saved many from unnecessary and health-damaging joint replacements. Just as there is a huge difference in physicians, so it is with any practitioner. And as usual, avoid folks with uni-focus. The "It's my way or the highway" demonstrates lack of awareness for the **therapeutic necessity of a multi-disciplined practitioner**. In the Sarasota, Florida area we have an **excellent yoga/trigger point/cranial sacral/myo-fascial release/ massage therapist, Linda Lee** (healthdoesmatter@comcast.net, 941-365-72270). If you find someone this dedicated and multi-talented, you have hit the jackpot. The *Total Wellness* newsletter will be going into more aspects of this very important contribution to aging. For it's this chronic pain and physical limitation that so seriously saps people of the energy needed to get themselves motivated in empowering themselves to heal.

In my experience it is better to avoid therapists (and physicians) with only one discipline, who can't explore beyond their own box. They tend to think the answer to everyone's problems lies exclusively in their particular therapy. They are clueless about the integral mechanics, toxicities and molecular biochemistry of the human frame and the effectiveness of combining resources for maximum healing. You are too smart to fall the uni-focused practitioner, since healing anything eventually involves attention to the total load, not just one aspect. Also check to see *how healthy the practitioner is.*

As usual, I never leave anyone out. Even if you have no joint complaints, one of the tell-tale signs of accelerated aging is the hunched over, pitched forward attitude of the body as the person is walking. The hips do not lead (like a model's walk) nor do they freely swing with each step. They are locked. Just look at the way a 16-year-old walks down the street versus a 60-year-old. One has free movement of ankles, knees, hips, torso, elbows, neck and shoulders. The other is pitched forward and stiff. This is usually due to tightness that insidiously develops in the groin. That's why **the door-jam stretch is vital for everyone.** And since half the population has inferior vitamin D levels, this leads also to imbalances and falls, as well as bone and muscle weakening plus osteoporosis of the hips and other joints. If you are not loose but constricted in some body areas, you are more likely to break something. Does this explain the majority of folks you know? Just watch them walk and observe how they carry themselves. Are the shoulders proudly back and the body erect with fluid hips swinging freely? Does the body move like a teen-ager's or a stiff old geezer as though led by a carrot on a stick?

Deficiencies/toxicities/inflexibility/stiffness/poor balance/injuries all become a vicious cycle propelling folks who are lazy or unmotivated to empower themselves into a life of enormous body restrictions. They are forever in pain, unable to get into positions they used to navigate, and forever adding new medications and surgeries to their lives as they steadily go down-hill. No wonder they **don't have any energy left to learn about reversing** more serious diseases like diabetes!

It may be easier to start by learning stretching. It sounds strange, I know, or folks tell me they already stretch. But I find very few who do it correctly. For example, they only stretch a few muscles and not even all the fibers of those, as you can learn from the **Mattes Method** in the resources below. **Fascia**, the thin membrane, a specialized type of connective tissue, may not look too important, but **it's part of our electrical system**. The fascia develops adhesions which restrict movement as well as electrical flow (so don't forget from *TW* your **BioSil** and **Germanium 132** for the electricity). The result is stiffness and chronic pain. Multiple methods are needed to "unglue" these fascial sheaths.

Stretching, massage, yoga, cranial-sacral, myo-fascial release, trigger point therapy and other body work are essential ways of removing toxins via the lymphatic system as well as bringing nutrients and oxygen to important tissues, but there are three catches. You must (1) have the right chemistry (like cod liver oil, PC Powder, magnesium, etc.), (2) you must remove the heavy metals and other pollutants that damage the chemistry, and then (3) **detox the mobilized toxins** (detox enema in *Wellness Against All Odds*, detox cocktail, in *Detoxify Or Die*, then *The High Blood Pressure Hoax* and subsequent *TW* for newer modalities).

Meanwhile, the primary focus of medicine in terms of joint replacements is relieving as much pain and improving as much function as possible immediately. Orthopedists in general do not look for the **nutrient deficiencies and toxins that caused the joint problems** initially. This in part contributes to the epidemic of premature failure of joints, starting with failure to correct the deterioration of the surrounding attachment tissues. Then you have the premature **degeneration of the glues that cement the metal joints in**. But most lawsuits are focused just on the premature failure of the joint replacement itself, for now.

And most physicians are oblivious to the other problems caused by the implant, namely the eventual sequelae from disturbed meridians. After all, this ushers in problems that are seemingly unrelated. For just imagine: you have a huge hunk of metal smack dab in a multitude of nerve, lymphatic and fascial pathways disturbing the electrical flow that connects them to other body organs (dental map of tooth connections to body organs is in *Pain Free In 6 Weeks*). Somehow medical folks have forgotten that the body is a magnificent intercommunicating creation. In the *Bible* it reminds us about the interconnectedness of all the parts of the body: "If one part suffers, every part suffers with it" (*I Cor* 12:26).

Meanwhile, the local paper had a big ad by local personal injury attorneys pointing out the **FDA recall of the Depuy ASR Hip Implant.** The attorneys' advertisement asks: Have folks had loosening of their implants? Bone fractures around the implant? Dislocation of the implant? **Cobalt or blood poisoning**? Tumors around the implant? Or have they had to have revision surgery in less than five years? If so consult us today, the ad suggests.

Don't let yourself even think of getting that far. To over-simplify this, yet remind you of the unimaginably great successes of many of you readers, I might just say, **"Joint replacement or detox the body? It's your choice".**

References:

• Mattes A, *Active Isolated Stretching: The Mattes Method* and *Active Isolated Strengthening: The Mattes Method,* both available from 1-941-922-3232 or 1-941-922-1939, or 2932 Lexington St., Sarasota, FL 342 31-6118 or fax one-941-927-6121 or www.stretchingUSA.com

• Travell JG, Simon D, *Myofascial Pain and Dysfunction, Vol. 1 & 2*, Baltimore: Williams and Wilkins, 1992 (absolutely fantastic, should be required reading in every medical school instead of *Gray's Anatomy*)

• Davies C, *The Trigger Point Therapy Workbook*, www.newharbinger.com, 1-800-748-6273

• Carrico M, *Yoga Journal's Yoga Basics*, 1997, Henry Holt, NY (1-800-436-9642)

• Fuhr AW, *Activator Methods Chiropractic Technique*, Mosby, 1997

• Sauer S, Biancalana M, *Trigger Point Therapy for Low Back Pain*, www.newharbinger.com, 1-800-748-6273

• Mehta M, et al, *Yoga The Iyenger Way*, 1994, Random House, NY

• Oschman JL, *Energy Medicine, The Scientific Basis*, Phil./Lond, Churchill Livingstone, 2000

• Rasch PJ, *Kinesiology and Applied Anatomy*, 7th Ed., Philadelphia: Lea and Febiger 1989

• Floyd RT, et al, *Manual of Structural Kinesiology*, St. Louis: Mosby 1994

• Majjoni, et al, Effects of skeletal muscle fiber determination on lymphatic volumes, *Am J Physiology* 259 (6Pt 2): 1860-8, 1990

- Plotnikoff GA, et al, Prevalence of **severe hypovitaminosis D in patients with persistent, nonspecific musculoskeletal pain,** *Mayo Clinic Procs* 78; 12:1463-70, 2003

- Barnes, *Myo-Fascial Release* (*TW*, and more to come in *TWs*)

How to Stall Aging, Especially of Your Heart

Are you worried about dying from heart disease? For diabetics the danger is magnified. But more important than how old you are or how much diabetes you have or don't have is another factor. What matters is how long your **telomeres** are. These are little **protective caps on the end of your chromosomes or genes. They play a huge role in determining how long you live**. And the neat thing is that even if they are damaged and aging you rapidly, you can slow this down enormously and even repair them. How much fun is that?

In the *Journal of the American Medical Association,* they studied only men with proven coronary artery disease, all of whom had already had a heart attack or bypass surgery (and of course all were on statins already which had no effect on protecting the telomeres). Their fatty acids of EPA and DHA (as found in cod liver oil and fish) were measured. As you recall, good labs like MetaMetrix® will then give the range in quartiles or even better, quintiles. This tells you where you stand in comparison to everyone else. For men who had "normal levels" of DHA and EPA but were in the lowest quartile, after 5 years their telomeres had shortened. That's bad. For folks with **shortened telomeres (remember it means the ends of the gene are rotting off) have likewise a shortened ("rotting") life**. They die earlier.

Once more this confirms that **being in the low end of "normal" is not "normal".** In fact it can be deadly. Furthermore, this explains why many studies over the years have shown that **folks on higher doses of cod liver oil live much longer**, regardless of their cardiac status. On the flip side of this study, men in the **highest quartile of the omega-3 fatty acids had a walloping 32% reduction in**

telomeres shortening. *Their genes were programmed to keep them alive much longer.* Cod liver oil stopped rotting genes!

It confirms facts that have been known for decades. (1) For many nutrients you want to be in the top quartile or quintile, in other words the top of normal. This is further proof. **Just being in the normal range can be extremely dangerous**. Don't forget the government makes labs define normal as anybody who is alive and can give a blood specimen. This includes the dumbest people, on the most medications, and eating the worst diets. I've shown in previous *TW* articles how folks in the normal range of vitamin D3, for example, have four times the heart attack rate as those who are in the top range of normal.

(2) Also as I've shown you the evidence for in the past, this again confirms that **food and nutrients talk to and control our genes**. Docs who are just looking at your genetics and not the 13-page report of your molecular biochemistry that controls your genetics (**Cardio/ION**) are downright missing the chance to cure.

The part that bothers me is that the American Heart Association merely recommends people just eat more fish. But as you know much fish now is contaminated with mercury, depending upon where the harvesting takes place. And as I've referenced in the past, many fish nowadays are farmed which can give the wrong fatty acid chemistry. In some cases you might as well have a steak, because some farmed fish have been fed (and have) similar fatty acid chemistry to a cow. Real fish eat sea vegetables, plankton, seaweeds and other fish (n-3), whereas some farmed fish eat pellets resembling dog food which often are manufactured from genetically modified soybean and also contain trans fats (n-6).

A bothersome part for me is why did the patients in this study only have 32% reduction in telomere shortening? Why not 100%? That's easy. That's because the researchers have not looked at the total load or the total package. Again they try to use nutrients like a drug, solo. They ignore the harmony of the body's chemistry. As an example, another **important aspect for preserving the telomeres is an enzyme called <u>DNA polymerase</u>. But this enzyme must have <u>zinc</u> in order to keep our genes in the longevity phase.** And of course what lowers zinc but Lipitor for cholesterol, beta blockers for blood pressure and angina like Toprol, Lopressor, metoprolol, etc. and phthalates to extend release, etc. Another reason why medication shortens life.

But let's be sure you know that **there are also a multitude of other nutrients that also are required in harmony to keep telomeres in the longevity range.** These include vitamins D, C, E, phosphatidyl choline, folate and much more. The evidence is overwhelming and the solution is incredibly easy. If your diabetologist or physician is not measuring and tailoring these nutrients to you as an individual, what good is a dinosaur? If you can't afford the tests, use the nutrient suggestions here in this book.

So in the meantime, I hope this at least convinces you that you definitely do not want one of the prescription synthetic fatty acids drugs (like Lovaza®). You at least want a tablespoon every other day of the best quality **Cod Liver Oil** that I know of. As I've shown in the past, cod liver oil has many other benefits which include (but are not limited to) improving your chance of surviving a heart attack, slowing down getting other age-related diseases, reducing blood vessel stiffness and blood pressure, slowing down the aging of the brain and even macular degeneration (the number one cause of blindness over the age of 50). You really cannot afford to be without this. And if your gut isn't yet healthy you may consider some pancreatic enzymes with bile, like 1-3 **Digestive Aid #34** to temporarily improve the absorption.

So do you have a double "i" physician? If he is not up on this rudimentary information, he is" **i**nexcusably **i**gnorant" about the very fundamental facts of his only specialty. No drug has the power over your heart and body longevity that foods and nutrients do.

References:

- Farzaneh-Far R, et al, Association of marine **Omega-3 fatty acid levels with telomeric aging** in patients with coronary heart disease, *J Am Med Assoc,* 303; 3:250-57, 2010

- Epel ES, et al, The rate of leukocyte **telomere shortening predicts mortality** from cardiovascular disease in elderly men, *Aging* 1;1:81-88, 2008

- Lee JH, et al, **Omega-3 fatty acids for cardioprotection,** *Mayo Clinic Proc,* 83; 3:324-32, 2008

- Marchioli R, et al, Early **protection against sudden death by n-3** polyunsaturated fatty acids after myocardial infarction: time-course analysis of the results of the Gruppo Italiano per lo Studio della Sopravvivenza nell'Infarcto Miocardico (GISSI)-Prevenzione, *Circulation* (the American Heart Association's official publication), 105; 16:1897-1903, 2002

- Paul L, et al, Telomere length in peripheral blood mononuclear cells is associated with folate status in man, *J Nutr* 139; 7:1273-78, 2009

- Richards JB, et al, **Higher** serum **vitamin D** concentrations are associated with **longer** leukocyte **telomere** length in women, *Am J Clin Nutr,* 86; 5: 1420-25, 2007

Prepare for Cardiac Emergencies Now

Before we close this chapter on nutrition, let's make sure you are prepared for one of the worst nightmares of your life, a heart attack. Let's look at a recent reader consultation I had with a 54-year-old surgeon who thought he was in great health. When he had mild chest pain he presented to the emergency room where he immediately arrested. He had no heart beat, no breathing and was literally dead. Of course, they immediately cardioverted him with the paddles of 200 Joules. When that failed to give any response whatsoever on the EKG, they electrocuted him again, this time with 300 joules. They even did a third cardioversion attempt, 600 joules, which is unusual in a "dead" man. When I was an emergency room doc we rarely shocked folks more than 4 times. However in view of his young age they were even more desperate to save him.

What I found particularly staggering was that **it wasn't until the fifth cardioversion that they also gave <u>IV heparin and magnesium which immediately revived the dead man</u>.** My point is that as you will see, the evidence is overwhelming that these should have been given in the very beginning. Even more importantly **they should be given** in the ambulance and even

210

better, **at home**. For the studies clearly show that **the earlier a clot buster is given, the smaller the infarct (area of damage in the heart) and the greater the chance of survival**. Yet unfortunately this man is not alone. And even during his hospitalization, never was there a measure of or a thought to giving more magnesium or heparin. When I reviewed his blood work later, he was still dangerously low in magnesium (which could have been the main trigger for his sudden heart attack to begin with).

I've consulted with many others whereupon review of their hospital records (from some of the most prestigious cardiac ERs and clinics), the practice of emergency medicine highlighted similar staggering ignorance. Sadly these 2 inexpensive agents (magnesium and heparin) still are not in the emergency recommendations written by American College of Cardiologists and the American College of Emergency Physicians.

Because heart attack or myocardial infarction is the number one cause of death in diabetics (and all adults for that matter), I cannot leave this chapter without warning you about the treatment in the ambulance, emergency room and coronary care unit of the hospital. "What?! These are state-of-the-art!", you say. We all tend to think of these as the bastions of the highest treatment. But tell me what you think after you have seen this evidence. After over 40 years in medicine and having seen so many needless deaths that may have been preventable, I want to make sure you folks have the right things on hand to save your lives and the lives of those you love the most. Even folks who look extremely healthy and have never been sick are now suddenly dying of heart attacks in their 40s and early 50s. And often **they die merely because they were without adequate pre-the hospital protection**. Plus **diabetics are doubly vulnerable** for heart attacks by the very nature of their multiple deficiencies and toxicities creating the disease. So let's review some of the things that are very necessary for you to have on hand and the evidence for them.

I feel it's very important for you to know about this. There are, however, many more details and references in *TW* 2011 and *The Cholesterol Hoax* and I suggest you get that year and make sure you have all of those emergency medicines on hand. Like most of my instructions, it contains the references to convince any physician as well. Since that is not the focus of this book, I can't go into all of them, but let's look at three items most important for saving your life, magnesium and heparin and D-Ribose.

Why do you need to become an expert in this *TW* issue? Because in the official medical journal of the American Heart Association, *Circulation,* the "experts" gave the guidelines for all cardiologists on how to treat certain types of heart attacks. In doing so they blatantly stated on several pages that vitamins played no role.

Even more scary is that in this entire cardiac manifest there was not one mention of magnesium. Many people have died from atrial fibrillation or other arrhythmias, angina, a heart attack or sudden cardiac arrest, cardiomyopathies, or congestive heart failure, just because of lack of magnesium. And in this American Heart Association's guidelines issue even though they found that, for example, **giving heparin early can improve survival over 50%**, it's not included in their standard recommendations. And as you will see in the reference, these official recommendations also involved the American College of Emergency Physicians, as well as several other medical specialty organizations.

And that's exactly why I'm driven to bring all of this extremely important information to you. First, you need to have protective medications at home, for studies clearly show **the sooner you treat a heart attack, the better the chance of survival**. Second, when you end up in the emergency room *do not* expect the cardiologist and emergency room physicians to know about what you are about to learn. I have seen the records from prestigious medical centers and clinics where folks got into serious trouble or died because this information was not used. This is **a vital alert for all folks who don't want to be a statistic of the emergency**

rooms. Just like heparin, magnesium should be injected at the very first sign of a heart attack, not at the end after the horse has been let out of the barn. The longer you wait before giving any of these things when someone is beginning a heart attack, the more destruction of heart tissue there is (duTroit, Bolli). Let's look at a smattering of the evidence for each one.

References:

• Anderson JL, et al, ACC/AHA 2007 **guidelines for** the management of patients with unstable angina/non-ST elevation **myocardial infarction**: executive summary: a report of the American College of Cardiology/American Heart Association Task Force on Practice Guidelines (writing committee to revise the 2002 guidelines for the management of patients with unstable angina/non-ST elevation myocardial infarction). Developed in collaboration with the American College of Emergency Physicians, the Society for Cardiovascular Angiography and Interventions and the Society of Thoracic Surgeons: endorsed by the American Association of Cardiovascular and Pulmonary Rehabilitation and the Society for Academic Emergency Medicine, *Circulation* 116:803-77, 2007

• Woods KL, Long-term outcome after intravenous magnesium sulfate in suspected acute myocardial infarction: the second Leicester Intravenous Magnesium Interventions Trial (LIMIT-2), *Lancet* 343:816-19, 1994

• Oler A, et al, **Adding heparin** to aspirin **reduces** the incidence of myocardial infarction and **death** in patients with unstable angina, a meta-analysis, *J Am Med Assoc* 276:811-15, **1996**

• Boersma E, et al, **Early thrombolytic treatment in acute myocardial infarction** and reappraisal of **the golden hour**, *Lancet* 348:771-75, **1996**

• duTroit EF, et al, Modulation of severity of reperfusion stunning in the isolated rat heart by agents altering calcium flux at onset of reperfusion, *Circul Res* 70:960-67, 1997

• Bolli R, et al, Marked reduction of free radical generation and contractile dysfunction by antioxidant therapy begun at the time of reperfusion. Evidence that **myocardial "stunning" as a manifestation of reperfusion injury**, *Circul Res* 65:607-22, 1989.

• Teo KK, et al, Effects of intravenous magnesium in suspected acute myocardial infarction: overview of randomized trials, *Brit Med J*, 303:1499-1503, 1991

Stock Your Home Emergency Heart Attack Box With Heparin

Right from the *Journal of the American College of Cardiology* they showed that a paltry 4000 units of **heparin given right away can as much as triple survival from a heart attack**. But it's clear that the earlier a clot buster is given, the better the results. Instead there are many studies which waste millions of dollars of research money using the new patented heparin substitutes, which are often not even 2% better than the inexpensive time-honored heparin

(Gibson). And worse was the unscientific nature of this 2007 paper since the heparin-substitute drug was given for a longer period of time than the natural heparin was given to comparative folks. In 1988 in the *New England Journal of Medicine* they showed **heparin was five times better than aspirin (the ambulance and ER standard) for a sudden heart attack** (Theroux).

There were many other flawed, unscientific studies to make inexpensive heparin appear inferior to the new and highly expensive synthetic heparin substitutes. In fact I couldn't believe how they stacked the deck against heparin. Giving the heparin too late, and having the heparin group have seven times more hypertensives, three times more diabetics, more smokers, four times more prior heart attack victims, and five times more angina patients are some of the examples! Yet still when you compared the heparin patients with those receiving the "new" heparins, the death rate and heart attack rates were pretty much the same!

These new patented heparin substitutes are highly expensive, sometimes $3000 a dose, while heparin is cheap. And the sad fact is some of the newer heparin substitutes take a week before they will work at top capacity. And then they can take a week before they will wear off, which is important if you have surgical or dental emergencies. On the flip side, **you can quickly reverse heparin with an injection of vitamin K**. It's much more natural, infinitely cheaper, well researched, and much more controllable and predictable.

An injection of a tiny little vial of **heparin has decreased the death rate 33-58%**, in other words cutting the death rate in nearly half. And I intentionally repeat: multiple studies also show that **the earlier it is given the better are the results.** As with anything, once the horse is out of the barn and the damage begins, time is of the essence. And **just one hour can make a big difference in determining (1) who survives. And if they do survive, it determines (2) how big an area of the heart dies as a result of the heart attack.**

Plus heparin can be much better than a stent. Nowadays, a heart attack usually means you are rushed in for a stent. Yet Boden's report also showed that **an immediate stent is not better than dissolving the clot as soon as possible.** In fact, without prior fibrinolysis (dissolving of clot, as with heparin) the death rate is the same whether you go to a community hospital or a fancy "hub" medical center for a stent. And if folks were **transferred** (to a bigger hospital) **without giving a strong clot dissolver first, the death rate was tripled.** Oddly enough once they got to the second hospital to have their procedures, then they were given things like heparin. But this was *given far too late*, given after too much damage had been done.

Meanwhile, **stents are a mere hunk of chicken wire mesh which becomes a veritable clot magnet, guaranteeing reclotting.** And the "new" **drug-coated stents can have a 30% higher death rate**, as they should, since a form of chemotherapy is incorporated into them in attempt to quell the re-clotting. Plus they elute other chemicals like their methylacrylate (like "Crazy-Glue" and dental glues) and fluorinated (like Teflon) copolymer coatings. As evidenced prior, even drug treatments surpassed stents in long-term survival, whereas nutritional treatments actually repair the underlying process (*TW*).

Meanwhile, in some heparin studies the researchers were so unknowledgeable it was almost laughable. For example, some of them cautioned heparin should not be given because once it was stopped, the angina can return (Theroux). Ya think, DiNozzo? How ignorant can they get? And they had done nothing to repair the underlying cause of the angina as described for you in *Is Your Cardiologist Killing You?* Even folks who realize there is a persistence of coagulation abnormality in heart attack victims until it is repaired were obtuse when it came to defining the cause and cure of the heart attack (Merlini).

So what dose should be used? That must take into consideration your medical, dental, environmental, surgical history and

Cardio/ION findings. Studies from seven medical centers showed that heparin is the best, but **nothing overcomes too low a dose.** Unfortunately **doctors who have not read all the papers get scared off and use 5000 units or less when 7,500-10,000 gives better results followed by about 1000 every hour,** adjusting on average 200 units depending on the clotting time. If it's a modern facility and medical folks can check your aPTT (activated partial thromboplastin time) at the bedside, this saves about six hours and improves your chances of survival even more so (Becker).

I hope that when your physician does review these papers that he takes into consideration that these authors are clueless about the effects of proper levels of DHA, the *eight* forms of vitamin E, the amount of vitamins K2, D3 and others that people have on board. Also when you find an interested cardiologist, **make sure you have a copy of your most recent EKG to keep in your wallet** in case you do end up in an emergency room, since that also accelerates your treatment and improves your chances of survival.

So review *The Cholesterol Hoax* and *TW* for the rest of the emergency program and to **make sure you have a tiny vial of 5000-10,000 of heparin from your doctor (add a 1cc needle/syringe) to give to yourself immediately**. Obviously many parameters will affect the dose. For example, our readers would probably be on vitamin K so they would be more likely to need 10,000 units, whereas the average person with no nutrients on board would probably do better with 5,000. Meanwhile, a knowledgeable and dedicated cardiologist, internist or family physician can help you decide what dose would be better for you considering the rest of your total load and history (Curtis).

References:

• Boden WE, et al, Reperfusion strategies in acute ST-segment elevation myocardial infarction, a comprehensive review of contemporary management options, *J Am Coll Cardiol*, 50; 10:917-29, 2007

• Curtis JP, et al, **Efficacy and safety of two unfractionated heparin** dosing strategies with tenecteplase in acute myocardial infarction, *Am J Cardiol* 94:279-83, 2004

- Wallentin L, et al, Efficacy and safety of tenecteplase in combination with low molecular weight heparin enoxaparin or **unfractionated heparin in the pre-hospital setting**, *Circul* 108:135-42, 2003

- Weaver WG, et al, **Prehospital** initiated versus hospital initiated **thrombolytic therapy**. The Myocardial Infarction Triage and Intervention Trial, *J Am Med Assoc* 270:1211-6, **1993**

- European Myocardial Infarction Project Group. **Prehospital thrombolytic therapy** in patients with suspected acute myocardial infarction, *New Engl J Med* 329:383-9, **1993**

- Morrison LJ, et al, Mortality and **prehospital thrombosis** prophylaxis for acute myocardial infarction: a meta-analysis, *J Am Med Assoc* 283:2686-92, **2000**

- Danchin N, et al, Impact of **prehospital thrombolysis** acute myocardial infarction on 1-year outcome, *Circulation* 110:1909-15, 2004

- Curtis JP, et al, The prehospital electrocardiogram and time to perfusion in patients with acute myocardial infarction, 2000-2002: findings from the National Registry of Myocardial Infarction-4, *J Am Coll Cardiol*, 47:1544-52, 2006

- Stenestrand Ulf, et al, Long-term outcome of primary percutaneous coronary intervention versus prehospital and in hospital thrombolysis for patients with ST elevation myocardial infarction, *J Am Med Assoc* 296; 14:1749-56, 2006

- Gibson CM, et al, Percutaneous coronary intervention in patients receiving enoxaparin or unfractionated heparin after fibrinolytic therapy for ST- segment elevation myocardial infarction in the ExTRACT TIMI-25 Trial, *J Am Coll Cardiol*, 49:2238-46, 2007

- Becker RC, et al, A randomized, multicenter trial of weight-adjusted intravenous heparin doses, titration and point-of-care coagulation monitoring in hospitalized patients with active thromboembolic disease, *Am Heart J* 137:59-71, 1991

- Hassan WM, et al, Improved anticoagulation with a weight-adjusted heparin normogram in patients with acute coronary syndromes: a randomized trial, *J Thrombo Thrombolysis* 2; 3:245-9, 1995

- Theroux P, et al, **Aspirin, heparin, or both to treat acute unstable angina**, *New Engl J Med* 319:1105-1111, **1988**

- Theroux P, et al, Reactivation of unstable angina after the discontinuation of heparin, *New Engl J Med* 237:141-5, 1992

- Merlini PA, et al, Persistent activation of regulation mechanism in unstable angina and myocardial infarction, *Circulation* 90:61-68, 1994

Magnesium a Must for Emergencies

At the start of a heart attack, what is the most important thing? Time. Many studies prove that the time wasted at home, in the ambulance, and in the emergency room has a huge bearing on who dies. It also determines how big the infarct area is (the amount of heart muscle that is killed). And even though research papers for decades have borne all of this out, it's ignored because **research**

money stresses drugs that make billions of dollars a year. So let's look at just a smattering more of the evidence.

First, let's go back in time to show how long this information has been known and ignored. In one study **in the very prestigious** *Lancet* **nearly 20 years ago, researchers showed that you can cut the heart attack death rate by 21% by giving magnesium**. And they had lots of flaws in their treatment at that point in time. They did not give magnesium early enough, they did not give a high enough dose, and they didn't measure it to determine how much was needed. When they did an assay, they didn't use the proper test. And they did not look at any of the other nutrients that are needed in concert for magnesium to work its best. **Magnesium should not be treated like a solo act like a drug** (Woods). Still in spite of a huge amount of flaws, it proved that **it is imperative that magnesium be included in emergency heart attack treatments**. So you can just imagine how much more potent a life-saver it is in capable hands.

Giving magnesium is crucial for stopping not only coronary **spasm** (anginal chest pain), but is pivotal in stopping arrhythmias (irregular heartbeat) which are a major cause of death after a heart attack. **Just giving magnesium for the spasm and arrhythmias improved survival** in some studies **as much as 50%.** And of course magnesium does a lot more. It **decreases the amount of clot** as well (Hwang, Adams, Gertz, Smith, Teo). In other older studies magnesium cut the death rate 30%, and in others as much as 66%, especially since **it aborted the arrhythmias which are often the cause of death if someone survives the heart attack** (Smith, Abraham, Ceremuzynski). **For over 25 years it has been known that immediate magnesium is crucial for heart attack survival** (Canon). To fail to give it? BS (bad science)!

And you will notice how old these references are, re-affirming the lack of financial incentive these days for research on magnesium. That's why more doctors don't know about it and **the most up-to-date "prestigious" authoritative treatment guidelines don't**

even mention magnesium. This is very serious business. That's why I've loaded you with so many references so that you are armed to the teeth with evidence. And those treating you will be put on notice that you know *you deserve and expect the best* life-saving treatment, regardless of their lack of knowledge.

Magnesium deficiency is the norm, not the exception. Government studies show we get less than a third of what we need in a day. **A major side effect of magnesium deficiency is sudden cardiac arrest**, often even happening within a few days of having had a "perfect report" on a "complete physical". The important thing is that **magnesium should be given right away, before you get to the hospital,** for a number of reasons. First of all it cuts the death rate by more than 1/5th because of its strong anti-clotting properties, as well as anti-spasm protection for the coronary arteries. Many other studies showed **giving magnesium cuts the death rate 30-55% as well as eliminates the chance of serious arrhythmias as well as vastly reducing the size of the infarct** (the size of the dead area in the heart as a result of the heart attack.)

So stock your home emergency heart attack box with magnesium now to include prescription **Magnesium Chloride Solution** 200 mg/cc when you need the most concentrated oral form (windhampharmacy.com) and the prescription of two 2 gm vials of magnesium sulfate for injection (which is preferred. It stings so read the directions in *TW* 2011 and *The Cholesterol Hoax*).

Meanwhile, with this brief amount of evidence on the sad state of affairs of "modern medicine", is it any wonder that at my 40th medical school graduation reunion a couple of years ago, that over 15% of my class was already dead. And these are the "specialists" in health only in their mid-60's!

References:

• Ceremuzynski L, et al, **Threatening arrhythmias in acute myocardial infarction are prevented by intravenous magnesium sulfate**, *Am Heart J* 118:1333-4, **1989**

- Smith LF, et al, Intravenous infusion of magnesium sulfate after acute myocardial infarction: effects on arrhythmias and mortality, *Internat J Cardiol,* 112:175-80, **1986**

- Abraham AS, et al, **Magnesium in the prevention of lethal arrhythmias in acute myocardial infarction**, *Arch Med* 147:753-5, **1987**

- Canon LA, et al, Magnesium levels in cardiac arrest victims: **relationship between magnesium levels and successful resuscitation**, *Ann Emergency Med* 16, 1195-98, **1987**

- Hwang DL, et al, Effect of extracellular **magnesium on platelet activation** and intracellular calcium mobilization, *Am J Hypert* 5:700-06, 1992

- Adams JH, et al, The effect of agents for **modifying platelet behavior and of magnesium ions on thrombus** formation in vivo, *Thromb Haemost* 42:603-10, 1979

- Gertz SD, et al, Effect of **magnesium sulfate on thrombus formation** following partial arterial constriction: implications for coronary vasospasm, *Magnesium* 6:2 to 5-35, 1987

- Lau J, et al, Cumulative meta-analysis of therapeutic trials for myocardial infarction, *New Engl J Med* 327:248-54, 1992

- Horner SM, Efficacy of **intravenous magnesium in acute myocardial infarction in reducing arrhythmias and mortality**, *Circul* 86:774-79, **1992**

- Hearse DJ, et al, Myocardial protection during ischemic cardiac arrest, *J Thoracic Cardiovasc Surg* 75:877-85, 1978,

- Editorial: **Magnesium for acute myocardial infarction?** *Lancet* 338:667-68, **1991**

- Woods KL, Long-term outcome after intravenous magnesium sulfate in suspected acute myocardial infarction: the second Leicester Intravenous Magnesium Interventions Trial (LIMIT-2), *Lancet* 343:816-19, 1994

- Teo KK, et al, Effects of intravenous magnesium in suspected acute myocardial infarction: overview of randomized trials, *Brit Med J* 303:1499-1503, 1991

- Rasmussen HS, et al, **Intravenous magnesium in acute myocardial infarction,** *Lancet* 1:234-6, **1986**

D-Ribose for Your Emergency Drug Box

In preceding chapters I gave you important information about D-ribose. And now I want to make sure that you have it in your emergency drug box to improve your chances of surviving a heart attack. Evidence now is clear that we should add to this list **D-Ribose Powder**. It restores the energy to the heart, and nothing else can take the place of its functions. It also **makes the size of the infarct (area in the heart that is killed by the heart attack) much smaller**. And it **speeds the recovery time of the heart**. Fortunately, now it comes in a jar of loose powder and also in individual packets which are very handy for stuffing into your purse, pocket, glove compartment of the car, or gym bag. If you have the slightest evidence of chest pain or sudden shortness of breath I would definitely devour the contents of 2-4 of these packets immediately in a large glass of water.

And don't think ribose is needed just for the heart attack, or just for repair of the heart after stenting. You also need it *to get the radioactive thallium out after heart scans.* For ribose can not only get the thallium out after heart x-rays, but *it can revive "dead" heart* areas. Once you've had a thallium heart scan with injection of a radioactive metal that goes into every cell of your heart, what do you think happens to that toxic radioactive material after the scan? Some areas of the heart (if they are damaged enough) do not have the ability to get rid of the thallium. Fortunately, a scoop or two of **D-Ribose Powder** can facilitate this.

Not only that, but some areas of the heart that the unknowledgeable cardiologist would diagnose as "dead" on the scan after a heart attack are merely "hibernating" and can be revived with this same nutrient. But that only happens if he is smart enough to know this. If you are told heart areas are dead but he hasn't tried to "revive" them with ribose, I'd move on to one who offers this solution that has been known for over 20 years. There is no excuse for ignorance in one's own field of "expertise" when folks' lives depend on you. Again, BS (bad science)!

D-ribose is also absolutely crucial after a heart attack, any heart surgery, in anyone with congestive heart failure or angina or diastolic hypertension or in whom it takes several days to recover after exertion, as in chronic fatigue or fibromyalgia. Also it **is crucial for any of you who have diabetes or <u>mitochondrial poisoning</u>** diagnosed on the Cardio/ION. Clearly your cardiologist is a dangerous dude and dinosaur if he has not recommended **D-Ribose Powder** for any of these conditions or even diagnosed/assayed your nutrient needs.

References:

- Sami H, et al, The effect of **ribose** administration on contractile recovery following brief periods of **ischemia,** *Anesthesiol,* 67; 3A: A74, 1987

- Pliml W, et al, Effects of **ribose on exercise-induced ischemia** in stable coronary artery disease, *Lancet,* 340:507-10, 1992

- Wallen JW, et al., Pre-ischemic administration of **ribose to delay the onset of irreversible ischemic** injury and improve function: studies in normal and hypertrophied hearts, *Canad J Physiol Pharmacol,* 81:40-47, 2003

- Pauly D, et al, **D-Ribose as a supplement for cardiac energy** metabolism, *J Cardiovasc Pharmacol Therap* 5; 4:249-58, 2000

- Gradus-Pizio I, et al, Effect of **D-ribose on the detection of the hibernating myocardium** during the low dose dobutamine stress echocardiography, *Circul* 100; 18:3394, **1999**

- Wilson R, et al, **D-Ribose enhances the identification of hibernating myocardium,** *Heart Drug,* 3; 61-62, 2003

- Hegewald MG, et al, **Ribose infusion accelerates a thallium redistribution** with early imaging compared with late 24-hour imaging without ribose, *J Am Coll Cardiol* 18:1671-81, **1991**

- Angelo D, et al, **Recovery of myocardial infarction and thallium 201 redistribution using ribose,** *Am J Cardiol Imag* 3; 4:256-65, 1989

- Perlmutter NS, et al. **Ribose facilitates thallium-201 redistribution in patients with coronary artery disease,** *J Nucl Med* 32:193, 1991

- Omran H, et al, **D-Ribose improves diastolic function and quality of life in congestive heart failure patients**: a prospective feasibility study, *Eur J Heart Fail* 5:615-19, 2003

- Teitlebaum JE, et al, The use **of D-ribose in chronic fatigue syndrome and fibromyalgia**: a pilot study, *J Altern Complement Med,* 12; 9:857-62, 2006

- Ingwall JS, et al, Is the failing heart energy starved? On using chemical energy to support cardiac function, *Circul Res* 95:135-45, 2004

- Illie S, et al, **D-Ribose improves myocardial function in congestive heart failure** , *FASEB J,* 15; 5:A 1142, 2001

- Omran H, et al, **D-Ribose improves myocardial function and quality of life** in congestive heart failure patients, *J Mol Cell Cardiol,* 33;6: A173, 2001

- Gebhart B, et al, Benefit of ribose in a patient with fibromyalgia, *Pharm* 24; 11:1646-48, 2004

How to Cut Your Risk of Death 80%

What if there were a way to cut your risk of sudden death 81%? And what if this was an inexpensive non-prescription natural product? And what if this had been proven and published by Harvard physicians in a government-sponsored study in the *New England Journal of Medicine*? Wouldn't it just be common sense that *all* physicians would know about this and be counseling their

222

patients in it? And wouldn't it also be logical that insurance companies would cover it? And yet failure to use this information, over a decade old, is another example of what I consider the flagrant misguided practice of medicine. And the only reason it isn't malpractice? It's because the definition of malpractice is failure to do what the rest of the "herd" of physicians is doing. It has nothing to do with doing the best for the patient (I've given you the tort evidences for this in *TW*).

Meanwhile the nutrient? Simple cod liver oil. And you want to be sure that you have the best quality, which would be **Carlson's Lemon-Flavored Cod Liver Oil**. I like to avoid capsules because, as you recall, most people are concomitantly so deficient in other nutrients that any time we can substitute liquids, powders or sublinguals (absorbed under the tongue), it helps spare the body the work of one more capsule. In 2012 *TW* I gave you the evidence how **the levels of cod liver oil have dramatically changed in the very chemistry of the average human body by as much as 60 fold in the last century**. This in part is a major contributor to our epidemics of chronic diseases.

Another thing this study showed was that the average level of cut-off for "normal" levels of fatty acids are totally wrong. How do we know this? Because **people in the lower "normal" quintile had a markedly increased amount of sudden death**. And don't think that this paper is alone. The **prestigious *Lancet* just three years earlier showed an over 45% decrease in risk of sudden death with omega-3 oils.** And most of these studies grossly under-dosed with a teaspoon a day, and failed to measure the levels as well as measure the effect of the ubiquitous phthalates which poison the proper metabolism of all fatty acids. And of course they never give people in the trials phosphatidyl choline, ALC, or the eight forms of E, without which cod liver oil's effectiveness is markedly reduced (refer back here to your recipe for fixing this). It literally boggles the mind at how ignorant the medical field is when it comes to ignoring cost-effective cures. This is clearly at the expense of focusing on money-generating drugs and devices which merely perpetuate the patient's disease, as well as bring on new diseases which "require" new medications.

And I love how these researchers are always so arrogant that they think they are the first people to make their discoveries. Yet in the **prestigious *Lancet* over 30 years ago they showed omega-3 oils (as in cod liver oil, fish, etc.) reduce platelet adhesiveness and arteriosclerosis. And they've known for over 30 years that half the people who have a heart attack don't even have high cholesterol.** Furthermore, as you also learned in *The Cholesterol Hoax,* half the people who do have a sudden heart attack don't even live to find out what caused it. And as I've shown here (and in much more detail in previous *TW* issues), the right level of cod liver oil for the individual negates the need for many medications. For example, for over a decade and a half researcher physicians have known that **with the right levels of fatty acids you don't need calcium channel blockers**. You'll recall from *The High Blood Pressure Hoax* that **calcium channel blockers like Norvasc, Coreg, Cardizem, Dilacor, Caduet, Adalat, Procardia, Lotrel, Calan, Verelan, etc. have been shown to shrink the brain away from the skull within five years and rot the IQ.** But they are not needed if you repair the channels!

And of course none of these wonderful papers proving the benefits of cod liver oil (cloaked in such terms as omega-3, n-3 polyunsaturated oils, eicosapentaenoic acid, docosahexaneoic acid, etc.) talk about how you can give cod liver oil until the cows come home, but it won't work without the rest of the supporting nutrients that I have shown you. None of these researchers advise even measuring whether folks have sufficient balance of not only the essential oils, but all the other nutrients that must be included to make them work, as found exclusively in the **Cardio/ION**.

For example, if you don't have enough zinc (which is lowered by statins like Lipitor, Crestor, Zocor, etc.) you cannot metabolize the fatty acids (through the zinc-requiring enzyme delta-6-desaturase).

Or if you have too many phthalates on board (the #1 pollutant in the human body and at the highest levels), these poison beta-oxidation of the fatty acids so that you can't use the fatty acids. Plus statins also poison carnitine so you can't move the oil into the cell to work. Or if you have insufficient pancreatic enzymes to absorb the oils (i.e., suggested by an elevated Cardio/ION indican from a gut full of yeast from antibiotics or an elevated stool elastase), etc., the oil will do no good. **Knowledge-challenged researchers keep trying to use nutrients as though they were a solo act like a drug, one at a time and without even measuring** to see how much is needed for the individual patient or if there are concomitant deficiencies creating imbalances. They continually ignore the total package of the beautiful orchestration of God's molecular biochemistry of the human body.

I could write a whole book just on cod liver oil. You can appreciate how powerful it is with just the smattering of references I have given you here. For by correcting the ratio of oils in the nuclear (protects the genes) and mitochondrial membranes, you can do what no drugs can do, especially all at once. As just a teeny look at some of its incomparable advantages, cod liver oil reduces sudden death, lowers cholesterol, reduces clots, repairs calcium, sodium and magnesium channels as well as cell surface receptors, melts plaque, prevents or stops arrhythmias, reduces overall death rate, and ….oh yes, **reverses insulin resistance and is crucial for reversing diabetes**. *So now what do you now think of any dinosaur physician who does not at first want to know the status of your fatty acids? For without this, all healing is at a standstill. Anything else is BS (bad science)!*

My message here? First, this makes me seriously question the worth of any physician who is not focused on assaying your precious fatty acids. To quote from Albert's paper, "As compared with men with levels of long-chain **n-3 fatty acids** in the lowest quartile, those with levels in the highest quartile had an **81% lower risk of sudden death**." How much more proof do they need? For a decade it's been known that a tablespoon of cod liver oil cuts your death risk 81%! Do dinosaurs read any journals? Why aren't they up on this? And second, don't just think that cod liver oil is the answer to everything. Even though you must have the right ratios, you still need all the rest of the knowledge that we have been feeding you over the last three decades. Clearly this tiny sample of evidence gives you **one more important tool with which to differentiate a dinosaur doc from a dynamo doc.**

References:

- Albert CM, et al, Blood levels of long-**chain n-3 fatty acids and the risk of sudden death,** *New Engl J Med* 346:1113-8, **2002**

- Gissi-Prevenzione Investigators, Dietary supplementation with n-3 polyunsaturated fatty acids and vitamin E after myocardial infarction, *Lancet* 354:447-55, 1999

- Thorngren M, et al, Effects of 11-week increase in dietary **eicosapentaenoic acid on bleeding time, lipids and platelet aggregation,** *Lancet* 318; 8257, 1190-3, **1981**

- Xiao YF, et al, Suppression of voltage-gated L.-type Ca+ currents by polyunsaturated fatty acids and adult and neonatal rat ventricular myositis, *Proc Natl Acad Sci USA*, 94:4182-7, 1997

- von Shackey C, et al, The effect of dietary **w-3 fatty acids** on coronary atherosclerosis, *Ann Intern Med* 130:554-62, **1999** (also **lowers platelet aggregation,** had one third the cardiovascular events and **double the regression** compared with folks not on omega-3)

- Simopoulis A, **The importance of the ratio of omega-6/omega-3 essential fatty acids,** *Biomedicine Pharmacotherapeutics* 56; 8:365-79, 2002

- Mozaffarian D, Rimm EB, et al, Fish intake, contaminants, and human health. Evaluating the risks and the benefits, *J Am Med Assoc* 269; 15:1885-99, 2006

- Hu FB, Bronner L, et al, Fish and **omega-3 fatty acid intake and risk of coronary heart disease** in women, *J Am Med Assoc* 287; 14:1815-21, 2002

- Lombardo YB, et al, Effects of dietary polyunsaturated **n-3 fatty acids** on dyslipidemia and **insulin resistance** in rodents and humans. A review, *J Nutr Biochem* 17:1-13, 2006

- Albert CM, Campos H, et al., Blood levels of long-chain **n-3 fatty acids and the risk of sudden death,** *New Engl J Med* 346; 15:1113-8, **2002**

- Studer M, Briel M, et al, Effect of different anti-lipidemia agents and diets on mortality, a systematic review, *Arch Intern Med* 165:725-30, 2005

- Macchia A, et al, **Omega-3 fatty acid supplementation reduces one year risk of atrial fibrillation in patients hospitalized with myocardial infarction,** *Eur J Clin Pharmaco*l 64; 6:6 to 7-34, 2008

- Lee SH, et al, Blood eicosapentaenoic acid and docosahexaenoic acid as **predictors of** all **cause mortality** in patients with acute myocardial infarction -- data from Infarction Prognosis Study (IPS) Registry, *Circulation* 73; 12:20 to 50-70, 2009

- Einvik G, et al, A randomized clinical trial of n-3 polyunsaturated fatty acid supplementation and all cause mortality in elderly men at high cardiovascular risk, *Eur J Cardiovasc Prev Rehab* 17; 5:588-92, 2010

- Trebble T, Wootton S, et al., Prostaglandin E2 production and T cell function after fish oil supplementation: response to antioxidant supplementation, *Am J Clin Nutr* 78; 3:376-82, 2003

- Mori T, Beilin L, Omega-3 fatty acids and inflammation, *Curr Atheroscler Rep* 6; 6:461-7, 2004

- Simopoulis A, Omega-3 fatty acids in inflammation and autoimmune diseases, *Am J Clin Nutr* 21; 6:495-505, 2002

- Bralley JA, Lord RS, *Laboratory Evaluation in Molecular Medicine,* metametrix.com, 2005

- Von Shackey, Clemons, et al, The effect of dietary omega-3 fatty acids on coronary atherosclerosis, *Ann Intern Med*, 130:554-62, 1999

- Kottke TE, Wu LA, et al, **Preventing sudden death with n-3 (omega-3) fatty acids** and defibrillators, *Am J Prev Med* 31; 4:316-23, 2006

- Madsen T, Skou HA, et al, C-reactive protein, dietary n-3 fatty acids and the extent of coronary artery disease, *Am J Cardiol* 88; 10:1139-42, 2001

- Tai, CC, et al, **N-3 polyunsaturated fatty acids regulate lipid metabolism** through several inflammation mediators: mechanisms and implications for obesity prevention, *J Nutr Biochem*, 21; 5:357-63, 2010

- Wang L, et al, **Changing ratios of omega-6 to omega-3 fatty acids** can differentially modulate polychlorinated biphenyl toxicity in endothelial cells, *Chem Biol Interact* 172; 1:27-38, 2008

- Hennig B, et al, Using nutrition for intervention and prevention against environmental chemical toxicity and associated diseases, *Environ Health Persp* 115:493-5, 2007

- Hennig B, et al, **Nutrition can modulate the toxicity of environmental pollutants:** Implications in risk assessment and human health, *Environ Health Persp* 120:771-4, 2012

The Real World of Medical Cures Rest in Nutrients

This glimpse at the omega-3 chemistry hardly does it justice, yet I could do the same for dozens of other crucial nutrients. For example, magnesium and four of the eight forms of natural vitamin E, the tocotrienols, are also HMG CoA reductase inhibitors. That means they can do what statins like Lipitor do, but without the brain-damaging side effects (Khor). They also do so without damaging the genes or poisoning the liver's gene to make coenzyme Q10, or creating selenium, tocopherol and zinc deficiencies, as well as damaging the *tau* protein that leads to sudden amnesia, Alzheimer's, cancer, and much more, as do the statin drugs.

227

Or what about folks tortured with high blood pressure's low sodium diet? Sometimes all they need to do is fix the sodium channels in the membrane or use **Gamma-Tocotrienol**, a vitamin E homolog, as a **natriuretic hormone precursor**.

Clearly the wonderful world of nutrients is ignored. That's a major reason to catch up on past *TW*s. There are so many other things that you need to know. For example, macular degeneration is the number one cause of blindness in the age over 50. As the eye ages it runs out of certain nutrients especially lutein and zeaxanthine. We should be taking these every day, especially if you are diabetic, since this raises the odds for eye deterioration. I suggest either **Lutein** (containing zeaxanthine) or **Lutein with Kale** (Krinsky).

I know you feel on overload now, but wait! There is more for you to learn. You are doing a great job by exploring the world of healing, by bringing yourself into the realm of cure. Aren't you curious about what else you could do?

References:

- Khor HT, et al, Effects of administration of alpha-tocopherol and tocotrienols on serum lipids and liver HMGCoA reductase activity, *Internat J Food Sci Nutr* 51 (supple): S3-11, 2000
- Saito H, et al, **Gamma-tocotrienol, a vitamin E homolog, is a natriuretic hormone precursor**, *J Lipid Res*, 44:1530-5, 2003
- Krinsky NI, et al, Biologic mechanisms of the protective role of lutein and zeaxanthin in the eye, *Ann Rev Nutr* 23:171-201, 2003

NOTE: As this goes to press, Gamma E-Gems are back ordered by Carlson's. However, you can get **Natural Gamma-E** from Allergy Research Group. (allergyresearchgroup.com 800-545-9960)

In closing this brief proof of the many nutrient cures needed for diabetes, authors of a recent scientific paper from 2 major medical schools sum up the current concepts regarding diabetes. It is (1) genetically determined, and (2) due to a progressive failure of pancreatic function. They are so far behind they think they are first! Needless-to-say there was mention of only one nutrient, the n-3 fatty acids (as found in cod liver oil). And only you know why that alone failed to cure: they never measured, balanced, or added the other nutrients (PC, E-8, ALC, Mg, etc.) needed to make it work. These specialists appear clueless about God's orchestration, which is why you have to learn it to cure yourselves. So I bet you can't wait for the next chapter on another major neglected, yet curable cause of diabetes.

References:

• Kim J ,et al, Endocannabinoid signaling and energy metabolism: A target for dietary intervention, *Nutr*, 27: 624-32, 2011

• Kabir M, et al, Treatment for 2 mo with n-3 polyunsaturatd fatty acids reduces adiposity and some atherogenic factors but does not improve insulin sensitivity in women with type 2 diabetes: a randomized controlled study, *Am J Clin Nutr* , 86: 1670-9, 2007

Chapter VI

Dinosaur Diabetes Docs Do Not Detoxify

"What If I'm Still Not Cured?"

Then you need to know the rest of the causes. **Diseases classically have only two causes**. First, as we go through life we get progressively more nutrient depleted. You have just seen a smattering of the overwhelming evidence for that. One of the major causes is that the work of living in this world and **detoxifying our daily exposures uses up nutrients**. Plus the processing of foods lowers countless nutrients. The second cause of disease? **Toxicities**. Most people don't give it a second thought. But we have so polluted the world that even the polar bears in the Arctic now have human diseases like osteoporosis and hypothyroidism from our chemicals. And those magnificent creatures have the cleanest air, food, and water on the planet.

And *diabetes* and its precursor insulin resistance (Metabolic Syndrome X) are no exceptions. Both have been *proven to be caused by a variety of chemicals* in our air, food, and water that we can no longer avoid. And this has been *known for over 3 decades* (Toniolo, Carpenter, Lee). As a tiny example, folks with **diabetes are more sensitive and more likely to die** of a heart attack or arrhythmia **on days of high air pollution** exposure (Goldberg).

Like most pollutants, air pollutants can create disease in anyyone through multiple mechanisms. For example, **common chemicals like those found in auto exhaust make the blood more eager to throw clots** (Jacobs), **can create angina, arrhythmias, or a heart attack.** Each day we are asked to detoxify well over 500 chemicals. Those that fail to be eliminated slowly tank up in our bodies. When they reach a critical level of damage to our chemistry, we call this "disease". We tell folks they should have disease because they're old. So **even though diseases are caused by chemical overload, we "treat" them by throwing yet** another chemical at them, disguised as a drug. Or worse yet we replace the worn out part or just cut it out and throw it away. And chalk it all up to age.

References:

- Ruzzin J, et al, Persistent **organic pollutant exposure leads to insulin resistance** syndrome, *Environ Health Persp* 118:465-71, 2010

- Rignell-Hydbom A, et al, Exposure to persistent organochlorine **pollutants and type 2 diabetes** mellitus, *Human Exp Toxicol* 26; 5:447-52, 2007

- Carpenter D.O., **Environmental contaminants as risk factors for developing diabetes**, *Rev Environ Health* 23:59-75, 2008

- Toniolo A, et al, Induction of **diabetes by cumulative environmental insults** from viruses and chemicals, *Nature* 288:383-85, 1980

- Lee DH, et al, A strong dose response relation between serum concentrations of persistent organic **pollutants and diabetes**, *Diabetes Care*, 29:1838-44, 2006

- Goldberg MS, Associations between ambient **air pollution and daily mortality** among persons **with diabetes** and cardiovascular disease, *Environ Res* 100:255-67, 2006

- Jacobs L, et al, **Air pollution-related prothrombotic changes in persons with diabetes**, *Environ Health Persp* 118:191-6, 2010

The Plastic Plague

Let's take a look at just one toxic environmental chemical family that is in all of us. We literally cannot avoid it if we live on this planet. U.S. Government researchers have found them in all humans. Even when researchers drop helicopters into pristine road-less areas, far from industry, they find this pollutant in all species of life they examine, from fish and salamanders to the largest mammals. They are actually a family of man-made chemicals which define modern life as we know it, **the phthalates, better recognized by you as plastics and plasticizers. But they go far beyond** our concept of a plastic, because they add flexibility, durability, slow-release, cost-effectiveness, scent, light- and heat-protection, and many other properties to things we do not consider as plastics.

Phthalates (**plastic-derived carcinogenic chemicals made from petroleum**) are in your plastic water bottle and other food

231

containers (linings of cans, juice boxes, plastic wrap and Styrofoam trays), not to mention infant formula bottles. In fact, **baby bottles have some of the highest levels of phthalates, and this is made even worse by microwaving a baby's bottle** (von Goetz). Plus when the mother drinks out of plastic water bottles, the plastics cross the placenta and head for the fetus's brain and glands that produce hormones. And unfortunately **low doses have been shown to be more toxic than higher ones. Phthalates are in food containers of nearly every type** from soup to cereals, hidden in boxes, bags and beer, food and soda cans, or blatantly in Styrofoam trays and cups and plastic wrap, and plastic bottles and jugs. Phthalates are in dental fillings (composites), even the glues for dental crowns, the bags that hold "safe" saline breast implants, and are a large part of dental implants and joint replacement adhesives or glues and elute from coronary artery stents (methylacrylates).

Phthalates or plasticizers outgas from IVs, dental materials, vinyl floors, carpeting, mattresses, most furnishings (couches, chairs, mattresses, desks and tables), appliances, computers, home and office and construction materials, automobiles, the coatings of electric wires (nestled in the walls of every building outgas as they heat), PVC plumbing, etc. The list is endless. Clearly phthalates are **the most ubiquitously unavoidable pollutant in the human body.** The evidence is overwhelming. The phthalates ("plastics") permeate every aspect of our life, since they are ingredients in even cosmetics and toiletries, nail polishes, perfumes, deodorants, hair conditioners, lotions, and other personal care products as well as medications, especially those that are called "extended release" or "24 hour" or "time release" or "slow release". For it is the plastic coating that creates this property.

And if these were not dangerous enough by themselves, they are never alone. They are usually combined in products with equally or even more dangerous environmental pollutants like the phthalate cousin **BPA** (bisphenol A, often accompanies phthalates), **PBDE** (flame retardants), **PFOA** (stain resistant, water resistant, Teflon-type chemicals), **VOHs** (volatile organic hydrocarbons which include xylene, toluene, benzene, and hundreds more), **pesticides,** etc. All these are often called **POPs**, or persistent environmental pollutants, because most of them take decades to break down.

And now even animals in the wild have measurable levels in their systems. Yet they don't use styrofoam cups, plastic water and infant formula bottles, nor shrink-wrap their foods in plastic. Nor do they live in enclosed homes and offices with huge amounts of furnishings as well as appliances that outgas phthalates. Nor do they ride in toxic cars/trains/planes, in heavy exhaust, or work in polluted factories and offices made from an abundance of construction materials making them literal *phthalate cocoons*. We have truly changed the air on the planet Earth in this century. And worse, **we have changed the chemistry of the human body more than at any other time**.

The evidence now for phthalates being able to contribute to or directly causing every malady known is overwhelming. Babies are born with measurable levels, and if they have to spend time in the hospital to be on I.V.s (intravenous), or have catheters or gastric tubes, this raises their levels even further. Birth defects and lowered IQ, hypothyroidism, neurologic and especially brain dysfunctions are among the many spin-off diseases for the privilege of living in this world of convenient plastics. **Cancers**, from prostate, testicular and breast to brain and pancreatic, **can be programmed** in the genetics of babies while they are still **in the womb,** only to have their **emergence suppressed until adulthood** (Barker).

In many of the reports you will encounter the term **bisphenol A or BPA**. As a broadly used industrial chemical and polycarbonate and epoxy resin that also lines food cans, **BPA migrates directly from those containers into the foods, just as phthalates do**. Although BPA is not technically a phthalate, it is most of the time found combined with phthalates (from carbonless copy paper to cabinets) and has its own toxic properties in addition to those of the phthalates that it's connected with. Therefore since these two toxins are usually present as a combination, it is quite meaningless to separate their toxicities since they usually occur in combination. As well, they share several mechanisms of toxicity in the body. So **don't be hoodwinked by proclamations that a product is "BPA free". The manufacturers assume you are ignorant of the hidden phthalates.** Plus you don't know the assay cut-off used.

Meanwhile, remember phthalates and BPA are only two of thousands of chemicals that we are exposed to and minimally hundreds each day that our bodies are asked to detoxify. Even chemicals in cellophane and plastic windows of cookie boxes are proven to migrate into the foods that they do not even contact. We cannot escape them, nor can we detoxify or metabolize all that we are exposed to in a day.

And most importantly, phthalates can cause every aspect of diabetes from its precursors of obesity, insulin resistance, hypertension, lipidemia, heart disease, hypoglycemia, hyperthyroidism, NASH, etc., to full blown type I or II and their nasty and eventual fatal sequelae. No wonder diabetes has become a global public health problem, with over 150 million people worldwide. And the level is expected to double in the next decade. As of now **over 7% (1 in 14**, or 1 in 8, depending on whose study you read) **of the U.S. population has type II diabetes**. (Zimmet). This is truly an epidemic out of control. Luckily we know the causes and cures.

References:

• Koch HM, et al, **Human body burdens of chemicals used in plastic** manufacture, *Philosoph Trans Roy Soc*, 364:2063-78, 2009

• Hauser R, et al, **Medications as a source of human exposure to phthalates**, *Environ Health Persp* 112:751-3, 2004

• Xu Y, et al, Predicting residential exposure to **phthalate plasticizer emitted from vinyl flooring**: sensitivity, uncertainty, and implications for biomonitoring, *Environ Health Persp,* 118; 2:253-58, Feb 2010

- Barker DJ, **In utero programming of chronic disease**, *Clin Sci* (Lond.) 95; 2:115-128, 1998

- Schafer KS, et al, **Persistent toxic chemicals in the US food supply**, *J Epidemiol Commun Health* 56; 11:813-17, 2002

- Xu Y, et al, Predicting residential **exposure to phthalate plasticizer emitted from vinyl flooring**: sensitivity, uncertainty, and implications for biomonitoring, *Environ Health Persp* 118:253-8, 2010

- Welshons WV, et al, **Large effects from a small exposures**. I. Mechanisms for endocrine-disrupting chemicals with estrogenic activity, *Environ Health Persp* 111:994-1006, 2003

- Zimmet P, et al, Global and societal implications of the diabetes epidemic *Nature* 414:782-7, 2001

Why Are Phthalates So Important?

Phthalates are the backbone of diabetes. Phthalates or "plastics" create not only diabetes and metabolic syndrome X, but allergies, prostatic hypertrophy, endometriosis, breast cancer, hypo-testosteronism, hypothyroidism, infertility, animals mating with the same sex, inability to lose weight, asthma, birth defects, cancers, and infinitely more (Lopez-Carrillo, vom Saal). No wonder we have the most out of control disease epidemics in the history of this planet.

Why do I focus on this one as an example from thousands of other toxins? Because **phthalate levels in the human body are over 10,000 times higher than most other pollutants. No other pollutant comes close to (1) affecting this number of folks, (2) being at such unprecedentedly high levels, (3) being so overwhelmingly ubiquitous and unavoidable, and (4) capable of creating such a vast array of diseases.** They are not only a known cause of diabetes and insulin resistance, but pancreatic cancers, inability to lose weight, high cholesterol, high blood pressure, elevated triglycerides, NASH (non-alcoholic steatohepatitis, the most common liver disease now and a precursor to diabetes), arteriosclerosis, and a host of other maladies (Grun).

And you guessed it. **Phthalates poison the mitochondria** that you learned about in chapter 3. And that is just for starters, for they damage many other crucial areas in the body chemistry (Melnick, Winberg). Probably most devastating is that **they**

235

seriously poison fatty acid chemistry (van der Leij). And you will **recall fatty acids are the backbone of all membranes including those that protect the cell, the genetics, and make the mitochondria where energy is produced, plus the endoplasmic reticulum where detoxification takes place,** and more. But you get the picture without my having to make you a specialist in cell biology. My point that I hope you never forget: **Many will never heal diabetes or whatever they have because no one depurated their phthalates.** And folks on dialysis get **even higher levels** of phthalates because of the IV tubes (Pollack).

My goal is not so much to make you an expert in the phthalates, as to show you an example of how merely *one* of thousands of unavoidable environmental toxins produces such a wide range of hidden damages to the human system. And yet in spite of all of the overwhelming evidence that I'm merely giving you a smattering of, this is not taught in medical schools. Plastics among many problems cause the silent loss of zinc, needed to repair your genes or else they will give the message for cancer. Zinc is needed to metabolize the fatty acids for all membrane repair via delta-5-desaturase, needed to convert B6 to its active form P5P, needed to convert B-carotene to vitamin A, etc. And phthalates damage sulfation detoxification pathways (another mechanism that can lead to cancer) as examples. The *good news* is we know how to get them out of the body and thereby reverse diseases.

Meanwhile, do you think government regulatory agencies are up to snuff on all this chemistry? I hope you don't. Not when **the dose used to create diabetes is 5000 times <u>below</u> the lowest "official" EPA level assumed to not cause any effect!** Yes, you read that right. **An amount 5000 times below the government "safe" level of phthalates is used to create diabetes in lab animals.** And the **researchers can create diabetes with phthalates in just <u>four</u> days** (Alonso-Magdalena). Government studies show that over 95% of the US population has measurable levels of these and not only are all of the diseases that these chemicals create worrisome, but **they damage the brain and the IQ**, and can be the backbone for a plethora of other diseases. But in "modern" medicine when there is no drug to throw at the symptoms, we merely tell folks "there is no known cause and no known cure". How wrong this is. You should never fall for this again.

References:

• Alonso-Magdalena P, et al., The estrogenic effect of **bisphenol A disrupts pancreatic B-cell** function *in vivo* and **induces insulin resistance**, *Environ Health Persp* 114:106-12, 2006

• Von Goetz N, et al, Bisphenol A: how the most relevant exposure sources contribute to total consumer exposure, *Risk Analysis* 30; 3:473-87, 2010

• Melnick RL, et al, **Mitochondrial toxicity of phthalate** esters, *Environ Health Persp* 45:51-6, **1982** (NOTE: known over 30 years)

• Winberg LD, et al, Mechanism of **phthalate-induced inhibition of hepatic mitochondrial beta-oxidation**, *Toxicology Letters* 76:63-69, **1995**

• Wanders RJA, Peroxisomes, lipid metabolism, and peroxisomal disorders, *Molec Genet Metabol*, 83:16-27, 2004

• Jaakkola JJK, et al, The role of exposure to **phthalates from polyvinyl chloride products** in the development of **asthma and allergies**: A systematic review and meta-analysis, *Environ Health Perspect* 116:845-53, 2008

• vom Saal FS, et al, **Large effects from small exposures**. II. The importance of positive controls in **low-dose research on bisphenol A**, *Environ Res* 100:50-76, 2005

• van der Leif FR, et al, Gene expression profiling in livers of mice after acute inhibition of beta oxidation, *Genomics* 90:680-9, 2007

• Pollack GM, et al, **Circulating concentrations** of di (2-ethylhexyl) **phthalate** and its de-esterified phthalic acid products following plasticizer exposure **in patients receiving hemodialysis**, *Toxicol Appl Pharmacol* 79:257-67, 1985

• Grun F, et al, Endocrine disruptors obesogens, *Molecul Cell Endocrinol* 304:19-29, 2009

Do You Keep Hearing That the Phthalates Are Safe?

I know sometimes you might think I'm a lone wolf in the woods when it comes to the staggering medical dangers of phthalates or plasticizers and their related chemicals. So I thought I'd tell you about a landmark paper published in the United States government's most prestigious environmental medical journal and authored by re-nowned specialists representing 30 medical institutions across the globe. These scientists showed beyond a doubt how lopsided the FDA has been in determining its bisphenol A (BPA) position.

First these **prestigious scientists presented the incontrovertible evidence of how phthalates with or without their cohort BPA can create every disease, including our focus here of epidemic diabetes, metabolic syndrome with an inability to lose weight, and all aspects of heart disease.** And others have shown how the levels in babies actually program them for prostate and breast cancers when they reach adulthood. Then they showed how **the FDA has chosen to cling to two outdated industry-funded studies, done by the plastics industry decades ago when modern laboratory technology was not available.** This was greatly in favor of industry because it made the levels of phthalates look harmlessly low, since researchers were unable to detect them with their archaic lab methods. In addition the studies were done for too short a time to create diseases.

At the same time **the FDA has chosen to ignore the current proof from over 100 modern and highly technical research papers in making their decisions about phthalates. Phthalates are a man-made chemical (category) extremely foreign to the human body chemistry and <u>there is no safe level</u>.** Disease or accelerated aging emerge once phthalates reach a critical level in conjunction with the total load of a lifetime of acquired nutrient deficiencies and other toxicities.

And these concerned researchers are not alone. Other researchers have shown how **the FDA has clung to 19 industry-funded studies done with outdated technology while it chose to ignore 115 low dose studies** and how prestigious big-name universities have been funded by the American Plastics Council and not surprisingly came out in favor of the safety of plastics (vom Saal).

Polycarbonates (one of the many disguises of phthalates) are not safe. Furthermore, how can we believe any product that boasts "No BPA" when manufactures don't state how low the detection level was? Nor how much phthalate was present? It's sort of like the trans fatty acids story where Harvard researchers warned the government for decades that there is no safe level. Yet they were ignored and disease-producing trans fats still permeate the American diet. Likewise, Harvard researchers warned decades ago that **there is no safe level of phthalates, and that these man-made foreign chemicals have no role in the metabolism of the human body, in fact they damage it**. We get such a huge amount every day unavoidably from our air, food and water that we can't possibly detoxify it all. So they slowly accumulate and tank up in our cells where they damage just about every normal cell/body function in some way.

And what about the recycling craze? Unfortunately **when plastics are <u>recycled this raises the level of phthalates</u> and concentrates the problem even further**. And bottles that are subjected to boiling, brushing, dishwashing can leach even more phthalates from them. This is particularly important for **baby plastic bottles which have higher levels than others.** This is partly responsible for our current generation of infants and young children and even teens who have more obesity, diabetes, more cancers, allergies, auto-immune disorders, more "adult diseases" like high cholesterol, not to mention lower IQ and less motivation oftentimes (compared with what would be expected from knowing their parents' accomplishments).

And unfortunately **low doses can sometimes even be more deleterious than high doses** because they allow the person to slowly tank up without perceiving any ill effects until the fateful day when they suddenly have diabetes, a heart attack or cancer, or whatever. And if they are so safe, why are polar bears in the pristine wild (who are not drinking out of Styrofoam® cups, living and working in cocoons of plastic or taking medications for every ailment) now having human diseases like hypothyroidism and osteoporosis?

And remember that this is only one of over 3,000-8,000 chemicals that we are potentially exposed to, and many of them persist much longer in the human body. Just think about it. Your food is prepared by people who wear plastic gloves, as your dentist does. Yet they outgas so much phthalate that they have been prohibited by the Japanese government. I remember the good old days in the 1970s when as an emergency room physician I and other ER docs routinely sutured folks wearing no gloves. But between overuse of antibiotics creating resistant bacterial strains and folks with impaired immune systems, lacking such essential vitamins as D and E (as examples of documented epidemic deficiencies in this land of plenty), folks are more vulnerable for infections.

Furthermore, **studies prove that phthalate levels far exceed what we used to think was safe.** And the more studies that are done, the more scientists find they have grossly underestimated phthalate levels in the environment (Itoh). And keep remembering this is only one pollutant. And as you have **learned, "No BPA" can be as serious a misconception as "No trans fats".** In addition, our total daily human exposure just to even BPA is much higher than previously assumed (Taylor). Bisphenol A, like phthalates has been shown to contribute to not only diabetes, but NASH, heart disease, and more (Lang).

Plus the hidden dangers do not stop with diabetes. **Phthalates make cancers resistant to chemotherapy**. Plus they poison fatty acid chemistry and damage calcium channels in cell membranes leading to high blood pressure, cholesterol, arrhythmias like atrial fibrillation, coronary heart disease, heart failure, and more. Yet in spite of triggering cancers, would you believe that in this era <u>there still is no FDA standard for the amount of phthalates that can be used in plastic bottles?</u> **Even baby bottles!** Meanwhile, carcinogenic chemicals like the **fire retardant PBDE were actually legislated by our government into mattresses**, car seats, airplane seats, babies' cribs and **are also found in plastics**. Since the U.S. was unique in legislating the fire retardant (PBDE) <u>into</u>

mattresses, levels of diabetes-causing PBDE in U.S. folks are twice as high as other folks in countries that were not as blatantly misguided. And as *USA Today* showed, our levels are doubling in the human body every few years (*TW*). These are among our most potent environmental endocrine disruptors and lead to obesity that will not budge, thyroid and vitamin A destruction, low IQ, ADD, etc., plus breast, prostate, thyroid, adrenal, brain and other cancers as well as chemotherapy-resistant cancers which rapidly metastasize and kill (Brun, Lim, Ellis-Hutchings, Hoppe). **And PBDE flame retardants can create diabetes and its precursor diseases and side effects.** If you think you don't have them in you, guess again. **Even the seagulls, Beluga whales and Arctic polar bears harbor them** (Verrault).

Clearly, we all must continually get rid of our unavoidable accumulation. **It's especially important for young folks who are planning a family to detoxify for a year or so before they conceive.** It would reduce the huge amount of birth defects as well as ADD, ADHD, PDD, autism, and children with a lowered IQ. Make sure you give newly married couples *Detoxify Or Die* and encourage them to at least have a **far infrared sauna** at home or at some community outreach such as a church, synagogue, AA, athletic and social clubs, or other organizations. Raising a child with birth defects is enormously stressful and expensive and has dissolved many a marriage. Yet detoxification of the couple for one year coupled with the knowledge in *DOD (Detoxify Or Die)* about even simple things like not using plastic baby bottles, crib mattresses and bumpers, or avoiding loading the child's environment up with plastic toys has a bearing on his future health.

References:

• Winberg LD, et al, Mechanism of **phthalate-induced inhibition** of hepatic **mitochondrial B-oxidation**, *Toxicol Lett* 76:63-69, 1995

• Alonso-Magdalena P, et al, The estrogenic effect of **bisphenol A disrupts pancreatic** B-cell function in vivo and induces **insulin resistance**, *Environ Health Perspect* 114:106-12, 2006

- LaPensee EW, et al, **Bisphenol A at low nanomolar doses confers chemoresistance in estrogen receptor-a-positive and -negative breast cancer cells,** *Environ Health Persp* 117:175-180, 2009

- Dooley EE, Better oversight for bottled water, *Environ Health Persp*, A 347, 117; 8: Aug 2009

- Verrault J, et al, **Flame retardants** and methoxylated and hydroxylated polybrominated diphenyl ethers **in** two Norwegian Arctic top predators: glaucus **gulls and polar bears,** *Environ Sci Technol* 39:6021-28, 2005

- Law RJ, et al, Levels and trends of polybrominated di-phenyl ethers and other brominated **flame retardants in wildlife,** *Environ Int* 29:757-70, 2003

- Meerts IATM, et al, In vitro **estrogenicity of** polybrominated diphenyl ethers, hydroxylated **PBDEs and** polybrominated **bisphenol A** compounds, *Environ Health Persp*, 19:399-407, 2001

- Kojima H, et al, Nuclear hormone receptor activity of polybrominated diphenyl ethers and their hydroxylated and methoxalated metabolites in transactivation assays using Chinese hamster ovary cells, *Environ Health Persp* 117; 8:1210-18, 2009

- Zhou T, et al, Effects of short-term in vivo exposure to brominated diphenyl ethers on thyroid hormones and hepatic enzyme activities in weanling rats, *Toxicol Sci* 61:76-82, 2001

- Shafer T., et al., Effects **of pyrethroids on voltage-sensitive calcium channels**: a critical evaluation of strengths, weaknesses, data needs, and relationship to assessment of **cumulative neurotoxicity.** *Toxicol Appl Pharmacol* 196:303-318, 2004

- Jaakkola JJK, et al, The role of exposure to phthalates from **polyvinyl** chloride products in the development of **asthma and allergies**: A systematic review and meta-analysis, *Environ Health Perspect* 116:845-53, 2008

- Lombardo YB, et al, Effects of dietary polyunsaturated **n-3 fatty acids on dyslipidemia and insulin resistance** in rodents and humans, A review, *J Nutr Biochem*, 17:1-13, 2006

- Myers JP, et al, Why public health agencies cannot depend on good laboratory practices as a criterion for selecting data: The case of bisphenol A, *Environ Health Persp* 117:309-15, 2008

- Welshons WV, et al, Large effects from small exposures III. Endocrine mechanisms mediating effects of bisphenol A at levels of human exposure, *Endocrinol* 147 (6 supple): 56-69, 2006

- Wanders RJA, Peroxisomes, lipid metabolism, and peroxisomal disorders, *Molec Genet Metabol*, 83:16-27, 2004

- Von Goetz N, et al, Bisphenol A: how the most relevant exposure sources contribute to total consumer exposure, *Risk Analysis* 30; 3:473-87, 2010

- Itoh H, et al, Quantitative identification **of unknown exposure pathways of phthalates** based on measuring their metabolites in human urine, *Environ Technol* 41:4542-7, 2007

- Taylor JA, et al, Similarity of bisphenol A pharmacokinetics in rhesus monkeys and mice: relevance for human exposure, *Environ Health Persp* 119:422-30, 2011

- Lang IA, et al, Association of urinary **bisphenol A concentration with medical disorders** and laboratory abnormalities in adults, *J Am Med Assoc*, 300; 11:1303-1310, 2008

- Lee, DH, et al, **Low dose of some persistent organic pollutants predicts type II diabetes**: a nested case-controlled study, *Environ Health Perspect* 118; 9: 1235-42, 2010

- Lee HJ, et al, **Anti-androgenic effects of bisphenol A** and nonylphenol on the function of androgen receptor, *Toxicol Sci*, 75:40-46, 2003
- Vom Saal FS, et al, An extensive new literature concerning **low-dose effects of bisphenol A** shows the need for a new risk assessment, *Environ Health Persp*, 113:926-33, 2005

242

- Le HH, et al, **Bisphenol A is released from polycarbonate drinking bottles and mimics the neurotoxic actions** of estrogen in developing cerebellar neurons, *Toxicol Lett*, 176:149-56, 2008

- Nadal A, et al, The **pancreatic B-cell as a target of** estrogens and **xenoestrogens**: implications for blood glucose homeostasis and **diabetes**, *Mol Cell Endocrinol*, 304; 1-2:63-8, 2009

- Nadal A, et al, The role of **estrogens in the adaptation of islets to insulin resistance**, *J Physiol*, 587 (pt 21): 5031-37, 2009

- Carwile JL, et al, **Polycarbonate bottle** use and urinary bisphenol A concentrations, *Environ Health Persp* 117 1368-72, 2009

- Brede C, et al, **Increased migration of bisphenol A from polycarbonate baby bottles after dishwashing, boiling and brushing**, *Food Addit Contamin* 20:684-89, 2003

- Durando M, et al, **Prenatal bisphenol A exposure induces pre-neoplastic lesions in the mammary gland** of Wistar rats, *Environ Health Persp* 115:80-86, 2007

- Wozniak AL, et al, **Xenoestrogens at picomolar to nanomolar concentrations trigger** membrane estrogen receptor-alpha-mediated Ca2+ fluxes and prolactin release in GH3/B6 **pituitary tumor cells**, *Environ Persp* 113:431-39, 2005

- Stahlhut, R, et al, **Bisphenol** A data in NHANES **has longer than expected half-life**, substantial non-food exposure, or both, *Environ Health Persp* 117; 5:784-89, 2009

- Matsushima A, et al, Bisphenol A is a full agonist for the estrogen receptor ER*a* but highly specific antagonist for ER*b*, *Environ Health Perspect* 118; 9: 1267-72, 2010

- Mendiola J, et al, Are environmental levels of bisphenol A associated with reproductive function in fertile men? *Environ Health Perspect* 118; 9: 1280-85, 2010

- Petersen JH, et al. **Plasticizers in** total diet samples, **baby food and infant formulas**, *Food Addit Contam* 17; 2:133-41, 2000

- Midoro-Horiuti T, et al, Maternal bisphenol A exposure promotes the development of experimental **asthma** in mouse pups, *Environ Health Persp,* 118; 2:273-77, Feb 2010

- Kabuto H, et al, Exposure to **bisphenol** A during embryonic/fetal life and infancy and increases oxidative injury and causes **under-development of the brain and testes** in mice, *Life Sci* 74:2931-40, 2004

- Schonfelder G, et al, Parental **bisphenol and accumulation in the human maternal-fetal-**placental unit, *Environ Health Perspect* 110:A703-07, 2002

- Barker DJ, **In utero programming of chronic disease**, *Clin Sci* (Lond.) 95; 2:115-128, 1998

- Bouskine A, et al, **Low doses of bisphenol A promote human adenoma** cell proliferation by activating PKA and PKG via a membrane G-protein-coupled estrogen receptor, *Environ Health Persp* 117; 7:1053-58, 2009

- Ikezuki Y, et al, Determination of **bisphenol A** concentration in human biological fluids reveals significant **early prenatal exposure**, *Hum Reprod* 17; 11:2839-41, 2002

- Vanderburg LN, et al., Exposure to environmentally relevant doses of the xenoestrogens **bisphenol A alters development of the field mouse mammary gland**, *Endocrinology* 148; 1:116-27, 2007

- Maffini MV, et al, **Endocrine disruptors** and reproductive health: the case of **bisphenol A**, *Molec Cell Endocrin* 254-5: 179-86, 2006

- Ho SM, et al, Developmental exposure to estradiol and **bisphenol A increases susceptibility to prostate carcinogenesis** and epigenetically regulates phosphodiesterase type 4 variant 4, *Cancer Res* 66:5624-32, 2006

243

- Seo KW, et al, Comparison of oxidative stress and **changes of xenobiotics metabolizing enzymes induced by phthalates** in rats, *Food Chem Toxicol* 42:107-14, 2004

- Liu PS, et al, Comparative **suppression of phthalate** monoesters and phthalate diesters **on calcium signaling** coupled to nicotinic **acetylcholine receptors**, *J Toxicol Sci*, 34; 3:255-63, 2009

- Liu PS, et al, **Phthalates suppressed the calcium signaling** of nicotinic acetylcholine receptors **in** bovine **adrenal** chromaffin cells, *Toxicol Appl Pharmacol*, 183:92-98, 2002
- Liu PS, et al, Butyl benzyl **phthalate blocks Ca2+ signaling and catecholamine** secretion couples with nicotinic **acetylcholine** receptors **in bovine adrenal** chromaffin cells, *Neurotoxicol* 2497-105, 2003

- Main KM, et al, **Human breast milk contamination with phthalates** and alterations of endogenous reproductive **hormones in infants** three months of age, *Environ Health Persp* 114:270-276, 2006

- Lim JS, et al, Association of brominated **flame retardants with diabetes and metabolic syndrome** in the United States population: 2003-2004, *Diabetes Care* 2008

- Hoppe AA, et al, **Polybrominated biphenyl ethers as endocrine disruptors of adipocyte** metabolism, *Obesity* (Silver Spring) 15:2942-50, 2007

- Ellis-Hutchings RG, et al., Polybrominated biphenyl ether **(PBDE)-induced alterations in vitamin A and thyroid hormone** concentrations in the rat during lactation and early postnatal development, *Toxicol Appl Pharmacol* 215:435-45, 2006

If Your Weight Is Stuck, It's Because Your Chemicals Are Stuck

Not only is diabetes associated with obesity, but so are its precursors (like metabolic syndrome X) and complications (like heart disease and high blood pressure). **A major cause of the obesity epidemic is the unprecedented level of phthalates or plasticizers, which according to the last decade of U.S. government surveys is the number one pollutant in the human body and in over 98% of folks.**

Instead of healing folks, however, the medical focus is on fat-blasting devices (*WSJ*, D1, 9/14/10), prescribing diet drugs that are barely effective but raise the risk of cancer, heart disease and depression (*WSJ* B4 9/16/10), or locating a virus that is found in higher amounts in fat folks (*WSJ* D6, 9/21/10). Obviously the researchers forgot that our **fat stores a huge amount of our chemicals. So the fatter you are the more chemicals you have on board.** Another thing these chemicals do is change your cytokines, so it makes you more vulnerable for viral infections, auto-immune diseases like lupus, MS, arthritis, and cancers.

Phthalates are now so pervasive that **children six years of age have levels that used to take adults until the age of 40 to accumulate**. A huge amount of government as well as other scientific and medical literature confirms how these plasticizers stockpile in the body and overwhelm our ability to detoxify them. No wonder **obesity only appears unsolvable to physicians who are unschooled in phthalate toxicity**. In fact a simple test is to ask your doc what role phthalates play in creating your diabetes.

We can measure phthalates and the damage that they have created so that we can show folks how to heal obesity, syndrome X, diabetes, NASH, arteriosclerosis, allergies, and much more. In fact **the name or label that a disease has is now inconsequential. All we care about is what *caused* the disease and what biochemical corrections and detoxifications are necessary to get rid of it and actually bring about *cure*,** a word you rarely hear in drug-oriented medicine.

As a quick example of their far-reaching effects in the human body, not only the **phthalates and BPA, but pesticides, heavy metals and many other pollutants fall under a category called EEDs or environmental endocrine disruptors**. These chemicals make a beeline for hormones and glands. As referenced in *TW* as one example, they can damage the thyroid without damaging the tests that doctors usually use to diagnose hypothyroidism. Therefore you can have not only obesity, but exhaustion, depression, constipation, high cholesterol, hair loss, and other symptoms of hypothyroidism, but be told that your thyroid is "normal". You must have a sensitive TSH (thyroid stimulating hormone) below 2.0 (not the antiquated and dangerous cut-off of 4.5 of conventional lab reports) and also have thyroid auto-antibodies checked (*TW* 2010 for details and documentation).

And if you are silently hypothyroid during pregnancy then your baby is also. This seriously retards the normal development of the brain. And even more important is the fact that a pregnant mother's phthalate levels (look at how many are unknowingly drinking from plastic water bottles, thinking that it's something healthful) hugely influence not only the development of the child's brain and glands, but even future sexual preferences, fertility and cancers in the unborn children not to mention, of course, obesity. That's why I wrote *Detoxify Or Die*. **The evidence is now incontrovertible that folks need to detoxify** *before* **they conceive to decrease the chances of passing their unavoidably unprecedented level of toxins on to the unborn.** For remember the newborn in this era is exposed to many more toxins than his parents were.

(For physicians: How else do the plastics damage the chemistry that brings on diabetes, plus obesity and many other chronic diseases? First by damaging areas inside the cells that regulate all the chemistry of the body called peroxisomes and their receptors called PPAR (peroxisome proliferator-activated receptors). Diabetes, insulin resistance, inability to lose weight, high blood pressure or cholesterol, arrhythmia, cancer, learning disability, autism, asthma, and other diseases start with **damage to the peroxisomes** and the **genes and chemistry that they control in the mitochondria** and elsewhere. And you've already learned that they also directly damage not just the genes, but the mitochondria themselves, and how that in itself can bring on a litany of "incurable" diseases. Incurable, that is, until someone looks for the cause and cure. No longer does it matter what the label of a disease is. What matters is what caused it and how you are going to fix it.)

The bottom line is many people will never lose weight or cure their diabetes or other medical problems simply because they have not gotten rid of the phthalates and other environmental pollutants that have damaged their chemistry and genetics.

References (just a smattering of some, and others are above):

• Alonso-Magdalena P, et al, The estrogenic effect of **bisphenol A disrupts pancreatic B-cell function in vivo and induces insulin resistance**, *Environ Health Perspect* 114:106-12, 2006

• Heindal JJ, **Endocrine disruptors and the obesity epidemic**, *Toxicol Sci* 76; 2:247-49, 2003

• Baillie-Hamilton PF, **Chemical toxins: a hypothesis to explain the global obesity epidemic**, *J Alt Complement Med* 8;2:185-92, 2002

- *The Hundred Year Diet* in the *Wall Street* (May 10, 2010, A15)

- Vom Saal FS, Welshons WV, **Large effects from small exposures**. II. The importance of positive controls in low-dose research on bisphenol A, *Environ Res*, 100;1:50-76, Jan. 2006

- Feige JN, et al, The **endocrine disruptor** monoethyl-hexyl **phthalate is a selective peroxisome** proliferator-activated receptor gamma modulator that **promotes adipogenesis**, *J Biol Chem* 282:19152-66, 2007

- Feige JN, et al, The pollutant diethylhexyl **phthalate regulates hepatic energy** metabolism via species-specific PPARa-dependent mechanisms, *Environ Health Persp,* 118; 2:234-41, Feb 2010

- Newbold RR, et al., **Environmental estrogens and obesity**, *Mol Cell Endocrinol*, 304; 1-2:84-89, 2009

- Newbold RR, et al., Effects of **Endocrine Disruptors on Obesity**, *Internat J Androl* 31; 2:201-8, 2008

- Clark K, et al, Observed concentrations in the environment. In: *The Handbook of Environmental Chemistry, Vol 3, Part Q: Phthalate Ester* (Staples CA, ed). New York: Springer, 125-177, 2003

- Hatch EE, et al, Association of urinary **phthalate** metabolite concentrations with a body mass index and **waist circumference**: a cross-sectional study of NHANES data, 1999-2002, *Environ Health* 7:27, 2008

- Seo KW, et al, Comparison of oxidative stress and **changes of xenobiotic metabolizing enzymes induced by phthalates**, *Food Chem Toxicol* 42:10 7-114, 2004

- Barr DB, et al, Assessing human exposure to phthalates using monoesters and their oxidized metabolites as biomarkers, *Environ Health Perspect* 111: 1148-51, 2003

- Winberg LD, et al, Mechanism of **phthalates-induced inhibition of hepatic mitochondrial B-oxidation**, *Toxicol Lett* 76:63-69, 1995

- Cani PD, Metabolic endotoxemia initiates obesity and insulin resistance, *Diabetes* 56; 7:1761-72, 2007

- Sun Q, et al, Ambient **air pollution exaggerates** adipose inflammation and **insulin resistance** in a mouse model of diet-induced **obesity**, *Circul,* 119; 4:438-46, 2009

- Hill JO, et al, Environmental contributions to the obesity epidemic, *Sci* 280;5368: 1371-74, 1998

- Meeker JD, et al, Di-(2-ethylhexyl) **phthalate metabolites may alter thyroid hormones** in men, *Environ Health Persp* 115:1029-34, 2007

- Kang SC, et al, DNA methylation of estrogen receptor alpha gene by phthalates, *J Toxicol Environ Health A* 68:1996-2003, 2005

- Boas M, et al, Childhood exposure to **phthalates**: Associations with **thyroid function**, insulin like growth factor I and growth, *Environ Health Persp* 118:1458-64, 2010

- Fukawatari T, et al, Elucidation of the toxic mechanism of the plasticizers, phthalate acid, putative endocrine disruptors: effects of dietary di(2-ethylhexyl)**phthalate on the metabolism of tryptophan to niacin** in rats, 66:705-10, 2002

- Clark K, et al, Observed concentrations in the environment. In: *The Handbook of Environmental Chemistry, Vol 3, Part Q: Phthalate Ester* (Staples CA, ed). New York: Springer, 125-177, 2003

247

• Jaakkola JJK, et al, The role of exposure to **phthalates from polyvinyl chloride products in the development of asthma and allergies**: A systematic review and meta-analysis, *Environ Health Perspect* 116:845-53, 2008

• Xu Y, et al, Predicting residential exposure to **phthalate plasticizer emitted from vinyl flooring**: sensitivity, uncertainty, and implications for biomonitoring, *Environ Health Persp,* 118; 2:253-58, Feb 2010

• Petersen JH, et al. **Plasticizers in total diet samples, baby food and infant formulas,** *Food Addit Contam* 17; 2:133-41, 2000

• Midoro-Horiuti T, et al, Maternal **bisphenol A exposure promotes** the development of experimental **asthma** in mouse pups, *Environ Health Persp,* 118; 2:273-77, Feb 2010

• Kabuto H, et al, Exposure to **bisphenol A** during embryonic/fetal life and infancy and increases oxidative injury and **causes under-development of the brain and testes** in mice, *Life Sci* 74:2931-40, 2004

• Grun F, et al, **Endocrine disruptors as obesogens**, *Molecul Cell Endocrinol* 304:19-29, 2009

• Schonfelder G, et al Parental bisphenol A accumulation in the human maternal-fetal-placental unit, *Environ Health Perspect* 110:A703-07, 2002

Begin by Boosting Phthalate Detoxification

Fortunately, *Someone up there* knew we were going to poison ourselves in this era. By design, many natural nutrients repair and rescue the peroxisomes and mitochondria from phthalate poisoning. Cod liver oil (especially its DHA, and its vitamins A and D) can rescue them. Many other nutrients and even the main adrenal hormone, DHEA, have a role in repairing the 21st century environmental damage to peroxisomes.

One of the main pathways for the body to detoxify plastics is glucuronidation. And because you have become so smart, you logically ask, "How can I rev up glucuronidation?". Fortunately, for once my answer is pretty simple and do-able by everyone. For we **rev up glucuronidation by eating more brassica vegetables** (broccoli, cauliflower, brussels sprouts, kale, collard greens, rutabaga, turnips, radishes, mizuna, arugula, cilantro, and more). And nutrients like two **IndolPlex** and one or two **Calcium-D Glucarate** each twice a day rev up glucuronidation, one of the pathways to detoxify plastics as they enter the body (*TW*).

Many nutrients and food actually repair the damage to peroxisomes done by plasticizers. For example, DHA (part of

248

cod liver oil) is needed to repair the damage of phthalates. In fact many people need it separately in the additional form of a daily **Super DHA** to bring their levels up into the fifth quintile (Yamamoto, Halade). As you might guess by now, in some folks just the repair of the cell membranes with the proper amount of cod liver oil has not only cleared syndrome X, hypertriglyceridemia, diabetes, repaired damaged mitochondria, improved insulin secretion, obesity, and coronary artery disease, but cancelled dialysis by healing kidney disease, and much more. You get the idea that **if a diabetologist is not assaying and repairing your fatty acids, he's an absolute dinosaur.** And even sadder is the evidence you have seen that **fatty acids repair the peroxisomes and do a better job than the diabetes medications.** Plus much of this has been known for decades! It's not new (Storlien).

References:

• Yu YH, et al, The function of porcine PPAR gamma and dietary **fish oil effect on** the expression of lipid and **glucose** metabolism related **genes**, *J Nutr Biochem* 20:171-186, 2011

• Storlien LH, et al **Fish oil prevents insulin resistance induced by high-fat feeding** in rats, *Science* 237:885-8, **1987**

• Lombardo YD, et al, Effects of dietary polyunsaturated **n-3 fatty acids on** dyslipidemia and insulin resistance in rodents and humans. A review, *J Nutr Biochem* 17:1-13, 2006

• Yamamoto K, et al, Identification of putative metabolites of **docosahexaenoic acid as potent PPAR gamma agonist and antidiabetic agents**, *Bioorg Med Chem Lett* 15:517-22, 2005

• Halade GV, et al, Combination of conjugated linoleic acid with **fish oil prevents** age-associated bone marrow **adiposity** in C57B1/6J mice, *J Nutr Biochem* 22:459-69, 2011

The Next Step for Getting the Phthalates and Other Toxins Out

Congratulations! You have learned a huge amount about the healing of the impossible that the average physician is clueless about. If in doubt, test him. As you have learned, **ALC Powder** and **R-Lipoic Acid** are just a few nutrients that are paramount in healing diabetic mitochondria. But **phthalates poison the production of these two priceless nutrients in the mitochondria. Zinc is likewise crucial** in not only restoring insulin secretion, protecting the genetic DNA, converting B6 and

B-carotene to more active forms, detoxification, converting fatty acids to build membranes, as well as being in 200 other enzymes. **But phthalates poison zinc, ALC, and Lipoate.** I could go on with dozens of pathways that are poisoned by phthalates, keeping cure at an arm's length. Obviously we need an easy way to get rid of phthalates, and to do so forever, since daily we fight off over 3 mg that we can get just in our foods.

The far infrared sauna fills the bill, and there is never wasted time, because you can read in there and get smarter. I gave the evidence for it in *Detoxify Or Die*. So let me just update you with studies that have come out since, adding evidence that **the far infrared sauna is an indispensable tool in healing diabetes and its complications, as well as reversing other diseases and slowing down aging.** After over 40 years in medicine, I can vouch for its incomparable and necessary inclusion in medical treatments for folks focused on actual healing. To neglect to get rid the lifetime accumulation of phthalates, pesticides, VOH, PCB, PFOA, PBDE, dioxins, heavy metals, and other pollutants is to be forever ill. But, choose your far infrared sauna provider carefully.

I'm frequently asked if any old type of sauna will do. So let me start with the fact that **heart failure patients are among the first folks to die when there's a heat wave. Saunas would be very contraindicated** for folks that sensitive to heat. Yet the far infrared technology was not only safe for them, but produced no side effects. Best of all, it accomplished what medicine was incapable of doing. In studies done on the worst heart patients at the Cleveland Clinic **the far infrared sauna actually reversed congestive heart failure in patients for which medicine had nothing more to offer.** Furthermore, other parameters improved, like ejection fraction (strength of the heart beat), and **folks got off medications**. This rarely happens in the real life clinical situation.

Usually once a person is diagnosed with heart failure, specialists keep piling on medications. Even then heart failure only has a median survival of five years (making it worse than cancer with a

250

median survival of 6 years). These folks rarely get rid off any medications (and this chronic disease is not a deficiency of drugs anyway). Clearly, finding and fixing the underlying cause is not the focus of their physicians. Yet isn't it sad that something as simple as a far infrared sauna has reversed an epidemic "incurable" disease (CHF) that has a worse prognosis than cancer? And to make it even more implausible the studies were done at the Cleveland Clinic. Yet when I consult with readers and review their medical records from this very same clinic, these heart failure patients have *never* been advised of a far infrared sauna. But the research was done under their physicians' roof!

I must caution however, that if you're on **medications like beta blockers for hypertension as just one example, you may block your own sweating**. If you are on one you need to read *The High Blood Pressure Hoax* to learn how to counter them. Meanwhile, be sure to follow the protocols in *Detoxify Or Die* and **be sure you at least have an RBC magnesium that is in the third or higher quintile before you start any sauna**. Most people are dangerously low in magnesium and don't even know it. **There's no point in sweating out your last bit of magnesium and causing an arrhythmia, seizure or heart attack.** Another **common reason for not being able to sweat is previous pesticide poisoning.** I drove the tractor and sprayed the atrazine on our cornfields, so I didn't sweat for months, but these days I drench a beach towel in one hour in my FIR. I hope you can work into your schedule a daily **far infrared sauna** (FIR) forever. And look how much smarter you will become with that committed reading time.

References:

• Beever R, The effects of repeated thermal therapy on quality of life in patients with type II diabetes, *J Altern Compl Med*, 16; 6:677-81, 2010

• Kihara T, et al, Effects of repeated sauna treatment on ventricular arrhythmias in patients with chronic heart failure, *Cardiol J* 68:1146-51, 2004

• Beever R, **Far infrared saunas for treatment of cardiovascular risk factors**: Summary of the published evidence, *Can Fam Phys* 55:691-6, 2009

- Masuda A, et al, The effects of repeated thermal therapy for patients with chronic pain, *Psychother Psychosom* 74:288-94, 2005

- Kihara T, et al, Repeated **sauna treatment improves the vascular endothelial and cardiac function** in patients with chronic heart failure, *J Am Coll Cardiol*, 39:754-9, 2002

- Sugahara Y, et al, Efficacy and **safety** of thermal vasodilatation therapy by **sauna in infants with severe congestive heart failure** secondary to the ventricular septal defect, *Am J Cardiol* 92:109-113, 2003

- Miyamoto H, et al, Safety and efficacy of repeated sauna bathing in patients with chronic systolic heart failure: a preliminary report. *J Cardiac Failure* 11:432-6, 2005

- McCarty MF, et al, Regular **thermal therapy may promote insulin sensitivity** while boosting expression of endothelial nitric oxide synthase -- Effects comparable to those of exercise training, *Med Hypoth* 73:103-5, 2009

- Nguyen Y, et al, Sauna as a therapeutic option for cardiovascular disease, *Cardiol Rev* 12:321-4, 2004

- Masuda A, et al, Repeated **sauna therapy reduces urinary 8-epi-prostaglandin** F2a, *Jpn Heart J*, 45:297-303, 2004

- Imamura M, et al, Repeated thermal therapy improves impaired vascular endothelial function in patients with coronary risk factors, *J Am Coll Cardiol* 38:1083-8, 2001

- Roehm DC, Effect of the program of **sauna** baths and megavitamins on adipose DDE and PCBs and on **clearing symptoms of agent orange (dioxin) toxicity**, *Clin Res* 31:243, 1983

- Biro S, et al, Clinical implications of thermal therapy and lifestyle-related diseases, *Exper Biol Med* 228:1245-49, 2003

- Perreault M, et al, Mechanism of impaired nitric oxide synthase in skeletal muscle of streptozotocin-induced diabetic rats, *Diabetologia* 43:427-37, 2000

- Kawaura A, et al, The effect of leg hyperthermia using **far infrared rays in bed-ridden subjects with type 2 diabetes mellitus**, *Acta Med Okayama*, 64; 2:143-7, 2010

- Kokura S, et al, **Whole body hyperthermia improves obesity-induced insulin resistance in diabetic** mice, *Internat J Hyperthermia* 23:259-65, 2007

- Davi G, et al, In vivo formation of **8-iso-prostaglandin F2a and platelet activation in diabetes mellitus**, *Circulation* 99:224-9, 1999

What About the Other Pollutants?

A vast number of toxins can cause diabetes, and in fact many diseases (Grun). Every cardiac abnormality can be caused by environmental pollutants (Park). Our PCBs, dioxins, VOH volatile organic hydrocarbons, PBDE flame retardants (foolishly legislated into mattresses), PFOA (Teflon®-type stain-resistant, non-stick chemicals, a known cause of not only diabetes, but recalcitrant obesity, hypothyroidism, high cholesterol, cancer, and many others) **make us the most polluted population in the history of**

the planet. And it is ever increasing for we don't even think about the electronic waste (E-waste) that has emerged as a critical global environmental health issue. Incineration of keyboards, computers, printers, copiers, laptops, etc., puts huge amounts of lead, mercury, and cadmium, as well as chromium, flame retardants, PBDE's, PCB, PAH, and much more as well as plasticizers into the air. And they all have the capacity to cause not only diabetes but damage brain function (Chen, Brun). And think of the disease-potential when *several* of these are combined in the body, *as happens in real life.* Only lab animals are given *one* pollutant at a time. No wonder inferior studies proclaim safety.

Environmental chemicals have such a huge range of damage in the human body that Luscious has organized five rooms of data for me. **Environmental chemicals** especially damage glands, not only pancreas, but thyroid, adrenal, pituitary, testes, ovaries and more. Clearly they **can cause every disease including diabetes** (Cox). They **are inescapable** in the air we breathe and the foods we eat (Schecter). Even the very medications that physicians prescribe can accumulate as toxic residues long after we have stopped them, when they are incompletely detoxified (Cecchini).

Dozens of countries have produced beautiful research which shows time and again that **the sudden worldwide epidemic of diabetes is caused at least in part and in many people by mere environmental pollutants** (Ruzzin). Remember, I focus on phthalates because they are the most ubiquitously unavoidable pollutants, and in the heaviest amounts in all humans. But unfortunately there are literally thousands of other chemicals. **And I repeat many facts for you here because this book is most probably the most thorough documentation of the dangers of environmental pollutants that you will find anywhere**. I certainly have not seen anything that even comes close. Yet because you are not chemists, I am trying to make learning as easy as possible for you. *I'm so proud of you because you now know* *more about the healing of diabetes and other "incurable" diseases than 99% of physicians.*

Some scientists merely call environmental toxins **POPs** (persistent organic pollutants), but they include everything from industrial dioxins to pesticides, and much more. These all **clearly poison membrane mitochondrial and peroxisome functions, creating diabetes, insulin resistance, obesity (that will not move) and even some of the newer diseases like NASH** (non-alcoholic steatohepatitis or fatty liver syndrome). These diseases are all diabetes precursors and have all reached alarming worldwide proportions. Yet **scientists unschooled in environmental medicine are perplexed as to the origin of these epidemics**, as countless newspaper and medical journal articles repeatedly prove.

Not only do the phthalates clearly damage pancreatic cells and create insulin resistance, but **diabetics have far more chemicals on board than the average** person (Lee). That's why I was strongly motivated to write a book for not only dynamo physicians but dynamo lay people to show them how to get these chemicals out. It's the only way to reverse disease and **turn back the hands of time**, making many people (myself included) even healthier than we ever were before. It's absolutely essential at this point in time on this planet, and needs to be continued for a lifetime.

Another deadly common unavoidable pollutant in the human body is a category called **PCBs** which have a half-life in the human body of 10 to 15 years (Ritter). And just something as simple as diesel exhaust not only can raise diabetic "danger" indicators, but create inflammation in other organs like the lung, not to mention neurodegenerative disorders like Alzheimer's, arteriosclerosis, and other inflammatory diseases (Reynolds). Or **triclosan** is also in most all humans and can cause anything from diabetes or lung cancer to dementia or allergies, and much more. Even though most have never heard of it, **triclosan is commonly used to prevent bacterial and mold growth in consumer products like soaps, laundry detergents, toothpaste, deodorant, facial tissues, and**

254

plastic kitchen utensils (Clayton). Do you get the picture? Their secret accumulation is unavoidable.

In brief, **most common disease begins with nutritional deficiencies** that you've learned about, especially minerals, vitamins and fatty acids. **The next most common causes are the world's toxins** like plasticizers, pesticides, industrial exhaust hydrocarbon fumes, heavy metals, etc. And don't forget that **many prescription drugs damage pancreatic function**. For example, some drugs for schizophrenia trigger diabetes, while Trilipix for triglycerides can not only have a side effect of pancreatitis but pancreatic cancers. And of course any long-acting medications, dental glues, as well as stents are usually impregnated with a plastic (phthalate, methacrylate) polymer.

Not only environmental chemicals like air pollution from traffic, but infections, molds and allergies as well as many other triggers can contribute to the widespread damage in the human body that we call diabetes. You can name any common pollutants and find proof that they can damage the body chemistry sufficiently to create diabetes, just alone by themselves (not to forget that we have hundreds in combination in us). For example, Air Force veterans who were exposed to dioxins, or folks who consume fish from the Great Lakes are more contaminated with organochlorines pesticides which can raise their vulnerability and multiply the damage produced by other pollutants. The evidence is endless.

References:

• Lee, DH, et al, **Low dose of some persistent organic pollutants predicts type II diabetes**: a nested case-controlled study, *Environ Health Perspect* 118; 9: 1235-42, 2010

• Ritter R, et al, Intrinsic human limitation half-lives of polychlorinated biphenyls derived from the temporal evolution of cross sectional biomonitoring data from the United Kingdom, *Environ Health Persp* 119:225-31, 2011

• Reynolds PR, et al, Diesel particulate matter induces receptor for advanced glycation end-products (RAGE) expression in pulmonary epithelial cells and RAGE signaling influences NF-kB-mediated inflammation, *Environ Health Persp* 119:332-6, 2011

• Clayton EMR, et al, The impact of bisphenol A and **triclosan on immune** parameters in the U.S. population, NHANES 2003-2006, *Environ Health Persp* 119:390-6, 2011

• Post GB, et al, Occurrence and potential significance of perfluorooctanoic acid (**PFOA**) detected in **New Jersey public drinking water systems**, *Environ Sci Technol* 43:4547-54, 2009

• Schecter A, et al, **Polybrominated diphenyl ethers (PBDE)** and hexabromocyclodecane (HPCD) in composite **US food** samples, *Environ Health Persp* 118:357-62, 2010

• Schecter A, et al, **Perfluorinated compounds, polychlorinated biphenyls, and organochlorine pesticide contamination in composite food samples** from Dallas Texas USA, *Environ Health Persp* 118:796-802, 2010

• Cox SK, et al, Prevalence of self-reported diabetes and exposure to organochlorine pesticides among Mexican Americans. Hispanic Health and Nutrition Examination Survey 1982-1984, *Environ Health Persp* 115:1747-52, 2007

• Van Leeuwen SPJ, et al, Halogenated **contaminants in farmed salmon, trout, tilapia,** pangasius, and **shrimp,** *Environ Sci Technol* 43:4009-15, 2009

• Chen A, et a, Developmental **neurotoxins in e-waste**: an emerging health concern, *Environ Health Persp* 119:431-8, 2011

• Park SK, et al, Particulate **air pollution, metabolic syndrome and heart rate** variability. The multi-ethnic study of atherosclerosis (MESA), *Environ Health Persp* 118:1406-11, 2010

• Jones OA, et al, **Environmental pollution and diabetes**: a neglected Association, *Lancet* 371; 9609:287-88, 2008

• Lopez-Carrillo L, et al, Exposure to **phthalates and breast cancer** risk in Northern Mexico, *Environ Health Persp* 118:539-544, 2010

• Lee DH, et al, A stronger dose-response relation between serum concentrations of persistent organic **pollutants and diabetes**: results from the National Health and Examination Survey 1999-2002, *Diabetes Care*, 29; 7:1 1638-44, July 2006

• Remillard RB, et al, **Linking dioxins to diabetes**: epidemiology and biologic plausibility, *Environ Health Persp* 110; 9:853-8, 2002

• Lang IA, et al, **Association of urinary bisphenol A concentration with medical disorders** and laboratory abnormalities and adults, *J Am Med Assoc* 300; 11:1303-10, 2008

• Cecchini M, et al, **Drug residues stored in the body** following cessation of use: impacts on neuroendocrine balance and behavior -- use of the Hubbard **sauna regimen to remove toxins and restore health,** *Med Hypoth* 68; 4:868-79, 2007

• Fujiyoshi PT, et al, Molecular epidemiologic **evidence of diabetogenic effects of dioxin** exposure in US Air Force veterans of the Vietnam War, *Environ Health Persp,* 114; 11:1677-83, 2006

• Hyman M, **Environmental toxins, obesity, and diabetes**: an emerging risk factor, *Altern Therap* 16; 2:56-8, Mar/Apr 2010

• Longnecker MP, et al, Serum **dioxin levels in relation to diabetes mellitus among Air Force veterans** with background levels of exposure, *Epidemiol,* 11; 1:44-8, 2000

• Turyk M, et al, Organochlorine exposure and incidence of diabetes in the cohort of Great Lakes sport fish consumers, *Environ Health Perspect,* 117:1076-82, 2009

• Alonso-Magdalena P, et al, **Bisphenol A exposure during pregnancy disrupts glucose** homeostasis in mothers and **adult male offspring**, *Environ Health Perspect* 118; 9:1243-50, 2010

• Fernandez, M, et al, Neonatal exposure to **bisphenol A** and reproductive and **endocrine** alterations resembling the **polycystic ovarian syndrome** in adult rats, *Environ Health Perspect* 118; 9: 1217-22, 2010

256

- Codru N, et al, **Diabetes in relation to serum levels of polychlorinated biphenyls and chlorinated pesticides** in adult Native Americans, *Environ Health Persp* 115; 10:1442-7, 2007

- Turyk M, Prevalence of **diabetes and body burdens of polychlorinated biphenyls, polybrominated diphenyl ethers and p,p-diethyldichloroethane in Great Lakes sport fish consumers**, *Chemosphere* 75; 5:674-9, 2009

- Ruzzin J, et al, **Persistent organic pollutant exposure leads to insulin resistance syndrome**, *Environ Health Persp* 118:465-71, 2010

The Heavy Metal Connection

What else can cause diabetes? Anything that damages (1) pancreatic function, and (2) insulin receptors, and (3) the chemistry inside mitochondria where energy is made from sugars, and/or (4) the peroxisomes that control their genes. Heavy metals include arsenic, cadmium, lead, aluminum, and mercury (which I've written about extensively in *The High Blood Pressure Hoax*). They are the last bastion of environmental pollutants that must be removed in order to cure resistant diseases. In other words, **when folks are at their wits' end and cannot heal, it is usually because no one assayed and got rid of the heavy metals.**

As an example other than diabetes, heavy metals can create "undiagnosable" neurologic problems, like ALS, MS, Parkinson's, Alzheimer's, motor neuron disease, etc. And like all the other pollutants, they are ubiquitous and unavoidable, but they usually require more than just far infrared sauna. **Lead is one example of a heavy metal we all harbor that damages fatty acid chemistry** (plus it damages the phospholipids that carry the fatty acids piggy-back to the mitochondria, and more). This in turn damages the membranes and receptors, causing hypertension, kidney disease and other symptoms that never get better until you *get the lead out* (Patrick).

Lead is a good example that I have referenced voluminously where the government's "norm" of 10 mcg/dL has been shown to cause a drop in I.Q. and intelligence (Canfield). Or recall from *The Cholesterol Hoax*, and *TW*, and other examples where government standards for "norms" often lag decades behind the evidence in the scientific literature. For example, the government makes labs say that normal lead is up to 250 ppb, which is insanely archaic and literally flaunts the ignorance of everyone associated with that designation (this has been highly referenced in the previous *TW* issues). That is even more reason for the functional assays of the **ION Panel** (organic acids with quintiles) and **Porphyrins.** More on that later.

As another example of an unavoidable heavy metal, over 13 million Americans are exposed to higher levels of arsenic just through public water systems from industry, mining, etc. (Fu). Just this heavy-metal alone causes everything from cancer (that is resistant to chemotherapy) to arteriosclerosis, high blood pressure, and.... you guessed it, diabetes. And arsenic can cause insulin resistance. Plus just like other pollutants that have far-reaching damages through their induction of reactive oxygen species, arsenic is no exception. **Arsenic is an example of a heavy metal in all of us that can damage pancreatic function, impair insulin secretion, glutathione detoxification and leads to the many side effects of diabetes. And it damages the very mitochondria that are needed to regulate and heal the pancreas.**

References:

•   Navas-Acien A, et al, **Arsenic exposure and prevalence of type II diabetes** in US adults, *J Am Med Assoc* 300:814-22, 2008
•   Fu J, et al, Low-level **arsenic impairs glucose stimulated insulin** secretion in pancreatic beta cells: involvement of cellular adaptive response to oxidative stress, *Environ Health Persp* 118:864-70, 2010

•   Navas-Acien A, et al, **Arsenic exposure and type II diabetes**: a systematic review of the experimental and epidemiologic **evidence**, *Environ Health Persp* 114:641-48, 2006

•   Diaz-Villasenor A, et al, Sodium **arsenite impairs insulin secretion** and transcription in pancreatic beta cells, *Toxicol Appl Pharm* 214:30-34, 2006

•   Paul DS, et al, Molecular mechanisms of the **diabetogenic effects of arsenic**: inhibition of insulin signaling by arsenite and methyl arsonous acid, *Environ Health Persp* 115:734-42, 2007

•   Wollheim CB, et al, Beta cell **mitochondria and insulin** secretion: messenger role of nucleotides and metabolites, *Diabetes 51* (supple 1): S. 37-S. 42, 2002

•   Chen CJ, et al, **Arsenic and diabetes and hypertension** in human populations: a review, *Toxicol Appl Pharmacol* 222:298-304, 2007

- Patrick L, Lead toxicity part II: the role of free radical damage and the use of antioxidants in the pathology and treatment of lead toxicity, *Altern Med Rev* 11; 2:114-127, 2006)

- Kramer U, et al, Traffic-related **air pollution and incident type II diabetes**: results from the SALIA Cohort Study, *Environ Health Perspect* 118; 9: 1273-79, 2010

- Brooke RD, et al., The relationship between **diabetes mellitus and traffic related air pollution**, *J Occup Environ Med*, 50:32-38, 2008

- Lockwood AH, **Diabetes and air pollution**, *Diabetes Care* 25:1487-88, 2002

- O'Neill MS, et al, **Diabetes enhances vulnerability** to particulate air pollution-associated impairment in vascular reactivity and endothelial function, *Circulation* 111:2 913-20, 2005

- Sun Q, et al, Ambient **air pollution exaggerates adipose inflammation and insulin resistance** in a mouse model of diet-induced obesity, *Circulation* 119:538-46, 2009

- Navas-Acien A, et al, Rejoinder: **Arsenic exposure and prevalence of type II diabetes**: updated findings from the National Health Nutrition and Examination Survey 2003-2006, 20:816-20, 2009

- Canfield RL, et al, **Intellectual impairment in children with blood lead concentrations below 10** mcg per deciliter, *New Engl J Med* 348; 16:1517-26, **2003**

- Lanphear BP, et al, **Low-level environmental lead exposure and children's intellectual function**: an international pooled analysis, *Environ Health Persp* 205 113; 7:894-99, 2005

- Shannon M, et al, Chelation therapy in children exposed to lead, *New Engl J Med* 345:16:1212-13, 2001

- Schnaas L, et al, **Reduced intellectual development in children with prenatal lead exposure**, *Environ Health Persp* 114; 5:791-7, 2006

- Chen A, et al, **Improving behavior of lead-exposed children**: micro nutrient supplementation, chelation or prevention. *J Ped* 147; 5:570-1, 2005

- Dietrich KN, et al, Effect of chelation therapy on neuropsychological and **behavioral** development of **lead exposed children** after school entry, *Ped* 114; 1:19-26, 2004

- Lin-Tan DT, et al, Long-term outcome of repeatedly chelation and therapy in progressive non-diabetic chronic kidney diseases, *Nephrol Dialysis Transplant* 2007

Treatment of Hypertension
Without Attention to Heavy Metals is Archaic

Here is a question submitted by a reader for *TW*:

Q. I asked my doctor to check my cadmium and other heavy metals because I have high blood pressure in addition to my diabetes. I really do not want to take the medications he prescribed because they make me feel awful. I can't think straight and ache with the Lipitor, I'm weak and have palpitations when I take the diuretic, and the beta blocker atenolol makes me depressed. Help me convince him.

259

A. It is dangerously archaic to ignore finding the correctable causes of hypertension in this era with all that is known, and heavy metals are a huge cause of it. But remember a vast majority of folks can permanently cure their hypertension with lot simpler things such as the **Arginine Powder** and **Chelated Magnesium**. Many others may need to add the membrane "oil change" nutrients, so fundamental to healing, that you learned about here. Of course the **Cardio/ION** is the best test for identifying those deficiencies, all at once. Then once you have normalized your pressure you won't need medications and you can take your sweet old time in getting rid of the heavy metals yourself.

I recommend testing heavy metals (the protocols in *The High Blood Pressure Hoax*) *only* for folks and physicians who are highly unknowledgeable and need convincing. Since you are neither and we *all* carry heavy metals, I would just go ahead and start getting rid of the heavy metals beginning with the protocols in *Detoxify Or Die*. You may then want to use the gentler heavy-metal detox, **Pectasol** (see the kids' detox section), before progressing to the more aggressive protocols in *The High Blood Pressure Hoax*.

I added a few references for you so that you can prove to him that mercury, cadmium, lead, arsenic, aluminum, nickel, and many other heavy metals are frequently the root causes of hypertension. If not treated, they can progress to cause serious kidney disease which can entail a lifetime of dialysis and be lethal. As well, untreated heavy metals can then cause cancers. For example, **cadmium or arsenic can trigger prostate cancer and even make it chemotherapy resistant**. If he is still not convinced by this and lending him the book, I'd say you have a dead-end dinosaur and should keep shopping for a Dr. Dynamo-type guy, interested in helping you cure your hypertension.

References:

• Engel RR, et al, **Vascular effects of chronic arsenic** exposure: a review, *Epidemiol Rev* 16; 2:184-209, 1994

- Navas-Acien A, et al, **Lead exposure and cardiovascular disease** -- -- a systematic review, *Environ Health Persp* 115:472-82, 2007

- Houston MC, The role **of mercury and cadmium heavy metals in vascular disease, hypertension, coronary heart disease, and myocardial infarction,** *Altern Ther Health Med* 13;2: S128-S133, 2007

- Mordukhovich I, et al, Associations of toenail **arsenic, cadmium, mercury, manganese, and lead with blood pressure** in the Normative Aging Study, *Environ Health Persp* 120:98-104, 2012

- Vinceti M, et al, Case-controlled study of toenail **cadmium and prostate cancer** risk in Italy, *Sci Total Environ* 373; 1:77-81, 2007

Nix on IV Chelation

Just because we are all loaded with heavy metals, don't fall for IV chelation. As described in more detail in *The High Blood Pressure Hoax*, **(1) non-IV chelation described there is actually five times cheaper, and (2) safer than IV, (3) does not require a prescription, and (4) can be individually-tailored to the person's chemistry.** And most importantly this protocol **(5) does not load you up with diabetes-producing phthalates (plasticizers) and heart-damaging cyclohexanones, both of which come out of chelation IV tubing.** One caveat is that recently the FDA has made the non-prescription detox suppositories in that book prescription. So your physician can use any of the many compounding pharmacies in former books and *TW* to make them. Why the ruling changed in this era of unprecedented insidious heavy metal poisoning boggles the mind, since this has been an FDA-approved food additive for over 50 years. Such is the politics of medicine.

And even though chelators like EDTA can slow down unwanted clotting and reduce calcification in arteries, the combined effect of many nutrients like vitamins K2, D3, magnesium, enzymes, and much more are essential in reducing arterial calcifications (details described in *The Cholesterol Hoax*). Another adverse effect of IV chelation with EDTA that I did not detail in *The High Blood Pressure Hoax* is that **EDTA given by IV push can break up biofilms, thereby releasing millions of organisms into your system at once.** If you have not been properly prepared to fight

261

them before-hand, you can end up being much worse (details in *TW* 2011). There's no substitute for a properly trained, well-read and motivated physician (which is why I've supplied you with many surreptitious tests of his knowledge for you in here).

Most chelations cost about $150 per session, are done 2-4 times a week over 1-4 hours (depending on technique), and force usually 3000 mg of EDTA through your brain, liver, etc., whether you are a 120 lb. woman or 230 lb. man. Then to make matters worse, most chelators give a standard cocktail afterwards of low-dose minerals, but do not measure the RBC minerals to see if they are correct for that person. They rarely **do a Cardio/ION beforehand**, either, **to determine if the patient's detox system is properly repaired in order to withstand the chelation without harm**. There have been deaths from IV chelation (references in 2010 *TW*). The bottom line? Suppository and oral forms are far preferable to IV, plus they are cheaper, safer, save time, and are more individualized.

Furthermore, new dangers have been discovered from the plastics of intravenous (IV) tubings: they hasten death in another way. When folks are on death's doorstep they're given IV (intravenous) medications in ICU, cardiac bypass surgery, or renal dialysis (kidney bypass). These life-saving procedures always require a lot of plastic bags and plastic tubing and plastic connectors. Researchers at Johns Hopkins University School of Medicine have shown that **a chemical inside these harmless-appearing plastic IV tubes accelerates disease and death**. It raises blood pressure, poisons the heart, creates arrhythmias, body swelling and even heart death. It's worse than the phthalates.

The chemical is **cyclohexanone, which is an organic solvent used in making polyvinyl chloride (PVC) medical devices. It turns out it even <u>kills quicker than the plasticizers or phthalates</u> that IVs also contain and emit**. Remember that **the chelation protocols in *The High Blood Pressure Hoax* are safer, cheaper, non-prescription, and done at home. And they are done** without loading your body with plasticizers from IVs. Furthermore, on the flipside, IV chelation forces a huge dose that is not titrated to your system through your brain, liver and heart, as well as kidneys with the potential of damaging any of these crucial organs. I recommend it only in emergency situations.

For now clearly, IV chelation not only loads you up with phthalates, but cyclohexanone which is an even more potent organ killer. No wonder folks who enter the hospital in a depleted condition who have been on many IV medications often die there. Or when they get home they never seem to rally ever again. The chemicals from the IVs are the last straw that have broken the camel's back. This is all the more reason to do your daily detoxification in as many ways as possible. Periodically review *Detoxify Or Die*, then *The High Blood Pressure Hoax*, then The *Cholesterol Hoax* as well as keeping up with your *TW* newsletter. For example, remember to **use the disappearance of the odor of urine sulfurs to be your guide that it is safe to give your next dose of DMSA** (*TW*). Let your body's metabolism guide you, not the "one dose fits all" protocols. You need to keep yourself as updated, protected and detoxed as much as possible, because you never know when adversity like an auto accident might strike. And of course, a detoxed body is essential for slowing down aging and the development of any disease.

References:

• Thompson-Torgerson CS, et al, **Cyclohexanone contamination** from extracorporeal circuits impairs cardiovascular function, *Am J Physiol Heart Circ Physiol*, 296: H1926-32, 2009

• Gondry E, The toxicity of cyclohexylamine, **cyclohexanone**, cyclohexanol, **metabolites** of **cyclamates**, *Eur J Toxicol* 5:227-38, 1972

• Bunin E, et al, **Chelator-induced dispersal** and killing of Pseudomonas aeruginosa cells **in a biofilm**, *Appl Environ Microbiol*, 72; 3:2064-69, 2006

Detoxification For Kids and Fragile Adults

"Just give me something easy to do!". I hear this all the time. The best detox protocol is the oral DMSA (Captomer) and EDTA suppositories (Detoxamin, recently needing a compounding pharmacy's Rx, since the government has decided to repeatedly punish manufacturers of this food additive that the FDA itself has approved for 50 years!). The protocols are in *The High Blood Pressure Hoax*. But for adults who are yet too fragile for the ultimate detox protocols or who are unable to check their detox capability and mineral repleteness (that should precede those protocols), here is a gentler option.

Let's focus on kids' health and how we can safely begin their necessary detox, although this is just as applicable for the fragile adult. For as research has shown, children are on a faster track of deterioration than adults. **Kids now by age 6 often have toxin levels that it used to take us until ages 35-40 to accumulate**. Of course, everything you learn can be adapted to multiple types of folks. But this detox nutrient is especially applicable also to those whose bodies are just too toxic for the stronger protocols in *The High Blood Pressure Hoax*, or who are just not ready yet for such intensive heavy metal detox.

In the books and previous *TW*s I've presented the overwhelmingly clear evidence that resistant diseases of every type have a component of heavy metal toxicity. In fact for many folks, **getting rid of heavy metals has been the pivotal issue that has taken them out of the quagmire of illness into the realm of wellness**. Many of them, myself included, have experienced loss of lifelong symptoms that we had erroneously thought we were saddled with for the rest of our lives. They have ranged from allergies, osteoporosis, arthritis (even rheumatoid), colitis, arrhythmias, tremors, weakness and nerve pain to MS, Alzheimer's and cancer, as just a few examples.

For children, the problem is more urgent. Why? Because they are more toxic at an earlier age than we were. This reflects that our planet has the highest concentration of chemicals ever known. This is giving children diseases that used to be seen only in adults, like "adult onset diabetes". But more importantly, they are unprecedentedly toxic at a point in life when they can least handle it. **Their immune systems are immature and their brains need to be free of toxins as brain parts are developing that determine their futures.**

Caution: whenever there is the interference of heavy metals in children, enough to cause a disease label, this means the developing brain may not reach its full potential. In *TW* I've given huge evidence of the hidden lead toxicity in kids, partly perpetuated by government steadfastly erroneous "normal" values, that ignore years of research. We already see this in the offspring of accomplished folks whose kids are not "a chip off the old block", but under-achievers. Sometimes it's just a case of uninformed parents who have no idea that the steady diet of trans fats, canola oil, modified food starch, aspartame, corn syrup (HFCS) sodas and phthalates, Teflon, aluminum, etc., that they feed their children have any bearing on brain function. On the flip side, those wise enough to provide brain-generating foods and nutrients have no toxin-knowledgeable pediatricians to partner with them in detoxifying their children. So let's look at a safer solution.

When you peel an orange you pretty much leave the white inner peel or pulp behind, called citrus pectin. But this fiber has unique properties. D-galacturonic acid is the principal sugar in citrus pectin, yet is usually insoluble and a good source of fiber in the gut. When it is modified or broken down into smaller molecular form it can be absorbed and has even turned off cancer metastases (as Pienta referenced in the *Journal of the National Cancer Institute,* and more evidence in *TW* 2010).

265

Well, **modified citrus pectin (MCP)** has even more interesting properties. It **has reduced the absorption of heavy metals in the gut. And once absorbed into the system it produces negatively charged D-galacturonic acid residues that become cation chelators, pulling heavy metals out into the urine and stool.** The interesting part is that in *short-term* studies **it does not lower the "good" minerals, such as zinc and magnesium**, as examples, like more potent forms of chelation do.

Furthermore, combined with **alginates, better known as sea vegetables** or more exactly brown algae kelp (*laminaria* species), there is even **further intestinal removal of heavy metals**. And again this is accomplished with selective binding of heavy metals without binding of the essential minerals. In fact, nature uses algae in waters to clean them, while food manufacturers use them to remove heavy metals from food-grade oils. Furthermore, alginates have enhanced the removal of other nasty unavoidable disease-producing environmental toxins like dioxins, hidden in our air, food, and water.

So I can hear many of you saying "Enough already! Just give us the bottom line of how to use it". O.K. (see how pliable I am?). For starters, consider a child who is on something like the **Scooter Rabbit Chewable** multiple vitamin-mineral maintenance and a daily **Happy Bodies Detox Cocktail**. Adding 2-4 **PectaSol Chelation Complex** twice a day (containing this unique alginate and modified citrus pectin) could slowly and safely lower his heavy-metal burden. After devouring the evidence, I think kids in this unprecedentedly toxic era should be on this as soon as they can handle a capsule. And there is always the option of opening the capsule and mixing the powder contents with applesauce or other disguises. I have also observed older adults lowering their heavy metals slowly (and without adverse symptoms or dramatic lowering of their minerals, as can happen with chelation).

So there you have it. Most any adult can certainly handle 2-3 **PectaSol Chelation Complex** 2-3 times a day on an empty stomach. What could be easier? You can see from the smattering of overwhelming evidence here that we clearly have to detoxify forever (and I'll be keeping you updated in future *TW* issues on newer detoxification methods).

References:

• Zhao ZY, et al, The role of **modified citrus pectin as an effective chelator of lead in children** hospitalized with toxic lead levels, *Alternative Therapies* 14; 4:34-38, 2008

• Eliaz I, et al, The effect of **modified citrus pectin on urinary excretion of toxic elements**, *Phytotherapy Research*, 20; 10:859-64, 2006

• Eliaz I, et al, Integrative medicine and the role of **modified citrus pectin/alginate in heavy metal chelation and detoxification**---five case reports, *Forschende Komplementarmedizin* 14:358-64, 2007

• Pienta KJ, et al, **Inhibition of spontaneous metastasis** in a rat prostate cancer model by administration of **modified citrus pectin**, *Journal National Cancer Institute* 87:348-53, 1995

• Brown MJ, et al, Deaths resulting from hypocalcemia after administration of edentate disodium: 2003-2005, *Pediatrics,* 118; 2:e534-6, Aug 2006

• Centers for Disease Control and Prevention (CDC), **Deaths associated with** hypocalcemia from **chelation** therapy -- -- Texas, Pennsylvania, and Oregon, 2003-2005, *MMWR Morbidity Mortality Weekly Reports* 55; 8:204-7, Mar 2006

• Aozasa O, et al, Enhancement in fecal excretion of dioxin isomer in mice by several dietary fibers, *Chemosphere* 45:195-200, 2001

Slow Down Aging and Get Rid of Fatigue

Fatigue, tiredness, exhaustion, no libido, no interest, and no initiative are such common problems that they are often not even mentioned when someone has a physical. And why are physicians not focused on these? Because there are no drugs for them. And as an example of one hidden cause, in previous 2009 *TW* I showed you how most physicians are using the wrong cut-off, so they are missing the diagnosis of hidden hypothyroidism. Assuming that you have already read and taken care of your thyroid, let's look at another very common yet hidden cause of exhaustion.

Again it's another gland and again it's also poisoned mainly by the plasticizers. This time the gland is the **adrenal gland**, actually two, as one sits on top of each kidney, as you learned in Chapter 5. Also called the **stress gland**, adrenals make a number of hormones without which we absolutely cannot live. One hormone is **DHEA** (dehydroepiandrosterone), not to be confused with an extremely important omega-3 fatty acid that has cured Alzheimer's and heart disease, DHA (docosahexanoic acid).

Studies show that when researchers give rats **plasticizers to determine the effects in humans, plasticizers actually shrink the adrenal glands** (Seo). And of course the plasticizers in the studies did a lot more, such as **damage a specific gene (we measure it as 8-OHdG or 8-hydroxy-2-deoxyguanosine in the Cardio/ION) that leads to cancer**, as well as lower detoxifying glutathione, which also leads to cancer.

And as usual, **plasticizers can damage the adrenal or stress gland in more than one way**. They can damage calcium signaling so that we do not make enough stress hormone. When they simultaneously damage calcium signaling in the heart (creating high blood pressure or arrhythmia or heart failure), we just slap people on calcium channel blockers like Norvasc® (evidence in 2011 *TW*). Recall, those **drugs (calcium channel blockers) actually cause the brain to shrink within 5 years as the intellect rots away**. But no worry. Everyone just chalks it up to normal aging. And the plasticizers damage other receptors in the adrenal that normally enable adrenal gland cells to talk to one another. Unfortunately, research shows that this **adrenal gland damage occurs at very low doses of plasticizers, lower than the doses we get daily just in foods**.

So what can you do if you are chronically exhausted and you don't know if your adrenal gland has been poisoned by the plastics that are the most ubiquitously unavoidable pollutant in the human body? First you can measure its #1 hormone, DHEA (dehydroepiandrosterone). I like the **Adrenal Stress Panel,** a salivary test that can be done at home using just your saliva ("spit"), so no blood draw is necessary. Even though I would prefer that you measure your nutrient levels and fix what's broken so you can make more of your own hormone, there's nothing wrong with temporarily using 1-3 **DHEA 25 mg** daily while you get organized (but don't be on it for the test). There are a few caveats such as women can develop more facial hair as they may increase their testosterone levels, while men increase their estrogen levels. But both sexes improve the IGF-1 (insulin-like growth factor). Anyway, your doctor can easily measure your DHEA and other adrenal hormones via the **Adrenal Stress Panel**. You only need to have your doctor (or chiropractor) order the test (or order on your own through *directlabs.com*). A clue for low DHEA can also be a low testosterone and an elevated sex hormone binding globulin on your **Cardio/ION**.

You might also want to do a trial of **DHEA**. To determine how you feel, 25 mg once or twice a day is a normal starting dose and you can get it without a prescription (intensivenutrition.com or 1-800-333-7414). Because DHEA can also be metabolized into testosterone, it often helps libidos. But *if women get too much facial hair they definitely want to drop their dose back*. Best of all, **DHEA has also rescued the peroxisomes, those crucial gene/ cell/mitochondrial controllers poisoned by phthalates.**

One particular disease where **DHEA replacement can make a profound difference is diabetes. It lowers the amount of insulin some need, makes the blood vessels healthier, and can lower blood pressure.** And that is just for starters. Clearly if you have **fatigue** complicating any disease, you need to know the status of your adrenal secretions. **DHEA can lower the hemoglobin A1C** (Brignardello). Not only do we make less DHEA as we get older, but our nutrient deficiencies and toxicities accelerate this problem. As much as **77% of diabetics are deficient in DHEA** (Ponikowska), while **having a low DHEA triples the death rat**e (Cappola). And when you think about it, it is logical, since phthalates create diabetes as well as target *all* glands. A sluggish adrenal robs you of the joy of life.

Obviously you do not want to take a hormone indefinitely, since it gives you feedback inhibition on the gland (you stop making hormone because there is enough in your bloodstream from the pill). But using this as a diagnostic trial to tell you the adrenal has suffered is priceless. And it can tide you over while you **repair your gland and cell receptors** by detoxifying them. So since **the adrenal is another stealth target of environmental toxins**, if you are exhausted and nobody can figure it out, consider a hidden adrenal deficiency, …. and especially if you already have diabetes!

I've even seen **type I diabetics drastically reduce their insulin or type II diabetics even get rid of their medications with DHEA** supplementation, depending upon the individual. In a study even in the *Journal of the American Medical Association*, researchers showed how **DHEA is important in the prevention and treatment of metabolic syndrome** as well as abdominal obesity (Villareal). Yet I rarely see it measured in diabetics.

I know we've talked about this before, but the reason I bring it up again is **DHEA** also has another role. It actually activates or starts to **repair the peroxisomes damaged by phthalates. This in turn starts to improve the function of the mitochondria** and revs up the action of insulin and decreases the side effects of diabetes. In fact this is one of the mechanisms of many prescription diabetes medications, to boost the peroxisome receptors. But as with any medications, you saw the side effects. In contrast, nutrients and hormones merely have multiple good effects. Even though **the DHEA hormone level dwindles with age and is paramount to healing diabetes and other damaged metabolisms**, and even though this was published in the *Journal of the American Medical Association* nearly a decade ago, and the information has been known for over two decades, it shows you the power of the drug industry, since most dinosaur diabetes doctors never check it.

References:

• Ponikowska B, et al, Gonadal and **adrenal androgen deficiencies as independent predictors of increased cardiovascular mortality in men with type II diabetes mellitus** and stable coronary artery disease, *Internat J Cardiol*, April 21, 2009

270

• Brignardello E, et al, **Dehydroepiandrosterone** administration conteracts oxidative imbalance and advanced glycation product formation **in type II diabetic patients**, *Diabetic Care*, 30; 11:2922-7, 2007

• Cappola AR, et al, Trajectories of **dehydroepiandrosterone sulfate predict mortality** in older adults: the cardiovascular health study, *J Gerontol Bio Sci Med Sci* 64; 12:1268-74, 2009

• Medina MC, et al, **Dehydroepiandrosterone increases beta-cell mass and improves the glucose-induced insulin secretion by pancreatic** islets from aged rats, *FEBS Lett* 508; 1:285-90, Jan 9, 2006

• Kawano H, et al, **Dehydroepiandrosterone supplementation improves** endothelial function and **insulin sensitivity** in men, *J Clin Endocrinol Metab* 88; 7:3190-5, July 2003

• Boudou P, et al, **Hyperglycemia acutely decreases circulating dehydroepiandrosterone** levels in healthy men, *Clin Endocr* (Oxf), 64; 1:46-52, 2006

• Villareal DT, et al, Effect of **DHEA on abdominal fat and insulin action** in elderly women and men: a randomized controlled trial, ***J Am Med Assoc***, 292; 18:2243-8, 2004

• Liu PS, et al, DHEA attenuates catecholamine secretion from bovine adrenal chromaffin cells, *J Biomed Sci* 11:200-05, 2004

• Feldman HA, et al, Low dehydroepiandrosterone sulfate and heart disease in middle-aged men: cross-sectional results from the Massachusetts Male Aging Study, *Ann Epidemiol* 8; 4:217-28, May 1998

• Alwardt CM, et al, Comparative effects of dehydroepiandrosterone sulfate on ventricular diastolic function with young and aged female mice, *Am J Physiol Regul Intergr Comp Physiol*, 290; 1: R251-6, Jan 2006

• Lord RS, Bralley JA, eds. *Laboratory Evaluations for Integrative and Functional Medicine*, 2nd edition, 2008, Hormone Biotransformation (Detoxification) page 578, Dehydroepiandrosterone (DHEA), page 558, metametrix.com, Duluth, Georgia,

• Goldberg M., Are oral DHEA supplements safe? *Emerg Med* 137-8, 1998

• Belgorosky A, et al, **Sex hormone binding globulin response to testosterone. An androgen sensitivity test,** *Acta Endocrinol*, 130-38, 1985

• Seo KW, et al, Comparison of oxidative stress and **changes of xenobiotic metabolizing enzymes induced by phthalates** in rats, *Food Chem Toxicol* 42:107-14, 2004

• Villareal DT, et al, Effect of **DHEA on abdominal fat and insulin** action in elderly women and men, ***J Am Med Assoc*** 292; 18:2243-48, 2004

• Peters JM, et al, Peroxisome proliferator-activated receptor alpha required for gene induction by dehydroepiandrosterone-3 beta-sulfate, *Molec Pharmacol* 50:67-74, 1996

• Gulick T, et al, The **peroxisome** proliferator-activated receptor **regulates mitochondrial fatty acid** oxidation enzyme **gene** expression, *Proc Nat Acad Sci USA* 91:1101 2-16, 1994

• Costet P, et al, **Peroxisome** proliferator-activated receptor alpha-isoform **deficiency leads to** progressive **dyslipidemia** in sexually dimorphic **obesity** and steatosis, *J Biolog Chem* 273:29577-85, 1998

• Tenenbaum A, et al, **Peroxisome proliferator-activated receptor** ligand benzafibrate **for prevention of type II diabetes mellitus** in patients with coronary artery disease, *Circul* 109:2197-2202, 2004

• Haffner SM, et al, **Decreased testosterone and dehydroepiandrosterone sulfate concentrations are associated with increased insulin and glucose** concentrations in nondiabetic men, *Metabolism* 43:599-603, 1994

271

- Guerre-Millo M, et al, **Peroxisome** proliferator-activated receptor alpha **activators improve insulin sensitivity and reduce adiposity,** *J Biol Chem* 275:16638-42, 2000

Cholesterol Rising in Spite of Doing "All the Right Things"?

High cholesterol is often an accompaniment of diabetes as well as metabolic syndrome. Many folks who have read *The Cholesterol Hoax* have completely normalized their cholesterol (or LDL, triglycerides, LP(a), or other lipids) for years, only to recently find that the levels have risen over the last year. What you need to never forget is that we are the first generation with this enormously unprecedented level of pollutants that bring on all chronic diseases. Even though you heal, bear in mind that **every day we are slowly tanking up on more pollutants. It is an unending battle that few in medicine appreciate.** We need to detox forever.

For example, none of us can avoid the number one pollutant in the body, the **plasticizers or phthalates.** Since they are over 10,000 times higher than any others, they **are the number one culprit for a rising cholesterol** or other lipid abnormalities. They dangerously damage the body at an extremely fundamental level (*change the peroxisomes plus the genes that control all the body chemistry, especially beta-oxidation or conversion of cholesterol and all membrane fatty acids to their healthier forms*). In essence, plasticizers are **responsible for our unprecedented epidemics of not only high cholesterol, but diabetes, obesity, cancer, metabolic syndrome X, NASH** (non-alcoholic steatohepatitis, also called NAFLD or non-alcoholic fatty liver disease), and much more. Did I repeat this on purpose? For sure!

The solution? **We need to detoxify forever.** As many days a week as possible do the **far infrared sauna** for 1-2 hours, following the directions in *Detoxify Or Die*. Then do the non-prescription heavy metal detox protocols that are 5-times cheaper and safer than IV chelation and described in *The High Blood Pressure Hoax* (yes, even though you may not have high blood pressure). In fact these have enabled folks to heal chronic diseases

272

that they have been told have "no known cause and no known cure". Diabetes is no exception, in fact leads the list.

The bottom line? **If your cholesterol has risen again after you had it under control, consider this** a lucky warning that it is time to step up your lifetime detoxification. Remember, I'm no smarter than any other doctor, I was just sicker. And I'm not some big fancy researcher in a medical school funded by pharmaceutical firms. I'm just a solo practitioner who got so sick I realized nothing I learned in medical school could make me well. It forced me to learn how to heal (without surgery or drugs) over 2 dozen "incurable" maladies. At months from turning 70, I don't even have grey hair yet, much less any symptoms, major surgery (except tonsils & adenoids at 10), implants, or medications. God clearly designed the body to heal. And the evidence from thousands of researchers across the globe has been here for decades. It is only medicine that wants to keep it a secret, since (as I have voluminously referenced and keep finding new evidence for) well people do not support the drug industry, which in turn controls the business of the *practice of* medicine.

References: (plus more in *Detoxify Or Die, The High Blood Pressure Hoax, The Cholesterol Hoax,* and *TW* 2000-present):

• Winberg LD, et al, Mechanism of **phthalates-induced inhibition of hepatic mitochondrial B-oxidation,** *Toxicol Lett* 76:63-69, 1995

• Alonso-Magdalena P, et al, The estrogenic effect of **bisphenol A disrupts pancreatic** B-cell function in vivo and **induces insulin resistance,** *Environ Health Perspect* 114:106-12, 2006

It's Downright Silly to Neglect Silymarin

You have learned here about how important the integrity of the mitochondrial membrane is for determining whether or not we get *any and all* the diseases of aging like diabetes or even just run out of energy as we get older. So let's look at a simple solution. **Silymarin helps repair the mitochondria** and keep their electrical potential protected so that we can produce adequate energy. Remember, mitochondria create "life".

273

Although I'm much more in favor of nutrients than herbs, this one we cannot afford to ignore. Silymarin is a naturally occurring bioflavonoid with such strong antioxidant capacity that it **stops cancers from growing** in many studies, and has **stopped metastases**. This is via its ability to up-regulate or **enhance the expression of the P53 gene that makes cancer cells commit suicide (called apoptosis).** (There is more on reversing the p53 cancer gene so that it makes cancer cells kill themselves in *Wellness Against All Odds, TW* and *DOD*).

Silymarin also has **lowered cholesterol by lowering the HMG CoA, yet it also raises the good HDL** cholesterol. And since it **revs up the liver detoxification**, it's important for all of us. And if you were not among the three out of four whose arthritis or any type of joint pain was eliminated by stopping the nightshades (see *Pain Free In 6 Weeks*), or if you used the **Lumen** (*TW* 2005, 2011) for your chronic joint pain, but they were not enough, look further. For **silymarin increases your cytochrome C** which is the targeted enzyme that the **Lumen** revs up (also recall that this enzyme requires copper).

And if you're still silly enough to be on something like Celebrex, Motrin or other NSAID pain relievers, remember that they work by being anti-inflammatory drugs. But silymarin **also turns down inflammation**. Yet unlike NSAIDs like Celebrex that can increase your chance of a heart attack, stroke, high blood pressure, eye damage, blood clots or renal papillary necrosis (killing your kidneys), as well as damage cartilage and guarantee a joint replacement, silymarin works *without* these side effects. And unlike the popular anti-inflammatories like Celebrex, silymarin does not bring on food allergies, irritable bowel, GERD, asthma, high blood pressure, and the other side effects symptoms of pain medications.

Plus don't forget that **cancer, as well as diabetes and most diseases, begin with inflammation.** So natural anti-inflammatory substances are a good thing. In fact, Harvard researchers reported in the *Journal of the American Medical Association* (302:1186-94, 2009) on the effects of metformin (Glucophage®) or insulin on 500 people with type II diabetes. Metformin with or without insulin lowered the blood sugars. However neither medication lead to reductions of a CRP, a key marker of inflammation that is dangerously out of control. Once more, drugs do not fix what's broken; they only make specific lab tests look normal.

Diabetes is a precursor to cancer. It's clear now that **diabetes promotes inflammation and inflammation feeds diabetes, as well as promotes its complications**, one of which is cancer. In fact cancer and obesity share not only inflammation as a warning but other similarities, not the least of which is abnormal sugar metabolism. Clearly, obesity, insulin resistance, type II diabetes, NASH, cancers, plus cardiovascular and renal diseases are all linked (Sears). But silymarin **also turns down this inflammation, while it improves liver detoxification.**

My favorite form? No question. It's **Super Milk Thistle X** (because of the reasons I've referenced in past *TW* issues). You can use anything from 1 to 3 capsules 1 to 3 times a day, depending upon your needs. Since we all should be doing the heavy-metal detox protocols for the rest of our lives, it seems pretty clear to me that **Super Milk Thistle X** should be a part of our detoxification protocol forever. You can add it to your **Detox Cocktail** or **PectaSol Chelation Complex** or any other nutrients. Clearly it's silly to neglect the best form of silymarin.

References:

• Ramakrishnan G, et al, **Silymarin inhibited** proliferation and **induced apoptosis** in hepatic **cancer cells**, *Cell Prolif* 42;2:229-40, Apr 2009

• Sears B, Anti-inflammatory diets for obesity and diabetes, *J Am Coll Nutr* 28; 4:482S-91S, 2009

• Kahn S, et al, Mechanisms linking obesity to insulin resistance and type II diabetes, *Nature* 444:840-6, 2007

• Ramakrishnan G, et al, **Silymarin** down **regulates COX-2** expression and **attenuates hyperlipidemia** during NDEA-induced rat hepatocellular **carcinoma**, *Mol Cell Biochem* 313:53-61, 2008

Ending Epidemic Arrhythmias

Diabetics are even more vulnerable for irregular heartbeats than other folks. And these **cardiac arrhythmias can throw clots to the brain or lungs, becoming the cause of immediate death themselves.** Unfortunately, the standard is to throw drugs at the patient that can kill (like amiodarone), then try electrocuting the heart with cardioversion (200-600 joules of electricity), and finally ablation, which is permanent destruction of heart nerves and muscle via a laser threaded through a groin vessel up into the heart. Even though this does not have FDA approval for this indication, that doesn't stop interventional cardiologists. Yet unfortunately, even the biggest name clinics (when I see their records on readers who have consulted me on the phone) have not looked for even the most rudimentary cures for arrhythmias, like atrial fibrillation. If you have an arrhythmia, be sure to at least read *Is Your Cardiologist Killing You?* before letting anyone permanently destroy part of your heart forever.

Top of the list of the myriad of correctable causes of arrhythmias are fatty acid/mineral deficiencies, yet heavy metals also prevail. But never neglect our most common everyday exposures (*The E.I. Syndrome* addresses environmental illness causes, while *Depression Cured At Last!* explores many other hidden causes merely using depression as the example). A Harvard study, for example, shows that traffic pollutants adversely change the EKG in diabetics increasing the autonomic dysfunction and heart block, changing calcium channels (for which brain-damaging calcium channel blockers are prescribed), and causing not only arrhythmias but sudden cardiac death (Baja).

Some of our readers have said, *"My cardiologist says there's no evidence that things like auto exhaust and days of heightened air pollution from cloud cover accentuating industrial exhausts have a bearing on his field of expertise. He won't even order a **Cardio/ION**, much less **Phthalates** or **Volatile Solvents**."*

276

My response if that it's too bad that he's ignorant of the last 40 years of data. Sadly, even the EPA recently published an article where they thought they were the first folks to present a case report of an individual who actually got atrial fibrillation precipitated by exposure to an increase in air pollution. They thought this was a unique discovery. The only thing unique about it is that it shows they haven't read anything in the last 30 years, because we've all been dealing with (and healing) this that long.

In addition, we've been showing physicians at courses and in publications how to cure disease by (1) identifying and correcting the nutrient deficiencies that would impede detoxification, and then (2) how to avoid the pollutants and negate their effects once exposed, as well as finally (3) reducing the levels of accumulated toxins in order to reverse their induced cardiac vulnerability or arrhythmia. I've included a small sampling of the voluminous references for physicians just from the last few decades. If really interested in doing the best service for their cardiovascular patients, they'll at least read the last decade of *TW* and all of the books, beginning with *ICKY (Is Your Cardiologist Killing You?)*.

I remember when I was fresh out of medical school and like most recent graduates thought I was God's gift to medicine. Then one day a nurse presented at my office showing me how she had been rescued from the jaws of death when all the local physicians were powerless to help her. At Dr. William Rea's Environmental Health Unit in Dallas they could provoke not only arrhythmias but angina, skin mottling, and vascular shutdown with a variety of common pollutants. I eventually studied there, taught physicians and wrote about these methods beginning with *The E.I. Syndrome*, a short booklet *Chemical Sensitivity*, and further in *The Scientific Basis for Selected Environmental Medicine Techniques*, as well as publishing the in-office testing technique to provoke chemically-induced symptoms in the U.S. Government's (NIH) leading environmental medicine journal, *Environmental Health Perspectives* (1987!).

When knowledge-challenged physicians would deny that these techniques could actually diagnose and treat chemical sensitivity, we hired a private plane and flew to Pennsylvania where we filmed a double-blind study using not humans but horses. We could literally bring the horses to their knees with heaves (the horse equivalent of human asthma). Then with the proper neutralizing dose, the horses would stand up within seconds where our double-blinded veterinarian examined them and proclaimed them as now having totally clear lungs. The proof of the pudding was they were once again able to be ridden, and for many years (my horse was, too). Environmental antigens can turn on and off body functions.

We have exhaustively used the same techniques for decades to document with film (and show at medical meetings) as well as write about in medical papers for physicians, how **environmental pollutants can cause just about any disease** (see some of my medical publications below as an example of one solo country physician). As an example, we filmed one woman crippled with rheumatoid arthritis, who within minutes of the proper neutralizing dose of a common household environmental chemical from new furniture and carpeting was able to skip down the hall waving her arms with no pain or limitation of motion. We've done the same thing turning on and off within minutes schizophrenia, migraines, dysphonia, asthma, ADD, and even the flu (*TW*). Now you can appreciate how after spending thousands of dollars and hours writing dozens of medical papers for physicians that I have decided to devote my energies to helping you folks instead. After all, who has a more vested interest in your health than you?

The bottom line is that **ambient air pollution has been a major proven cause of any disease for decades**. It merely depends on the total load and biochemistry of the individual person. Who knows? This short article may be the impetus that your physician has needed all along to bring him into the 21st century of medicine. Then he, too, can have the fun and satisfaction in finding the cause and cure of cardiovascular and other consequences of diabetes, and not just resort to drugs and devices to perpetuate and accelerate disease.

Meanwhile, are you remembering to put your air handling system of your car on re-circulate, to avoid sucking in highway fumes ? And better yet would be a **Foust Car Air Purifier**, plus doing that **Detox Cocktail** when you arrive at your destination or even before leaving and during a long trip.

References:

• Dockery DW, Epidemiologic evidence of **cardiovascular effects of** particulate **air pollution**, *Environ Health Persp* 109 (supple 4): 483-6, 2001

• Forastiere F, et al, A case-crossover analysis of out-of-hospital **coronary deaths and air pollution** in Rome Italy, *Am J Resp Crit Care Med* 172; 12:1549-55, 2005

• Liungman PL, et al, **Rapid effects of air pollution on ventricular arrhythmias,** *Eur Heart J* 29; 23:2894-2901, 2008

• Peters A, et al, **Air pollution and incidence of cardiac arrhythmia**, *Epidemiology* 11; 1:11-17, 2000

• Rich D0, et al, Association of **short-term** ambient **air pollution concentrations and ventricular arrhythmias**, *Am J Epidem* 161; 12:1123-32, 2005

• Rosenthal FS, et al, Out of hospital **cardiac arrest and airborne fine particulate matter**: a case crossover analysis of emergency medical services data in Indianapolis Indiana, *Environ Health Persp* 116:631-6, 2008

• Zanobetti A, et al, The effect of particulate air pollution on emergency admissions for **myocardial infarction**: a multicity case-crossover analysis, *Environ Health Persp* 113:978-82, 2005

• Ghio AJ, et al, Case report: super **ventricular arrhythmia after exposure to** concentrated ambient **air pollution** particles, *Environ Health Persp* 120:275-77, 2012

• Liungman PL, et al, Rapid **effects of air pollution on arrhythmias**, *Eur Heart J* 29; 23:2894-2901, 2008

• O'Neill MS, et al, **Diabetes enhances vulnerability to particular air pollution** associated impairment in vascular reactivity and endothelial function, *Circulation* 111; 22:2913-20, 2005

• Park SK, et al, Traffic related particles are associated with elevated homocysteine: the normative aging study, *Am J Respir Crit Care Med* 178; 3:283-89, 2008

• Peters A, et al, Increased particulate **air pollution and the triggering of myocardial** infarction, *Circulation* 103; 23:2810-15, 2001

• Peters A, et al, Exposure to traffic and the onset of myocardial infarction, *New Engl J Med* 351; 17:1721-30, 2004

• Baja ES, et al, Traffic related **air pollution and QT interval: modification by diabetes**, obesity and oxidative stress gene polymorphisms in the normative aging study, *Environ Health Persp* 118:840-6, 2010

279

- **Rogers SA, Diagnosing the tight building syndrome,** *Environmental Health Perspectives,* 1987;76:195-98

- **Rogers SA,** Indoor fungi as part of the cause of recalcitrant symptoms of the tight building syndrome, *Environment International,* 17;4:271-2765, 1991

- **Rogers SA,** Zinc deficiency as a model for developing chemical sensitivity, *International Clinical Nutrition Reviews,* 10;1:253-259, Jan 1990

- **Rogers, SA,** Diagnosing the tight building syndrome or diagnosing chemical hypersensitivity, *Environment International* 15;75-79, 1989

- **Rogers SA,** Resistant cases, Response to mold immunotherapy and environmental and dietary controls, *Clinical Ecology, Archives for Human Ecology in Health and Disease,* 5;3:115-120, 1987/88

- **Rogers SA,** Diagnosing chemical hypersensitivity: Case examples, *Clinical Ecology* 6;4:129-134, 1989

- **Rogers SA,** Provocation-Neutralization of cough and wheezing in a horse, *Clinical Ecology,* 5;5:185-187, 1987/88

- **Rogers SA,** Is it chronic low back pain or environmental illness?, *Journal of Applied Nutrition,* 46:106-109, Nov. 4, 1994

- **Rogers SA,** Improvement in chemical sensitivity with the macrobiotic diet, *Journal of Applied Nutrition,* 48;3:85-93, 1997

- **Rogers SA,** A practical approach to the person with suspected indoor air quality problems, *Internat Clin Nutr Rev* 10;1:253-9, Jan 1990

- **Rogers SA,** Chemical sensitivity; Breaking the paralyzing paradigm, Part I, *Internal Medicine World Report,* 7;4:1, 15-17, Feb 1-15, 1992

- **Rogers SA,** Chemical sensitivity: Breaking the paralyzing paradigm, Diagnosis and treatment, Part II, *Internal Med World Rep,* 7;6:2, 21-31. Mar 1-15, 1992

- **Rogers SA,** Chemical sensitivity: Breaking the paralyzing paradigm. How knowledge of chemical sensitivity enhances the treatment of chronic diseases, Part III, *Internal Med World Rep,* 7;8:13-16, 32-33, 40-41, Apr 15-30, 1992

- **Rogers SA,** When stumped, think environmental medicine, *Internal Med World Rep* 7;13:3, July 1992

- **Rogers SA,** Is it senility or chemical sensitivity?, *Intern Med World Rep,* 7;13:3, July 1992

- **Rogers SA,** How cost effective is improving the work environments?, *Intern Med World Rep* 7;14:48, Aug 1992

- **Rogers SA, Is it recalcitrant arrhythmia or environmental illness ?,** *Intern Med World Rep* 7;19:28, Nov 1-14, 1992

- **Rogers SA,** Lipoic acid as a potential first agent for protection from mycotoxins and treatment of mycotoxicosis, p136-140, chapter 18 in *Molds and Mycotoxins,* Papers from an International Symposium, Kilburn KH, Ed., Heldref Publ, Wash DC, 2004

- **Rogers SA,** Environmental Medicine for Veterinary Practitioners, Chapter 29 in Schoen AM, Wynn SG, *Complementary and Alternative Veterinary Medicine, Principles and Practice,* **Mosby,** St Louis MO, 1998

Flagrant Cheating of the Cancer Patient is the Norm

Since cancer is yet another serious disease that is more prevalent in diabetics, let's explore more facts that will help you protect yourselves (and spur you on to learn more). I've shown you in December 2006 *TW*, the evidence for how one nurse given 48 hours to live with wildly metastatic cancer is radiantly healthy (now over a decade and a half later) and cured herself with mere diet. And this is after everything that medicine had to offer had failed. In prior issues I showed you a surgeon who refused to have surgery and also healed her cancer with another type of detox diet. In the **Macro Trilogy**, which begins with *You Are What You Ate* then progresses to the *The Cure Is In The Kitchen*, followed by *Macro Mellow* there are numerous other cancer case histories as well as the complete directions of how to pull it off yourself.

But in this era of unprecedented toxicity and damaged chemistry of the human body, we often need to go much further than mere diets. As I showed you, **some human cell membrane chemistry has changed as much as 60-fold in the last century in the human body**. And remember, the cell membrane is not just for holding the contents of the cell, but out of it emanates cytokines. These are God's magnificently orchestrated chemicals like *tumor necrosis factor* and *natural killer cells* that are designed to purposely fight cancers daily in our bodies and destroy cancer cells. Yet popular Rx meds like Embrel, Humira, and Remicade kill TNF (while nutrients like tocotrienols control it) !

One of the most crucial ingredients for repairing the cell membrane is docosahexaenoic acid (DHA) as found in **Super DHA**, and also as part of **Carlson' s Lemon-Flavored Cod Liver Oil**. The thing that scares me incredibly is that **DHA is also among scores of nutrients that play an important role in stopping cancer growth**, stopping cancer metastases, inhibiting cancers initially, and even *making cancer cells commit suicide* (that word *apoptosis* that you see in the references). You might think that this information is new, but **it's been known for over**

two decades. Plus a lot of the information has come right out of the *Journal of the National Cancer Institute*, which we as American citizens fund annually with billions of our tax dollars.

Then you would think that at least every oncologist would be measuring your DHA and balancing it and prescribing it with the dozens of other nutrients that we have shown the evidence for (in the past two decades of the *TW* newsletter) in being essential to stop cancer growth. But no. Even though the *Wall Street Journal* has shown us that there is as much as a 60% mark-up in cancer oncology offices and clinics for their chemotherapy drugs, and even though the average person spends well over $100,000 for the first year of cancer treatment, I have yet to consult on anyone whose oncologist or specialty cancer clinic has looked at any of the fatty acids much less DHA. This chemistry is crucial for cure.

And the sad thing is that if oncologists merely read this medical journal article and then measured DHA, or even just told patients to take the nutrients, that wouldn't be enough because they haven't measured the adipate and suberate to see if the resident phthalates have poisoned carnitine that caries the fatty acids like DNA into the cell (**ALC Powder**). **Without enough ALC no matter how much DHA you take, it cannot be incorporated into the cell and mitochondrial membranes.** And as well, most oncologists don't do the **Cardio/ION**, the 13-page assay that includes all of this and the majority of nutrients that you need. Plus it shows the balance that you need (can't they afford a dollar a week for a *TW* subscription, or even less for the electronic version?). Furthermore, this test often shows you how you were vulnerable enough in the first place to get your cancer, and what you need to do to correct this. I'm baffled by their oversight.

To fail to measure and give a fatty acid that has a huge role in stopping metastases seems like malpractice to me. But it is not in this era, because the definition of malpractice, remember, is if a physician is not doing what the "herd" is doing. It appears to me the herd is irresponsibly unschooled in the very essential molecular biochemistry that they as purveyors of their specialty should be experts in. I'm truly disgusted with the field of medicine for continuing to ignore the chemistry of healing. Clearly the evidence points to the fact that money rules.

There is another reason to check DHA. Cisplatin is a widely used form of chemotherapy. But in 30% of the people it kills their kidneys and they die from this effect of the drug. It actually changes the tumor suppressor p53 gene that is designed to make cancer cells commit suicide. Cisplatin actually mutates the p53 gene so that now it does the exact opposite of what God designed; it now becomes fertilizer for cancer cells.

But God always orchestrates a way out for us. You saw how high amounts of brassica vegetables (broccoli, cabbage, etc.) as in the macrobiotic diet, and concentrated in nutrients like **Indol Plex,** can stop chemotherapy from killing the kidneys. Yet where are the oncologists or cancer clinic doctors who have discussed diet and/or nutrients, much less measured them?

They should know that phytochemicals from foods actually make the cisplatin work better in killing cancer cells and inhibiting angiogenesis (meaning turn off metastases), for those who do choose to go the chemotherapy route. And this paper isn't alone. Although it is not the focus of this book, because diabetics are more prone to cancer, I've included a glimpse of the evidence. Did your oncologist read the studies where cod liver oil membrane repair stopped prostate cancer progression (Freidrichs), or cut prostate cancer risk 41% (Norrish), or cut breast cancer risk 25% (Patterson)? Has it anything to do with the *WSJ* article (C4, Oct 6, 2012) that some oncologists make $7 million a year?! Why is this information not used in oncology and at least in prevention? And who needs prevention of cancer more than the person who has already had it? (Remember in the references, apoptosis is cell death.)

Yes, I'm afraid we are in the scariest era of medicine ever. It makes the Ponzi scheme robbers who were splashed all over the newspapers in the last decade look like philanthropists. If I had a cancer? I would review all of my books and the last two decades of newsletters because I don't know of any other place where all of this information has been laid out, explained, collated, referenced, etc. I would want to give myself the most thorough refresher course/education in the workings of the human body as possible. At the risk of sounding self-serving I wish I did know of another source or person that I would trust. It would be so easy to just say, "Take over for me, they are all yours." Meanwhile, I would get a current **Cardio/ION**, interpret it myself, and take it from there.

References:

• D'Eliseo D, et al, **Docosahexaenoic acid inhibits invasion of human** RT112 urinary **bladder and PT45 pancreatic carcinoma cells** via down-modulation of granzyme B expression, *J Nutr Biochem* 23:452-7, 2012

• Serini S, et al, Dietary polyunsaturated **fatty acids as inducers of apoptosis**: implications for cancer, *Apoptosis* 14 135-52, 2009

• Merendino N, et al, **Induction of apoptosis in human pancreatic cancer cells by docosahexaenoic acid**, *Ann N Y Acad Sci* 1010:361-4, 2003

• Bougnoux P, et al, **Improving outcome of chemotherapy of metastatic breast cancer by docosahexaenoic acid:** a phase 2 trial, *Brit J Cancer* 101:1978-85, 2009

• Rose DP, et al., **Influence of diets** containing eicosapentaenoic or **docosahexaenoic acid on growth and metastasis of breast cancer cells** in nude mice, *J Natl Cancer Instit*, 87:587-92, 1995

• Yam D, et al, **Suppression of tumor growth and metastasis by dietary fish oil** combined with vitamins C and E and cisplatin, *Cancer Chemother Pharmacol* 47:34-40, 2001

• D'Eliseo D, et al, Granzyme B is expressed in urothelial carcinoma and promotes cancer cell invasion, *Internat J Cancer* 127:1283-94, 2010

• Guerrero-Beltran CE, et al, Sulforaphane, a natural constituent of **broccoli, prevents cell death** and inflammation in nephropathy, *J Nutr Biochem*, 23:494-500, 2012

• Kallifatidis G, et al, **Sulforaphane increases drug-mediated cytotoxicity** toward cancer stem-like cells of the pancreas and prostate, *Mol Ther* 19:188-95, 2011

• Hu R, et al, In vivo pharmacokinetics and **regulation of gene expression** profiles **by isothiocyanate sulforaphane** in the rat, *J Pharmacol Exp Ther* 310:263-71, 2004

• Freidrichs W, et al, **Omega-3 fatty acid inhibition of prostate cancer progression** to hormone independence is associated with suppression of mTOR signaling and androgen receptor expression, *Nutrition Cancer* 10:1-7, 2011

• Norrish AE, et al, Prostate cancer risk and consumption of fish oils: a dietary biomarker-based case-controlled study, *British Journal Cancer* 81; 7:1238-42, 1999

•   Courtney ED, et al, Eicosapentaenoic acid (**EPA**) reduces crypt cell proliferation and **increases apoptosis** in colonic mucosal in subjects with a history of colorectal adenomas, *Inter J Colorectal Dis*, 22; 7:765-76, 2007

•   Patterson RE, et al, Marine fatty acid intake is associated with breast cancer prognosis, *J Nutr* 141; 2:201-06, 2011

Do You Fully Appreciate the Clandestine Role of Environmental Pollutants?

Clearly **environmental exposures are a major cause of type II diabetes** as well as obesity and are capable of initiating any disease. But the lack of understanding has created a critical gap between what we know and what is being implemented in medicine (Thayer, Grun, Oh, Tai, Itoh, Achard, Boullu).

BPA is in hard and flexible, clear polycarbonate plastics widely used as food containers. In one study in Texas of 105 samples of fresh plastic wrapped foods, researchers found detectable levels of packaging chemicals in 60% of the foods. In some studies in terms of amounts, authors wrote that "migration from packaging material is the most important source: it exceeds most other factors by 100-1000." (Grob). **We know even from the *Journal of the American Medical Association* that food packaging chemicals can create just about any medical disorder or laboratory abnormality, yet it is ignored in medicine.** In fact in one *TW* 2012 referenced study families cut their phthalate levels in half in a mere week by just eating foods that were not packaged. But where are the public health officials who should be making this simple partial remedy known?

I could literally fill volumes of books with the evidence but I know you get the point now. And *TW* will take you even further with tests like **Volatile Solvents, Pesticides,** and even more importantly, **Porphyrins**, that all contribute to prove how seriously your body is poisoned and in which pathways. Then you know what screams to be repaired first, for the body has a definitive "pecking order". The bottom line is **if you are ever stuck with any disease, you know that you must eventually detoxify. And** a physician ignorant of the very fundamentals of phthalate toxicity may keep you from achieving wellness indefinitely.

References:

• Thayer KA, et al, **Role of environmental chemicals in diabetes and obesity**: a national toxicology program workshop review, *Environ Health Persp* 120:779-89, 2012

• Editorial, Our **food: Packaging and public health**, *Environ Health Persp*, 120;6:A232-7, 2012

• Grob K, et al, Food contamination with organic materials in perspective **packaging materials** as the **largest and least controlled source**: A view focusing on the European situation, *Crit Rev Food Sci Nutr* 46; 7:529-36, 2006

• Lang IA, et al, **Association of urinary bisphenol A concentration with medical disorders** and laboratory abnormalities in adults, *J Am Med Assoc* 300; 11:1303-10, 2008

• **Low dose of some persistent organic pollutants predicts type II diabetes**: a nested case-controlled study, *Environ Health Persp* 118:1235-42, 2010

• Rahimi R, et al, A review on the mechanisms involved in **hypoglycemia induced by organophosphorus pesticides**, *Pesticides Biochem Physiol* 88:115-21, 2007

• Tsang CH, The potential biological mechanisms of **arsenic-induced diabetes mellitus**, *Toxicol Appl Pharmacol* 187; 2:67-83, 2004

• Boullu-Ciocca S, et al, Post-natal diet-induced obesity in rats upregulates systemic and adipose tissue glucocorticoid metabolism during development and in adulthood: Its relationship with the metabolic syndrome, *Diabetes* 54:197-203, 2005

• Achard V, et al, **Perinatal programming of central obesity and the metabolic syndrome**: role of glucocorticoids, *Metab Syndr Relat Disord* 4; 129-37, 2006

• Itoh Y, et al, **Free fatty acids regulate insulin secretion from pancreatic beta cells** through GPRS 40, *Nature* 422:173-76, 2003

• Oh DY, et al, GTR 120 is a **Omega-3 fatty acid receptor** mediating potent anti-inflammatory and **insulin-sensitizing** effects, *Cell* 142: 687-98, 2010

• Tai CC, et al, N-3 polyunsaturated fatty acids regulate lipid metabolism through several inflammation mediators: mechanisms and implications for obesity prevention, *J Nutr Biochem* 21:357-63, 2010

Overwhelmed?

Meanwhile, are you overwhelmed? Don't be. I sometimes feel the same, as I discover the ever-mounting evidence that supports the "healing of the impossible". But we have the proof for how so many of you (and myself included) have been able to heal diseases that medicine is still teaching have "no known cause" and "no known cure". I believe I, for one, would be dead if it were not for this information. I have purposely given you a smattering of the multitude of options (and there are more in *TW* and the other books) to show you **there are *many* paths to health. But don't worry. You can't do everything in here, nor should you**. But with this new knowledge you can (with your health professional) choose the most likely start and the most "do-able" plans at this point in your life. **Health is a process. It is a continuing journey.** And consider yourselves lucky. I have not given you 1/10th of the information that I could have.

Clearly, we must get rid of toxins daily. Every night when we go to bed, we can reflect back **on our choices we made that day. Are we going to go to sleep with a body that is *better, same or worse* than the one we awakened with in the morning? The choice is totally up to you. You have seen a multitude of ways for getting these toxins out of the body. Clearly it is one of the keys for not only reversing diabetes and other diseases, but** turning back the hands of time and aging. *Why not focus on 4 priorities?*

(1) You can start by simply reducing the use of packaged foods, and especially plastic containers. Glass is preferred. Sure it is not 100% possible. Life isn't perfect. Yes, I have plastic wrap in my cupboards, but I use it as little as possible. We all just do the best we can with the limits we are given. But your new knowledge will help you make a lot more healthful decisions.

(2) A next step could be alkaline water, and (3) a few of your nutrients in Chapter 5. Later on you could add more nutrients. Just the detox cocktail, mitochondrial and membrane repair have rescued many. I know this from reader phone consults and gracious "thank you" cards, letters and gifts. (4) Soon you could be ready for the **far infrared sauna** and **PectaSol**. Now that's pretty simple, isn't it? After all, we are talking about the rest of your life. Why not choose to make it disease-free?

In the meantime, **should you stop your medications? Absolutely not**. You haven't done enough yet to make yourself well. And **how**

287

do you find a physician who knows this information? Probably the simplest thing would be to ask him if he has read this. And if not, would he be interested? Remember to use the analogy of a mechanic who would refuse to read the latest repair manual for your new car. Would you let him touch your precious car? And for ordering the blood tests, you might call MetaMetrix and see who in your zip code radius orders their tests, or use *directlabs.com* to order your own, plus *anylabtestnow.com* can direct you to the nearest lab to draw your tests. Take a breather, then in the next chapter I'll give you more easy starter tips.

So instead of being overwhelmed, I choose to have *overwhelming gratitude* for the researchers who dedicated their lives to giving us this information. Instead, pity the poor folks who surround you and me daily who will go to their graves never knowing what a healthful life they could have had. Some we can reach and educate, while others resist our kindest efforts. Meanwhile, anything you learn and apply, no matter how small a step it may be, is better than doing nothing. *Plus, the more you read, the more you will understand, and the easier it will become* to implement. And **once you learn something, it is yours forever**. What a gift! No one can take it away from you. Most of all, remember, the more you learn, the more *you set yourself up to be too smart to fail.*

You Have Become Clairvoyant

"Paging Doctor Claire Voyant, …… Paging Dr. Clair Voyant…". That's you, dear precious reader, for you have now become clairvoyant. You can see right through the misdirected ruses and deceptions that permeate conventional medicine and journalism. If you don't believe it, let's give your new talents a trial run.

Here's a current article from the *Wall Street Journal* (Landro, D1, D4, Aug. 14, 2012). The title brags "The Informed Patient: Wider Testing to Head Off Diabetes Before It Hits". It starts out teaching us that one in three American adults is pre-diabetic. In fact the National Institutes of Health says that on top of the **26 million**

Americans who have type II diabetes, 7 million don't even know they have diabetes, and 79 million more (ages 20 and older) are pre-diabetic. Clearly this disease will bankrupt our system. Anyway the article then goes on to tell that the A1C is used to diagnose pre-diabetics as well as diabetes out of control. So far so good. But then when it comes to treatment, they fail miserably. But only you can see through this herd of dinosaurs because you know now that diabetes is curable, not a disease that merely requires a hemoglobin A1C test every three months for monitoring. But it gets worse.

The article featured interviews with several leading diabetologists. But the crux of all their treatments was merely exercise, diet and losing weight. And when that fails, as it inevitably does, then the patients can go on medications. There's not one mention of fixing what's broken and repairing the system that is both deficient and toxic. They are literally pre-historic dinosaurs when you compare them with what you know, ... and you're not even a medical school-trained diabetes specialist. And you can bet that many pharmaceutical companies are willing to jump right in with money for these clinics. It's a marriage made in heaven. How does it make you feel when you see right through the glaring inadequacies of conventional medicine and journalism in light of all that you now know and are capable of curing? You're clairvoyant.

Let's try out your new talents for discerning the truth with another article. This *Wall Street Journal* article (Linebaugh, D1, D4, Aug. 7, 2012), entitled "Wrong Call: The Trouble Diagnosing Diabetes". The article focused on exactly what happens to folks when they don't find the cause and cure of their type II diabetes. They go on to metamorphose into type I diabetes, requiring lifelong insulin injections along with accelerated morbidity and mortality, not to mention toxic dialysis. Again, so far so good. Then we get into the BS (**b**ad **s**cience) that only you can see through.

They state that scientists have "scoured" the medical journals and are all baffled. They don't know what the trigger for diabetes is.

289

But you do. They are literally clueless. And the sad thing is without knowing the triggers, they will never know there is a cause and cure. But you do.

I guess these revered scientists don't have time to read the very literature in their own journals to know that for example, the phthalates (that are the number one pollutant in the human body repeatedly proven by the U.S. government for over a decade) are among dozens of everyday common toxins that can create diabetes just by themselves. And it happens even faster when toxins are in combination, as happens in real life. And even faster when coupled with the nutrient deficiencies that inevitably sneak up on folks. Even the *Journal of the American Medical Association* published that the phthalate cousin, bisphenol A, can cause diabetes five years ago (Wei). So there's really no excuse for such blatant ignorance. Is a major reason for this blind eye merely another example of how tightly medicine is controlled by the drug industry? Is that why the *WSJ* never printed my scores of replies?

And the dinosaurs don't give up. Check another article in a prestigious *Lancet* paper authored by Harvard Medical School cardiologists. The *Wall Street Journal* article, "New Study Fine-Tunes **Diabetes, Statin Link**" (Wang, A3, Aug. 10, 2012) started out showing that many diabetics **develop worse disease once they start taking the cholesterol-lowering statins** (Lipitor, Crestor, etc.). Only you are clairvoyant enough to know why. (1) They didn't fix the chemistry that gave them their diabetes in the first place, and now (2) they are ignoring fixing the causes and cures of their high cholesterol. And worse, (3) now with the addition of a new drug to deplete over half a dozen nutrients even faster from their already depleted bodies, of course these poor folks are going to be on an accelerated downhill course. But this all appears to be a "mystery" to the prestigious investigators of this 17,000-patient Jupiter trial. What a ridiculous waste of time and money and print space. Do you appreciate how really clairvoyant you are? You know more than the article authors, the prestigious physicians and researchers who carried out the studies. But it gets uglier when you learn of their ultimate decision from this costly study.

First they decided the enormously expensive study was "a positive contribution" because it showed which folks would go downhill and develop diabetes or worsen their existing diabetes when prescribed statin cholesterol-lowering drugs. In essence, that would be any patients who were pre-diabetic or overtly diabetic. But you already know that would be namely the folks who have never had the benefit of a dynamo physician who would look for the cause and cure of their pre-diabetes or overt diabetes to begin with, much less find the cause and cure of their new diagnosis of hypercholesterolemia. Obviously it's easier to push somebody over who's standing on one leg as opposed two. In fact that's one reason why it is rather inconsequential whether someone has type I or type II diabetes, since depending upon the nutritional/toxic situation, either one can metamorphose in either direction. But the next decision based on this study is even more disheartening.

This Harvard professor of medicine and cardiology has authoritatively decided that (I just have to quote from the article because it's too unbelievable) "The cardiovascular benefits simply outweigh the diabetes risk, even among those with the highest risk for diabetes." In other words, even though they haven't a clue as to why folks with pre-diabetes get worse on a statin medication (ignoring the deficiencies and toxicities they started with and then placing them on a medication that further enormously depletes nutrients), **they feel bludgeoning their cholesterol production is worth it, even when this means their diabetes will get much worse**. This alone sums up the direction of current medicine.

It shows you why I made sure once again that you understood about cholesterol, high blood pressure, arrhythmias, etc. in the earlier chapters. I would love to see the records of any diabetic from that clinic who has had even membrane and mitochondrial assays with corrections, much less assays for phthalates, or a Cardio/ION, etc. (Ren, Kim, Lowell, Nisoli, Kelley, Ritov). How many folks treated by these brilliant clinicians do you think will ever in their lifetimes be prescribed acetyl-L-carnitine, DHA, DHEA, phosphatidylcholine, the eight forms of vitamin E, or chelated chromium, manganese or zinc? Also even I don't have to be clairvoyant to show no surprise when I read that "The study was funded by Astra-Zeneca PLC, the maker of Crestor." No wonder the conclusion was go ahead and use the medication, no matter what the consequences are. Even though they knew diabetics would get worse with their drugs, it was recommended!

Oddly enough from their same institution, Harvard, the Harvard School of Public Health the year before published a great article showing that 75 volunteers who consumed 12 ounces of Progresso® canned vegetable soup a day for just five days in a row raised their urinary BPA (bisphenol A) levels over 1000% (Carwile). Sadly when these folks get their diabetes or whatever other disease is triggered, they will never know that (1) this was all condoned by the FDA in spite of the huge amount of evidence that you have read, and (2) worse, their physicians had the opportunity all along to find the cause and cure of their diabetes. This article about **innocent soup cans dangerously raising the level of BPA** also was published in the *Journal of the American Medical Association*, as was a 2009 *Journal of the American Medical Association* article showing **BPA as a cause of diabetes**. I guess cardiologists don't have time to read their colleagues' works, even when they are in the same journals that they publish in.

Decades ago, **the FDA had classified BPA as a food additive in 1988**, and in spite of all of the evidence that you have seen, established a safety threshold for oral exposure at 50 mcg per kilogram of body weight per day (Hunter), about 3.5 mg. But they have no idea about how much phthalates you and I are personally ingesting each day. I'm just about speechless when it comes to this flagrant disconnect. Clearly multiple U.S. government surveys over the last decade have consistently shown that around 95% of Americans have disease-causing levels. In the meantime, the FDA continues to torment small nutritional supplement and natural detoxification companies while procrastinating with decisions that surreptitiously allow multi-billion dollar pharmaceutical companies to maximize patent protection times to the tune of billions of dollars for each year of FDA procrastination..

And if that weren't enough, many base chemicals that go into the manufacture of medications come from China as the sole source, where the U.S. FDA has minimal oversight. We're all familiar with the industrial chemical melamine (used to make plastic dishes) that was intentionally added to milk by a Chinese dairy company in 2008 that killed many infants and caused illness in over a third of a million. This plastic was added intentionally to increase the weight of the product without having to use more milk. And even though the Chinese government, to save face, threatened punishment by death, subsequently Chinese companies continued this poisonous deceit. Meanwhile, this same company was found just a few months ago to have aflatoxins in their milk. This is one of the most potent cancer-causing chemicals (mycotoxin) on the face of the earth. It was caused by feeding the cows rotten mildewed hay (Ho). They have now resorted to TV ads with apologies. Big deal. Are these the kind of people you want to trust your health to? And with the predicted physician shortage, U.S. drug-driven medicine delivered by PA's, pharmacists, etc., will become an even more fulminant dictator of the medical scene (Goodman).

By now I'm sure you are infinitely more clairvoyant about how to "see through" articles in the news. It no longer matters how highly educated, "authoritative", and prestigious folks are. What matters is whether or not they know what you know: how to find the causes and the cures of diabetes, or any disease. In fact, I'd much rather have you treat me than them.

References:

• Wei M, **Association of bisphenol A with diabetes** and other abnormalities, *Journal American Medical Association* 301; 7:720-22, **2009**

293

- Shankter A, et al, Relationship between urinary bisphenol A levels and diabetes mellitus, *Journal Clinical Endocrinology Metabolism*, 96; 12:3822-6, Dec. 2011

- Ehrenberg R, Popular plastics chemical poses another threat: this time diabetes: bisphenol A blocks protective hormone in human tissue, *Science News* 174; 6:15, Sept. 13, 2008

- Carwile JL, et al, **Canned soup** consumption and urinary **bisphenol A**.: a randomized crossover trial, *Journal American Medical Association* 306; 20:2218-20, Nov. 2011

- Hunter BT, Packaging, plastics, and paper: The pervasiveness of bisphenol A, *Price-Pottenger Journal*, 36; 2:14-20, summer 2012 (www.ppnf.org, 1-800-366-3748)

- Ho P, et al, China dairy tries to lift taint, Mengiu pursues a deal to gain more control over supplies after 2008 contamination scandal, *WSJ*, D5, Aug. 15, 2012

- Goodman JC, Why the doctor can't see you, *WSJ*, A13, Aug 15, 2012

- Ren J, et al, **Mitochondrial** biogenesis in the **metabolic syndrome** and cardiovascular disease, *Journal Molecular Medicine* 88:993-1001, 2010

- Kim JA, et al, Role of **mitochondrial dysfunction in insulin resistance**, *Circulation Research* 102:401-14, 2008

- Lowell BB, et al, **Mitochondrial dysfunction and type II diabetes**, *Science* 307:384-7, 2005

- Nisoli E, et al, **Defective mitochondrial** biogenesis: a hallmark of the high cardiovascular **risk** in the **metabolic syndrome?**, *Circulation Research* 100:795-806, 2007

- Kelley DE, et al, Dysfunction of **mitochondria in human** skeletal **muscle** in type II diabetes, *Diabetes* 51:2944-50, 2002

- Ritov VB, et al, **Deficiency of** subsarcolemmal **mitochondria in** obesity and type II **diabetes**, *Diabetes* 54:8-14, 2005

A Proven Way to Lower Your Plastic Level

Okay, you have learned enough about placticisers (phthalates) that outgas from out food containers, medications, IV's, dental materials, furnishings, clothes, cosmetics, fragrances, appliances, computers, automobiles, planes, construction materials and even the wiring in the walls, as just a few examples.

By now you know they are (1) proven by government studies to be in all of us, because they are (2) unavoidably ubiquitous environmental toxins. And you know (3) that they can damage the human chemistry in a multitude of ways including creating diabetes and all of its complications. **Phthalates are a perfect example of how unavoidable environmental toxins can create every disease.** Clearly, plasticizers (phthalates and BPA) can cause everything from birth defects and learning disabilities to cancers, obesity, hyperthyroidism, metabolic syndrome,

Alzheimer's, coronary artery disease, NASH, insulin resistance, and ....diabetes.

And you have learned from *Detoxify or Die* **that the far infrared sauna is one of the best ways on the planet to reduce your levels and thereby reduce disease.** In fact, it is such a potent therapeutic tool that researchers at the Mayo clinic did the unthinkable. They put folks with end-stage congestive heart failure in the saunas. Normally even a heat wave kills off these folks. But because the far infrared technology is so different from a regular sauna, these folks improved so much that they were able to get off medications, something folks with heart failure never do as a rule. In fact median survival is about 5 years after diagnosis and that's with a dozen medications on board.

So wouldn't it be wonderful if we had another way to lower the level of phthalates? And wouldn't it be even greater if it didn't cost any money? Well, researchers have accomplished this dream. They took 5 families and educated them in how cans, packages, plastic bottles, plastic wrap and other food packagings as well as (especially!) eating out, contribute to high levels. Then for only 3 days the had them eat only "fresh foods" that were not packaged.

These **families lowered their levels of various phthalates and BPA's from 53 to 96% in 3 days.** There you have it folks, it doesn't get much more straight forward and simple than that. Recall the old original days of *The EI Syndrome* where many of us were so chemically sensitive that we had to use cellophane and glass refrigerator storage dishes.? Looks like that's still not such a bad idea. (Available NaturalLifestyleMarket.com 800-752-2775)

So with (1) common sense avoidance (or at least cutting back on plastic, especially concerning foods), (2) repairing and reving up the detoxification of our unavoidable plastics contamination from air, food and water, and (3) using your far infrared sauna to detoxify, you are so much further ahead than you were when you were younger. Now *you* understand why only *you* have the power to turn back the hands of time and reverse your diabetes.

Reference:

- Rudel RA, et al, **Food packaging and bisphenolA and** bis(#2-ethylhexyl) **phthalate exposure**: Findings from a dietary intervention, *Environ Heath Persp* 119:914-20, 2011

Cure Diabetic Kidney Disease

As I try to close this chapter, I'm inundated with evidences of cures that are so simple, yet far from the realm of conventional drug-driven medicine. As a tiny yet earth-shattering example, in this diabetic pandemic 40% of type I and 15% of type II could be eligible for renal dialysis. Not only is this detrimental as I've evidenced, but it could bankrupt the country. Yet two of the 8 forms of Vitamin E can stop the kidney failure from happening and reverse it once it has started. The problem is where are the docs who know to add 3 tocotrienols twice a day to the rest of the program?

And don't forget you have already learned how powerful and necessary vitamin B1 and DHA, PC, etc. are for preventing and curing diabetic nephropathy! Medicine is operating in the dark ages when all the answers are here for everyone.

Reference:

- Kuhad A, et al, **Attenuation of diabetic nephropathy by tocotrienol**: Involvement of NFkB signaling pathway, *Life Sci* 84: 296-301, 2009

Chapter VII

Dinosaur Doctors Deny Deity

Dinosaur Docs Don't Read

Millions of Americans across the United States have dangerous dinosaur doctors. Folks are unknowingly being robbed of life as well as money, merely because most in medicine have lazily taken the drug route as opposed to taking the time to learn how **God has miraculously designed the body to heal, ….. against all odds.**

I have a tough time letting you go, since there is so much more empowerment available to you. Remember I've only given you less than 20%. So let's look at some simple examples of common medical problems that are ineptly handled. Yet if the physician was reading the monthly referenced newsletter (I think he can afford 80□ a week for the electronic version!) and catching up on the previous books, he could turn his practice into one of actually curing diseases. He could step out of the mold of being a **3-D** **d**inosaur **d**octor (**d**rugs, **d**evices, and surgical **d**estruction/procedures as the main tools to temporarily stifle symptoms). He could become a dynamo and actually show folks how to heal (complete with scientific evidence).

Let's take a simple example of an epidemic disease that often accompanies diabetes. Suppose you've been diagnosed with **low thyroid, hypothyroidism or Graves' disease or Hashimoto's thyroiditis or auto-immune thyroiditis**. When thyroid function is low 3-D doctors immediately spring into action and prescribe thyroid. They fail to check minerals like **selenium, zinc, iodine** or others that have totally cured the thyroid gland so that it can once more function normally (depending on the individual person's deficiencies). However once you start taking thyroid pills then you get *feedback inhibition* which tells the gland "Don't bother making any thyroid because we already have enough on board". So eventually the gland burns out and you subsequently need higher doses of thyroid.

But also because he never checked the mitochondrial chemistry he doesn't know that you can take thyroid until the cows come home, but **if you don't make enough energy in the mitochondria inside your cells, then the thyroid and the cells it controls can't function.** In addition, as you have learned here, if you haven't repaired the cell membrane receptors for thyroid on the surface of cells, they won't properly accept the thyroid and allow it to turn on energy pathways. The dinosaur fails to check if you have toxic plasticizers, heavy metals, flame retardants, pesticides, etc. or deficiencies of fatty acids or phosphatidyl choline in the cell membrane (Vandenberg, Moriyama, Kitamura). In other words, **you can give thyroid until the cows come home, but it won't work until you repair and detox the receptors.** Meanwhile, dinosaurs are baffled when thyroid pills don't fix your symptoms or give you energy to rave about.

And so it goes, only because he totally neglected to find out *why* you were suddenly deficient in the thyroid in the first place. Recall as an example from the previous chapter that most environmental toxins, starting with the plasticizers, right on down to heavy metals, pesticides, VOH, etc. are **environmental endocrine disruptors.** Most toxins' destruction targets glands. And remember the thyroid is just an example of another gland, but not much different from the pancreas.

Why does a person become hypothyroid? For the same reasons one becomes diabetic. The gland can burn out for a multitude of reasons. One of the most common is from **the phthalates or plasticizers which are the strongest environmental endocrine disruptors in the human body and are the pollutant of highest level. They especially make a beeline to glands** to destroy slowly or quickly. When it happens slowly to the thyroid, you have "normal thyroid levels" but feel horrible. Yet your doctor doesn't know why because he didn't read about the newer cut-off levels of

TSH (thyroid stimulating hormone) in 2009 *TW*. In here we have put the proof that the cut-off for a "normal" level used by commercial labs lags over a decade behind the scientific research showing that it should be lowered to less than 2.

Another **common reason for thyroid destruction is a gut full of Candida that has led to irritable bowel, gas, bloating, indigestion**, alternating diarrhea and constipation, or heartburn. Often the gut symptoms are ignored, or worse yet, the less knowledgeable person takes acid inhibitors like Prilosec. But these turn off the stomach acid. That means there is less acid that was designed to kill Candida. And by killing acid secretion you also inhibit the absorption of the very nutrients you need in order to fight Candida. Meanwhile, once the Candida inflames the lining of the gut and creates the leaky gut syndrome, then you start making antibodies against the Candida which share similar physical properties with antigenic sites on your thyroid. Hence you now start making antibodies that attack your very own thyroid gland. We call this **auto-immune thyroiditis**. And it doesn't stop there, for many folks then **develop food allergies that they never had before, which masquerade as arthritis**, fibromyalgia, a bad hip, or other seemingly unrelated new diagnoses. You are on a roll as though you had joined the disease-of-the-month club. (How to heal the leaky gut is explained *No More Heartburn*).

Just as with hypothyroidism, when you are diagnosed with **diabetes,** immediately the doctor plunks you on the latest and greatest medication that he has been taught about by the pharmaceutical representative (called a detail man). You learned how **common drugs for diabetes actually lower nutrients like B12 and zinc, which then can slowly and silently create common complications of diabetes, like heart disease, exhaustion, infections, BPH, memory loss, Alzheimer's disease**, and much more. But I think this dinosaur should be fired from action if he has not even checked so much as your fatty acids, chromium, biotin, ALC, and vanadium, etc., since these rudimentary nutrients have a huge bearing on whether or not you actually *cure* your diabetes.

Or let's look at something more serious that affects diabetics more often than folks without diabetes, cancer. After surgery for **breast cancer** usually chemotherapy and/or radiation follow, then women often get breast implants (which of course are bags made of phthalates, while phthalates from other previous sources may have been the underlying cause of the cancer to begin with). Meanwhile, they are told "Everything looks fine" when they go for their check ups. And yet most of them have never had even the most rudimentary and simple test to show if they are silently on the road to metastases in the future. The **Estronex** test shows whether or not you have a good ratio (of about double the amount) of 2-hydroxyestrone (the good protective estrogen) versus the 16-a-hydroxyestrone (the one that triggers breast cancers and metastases). And you have total control over those ratios.

The **Estronex Test** is extremely simple because your physician merely writes a prescription for it (or you go to directlabs.com for yourself). Then you call the lab (MetaMetrix.com) and get the kit, put your urine in it and send it back in the Fed-Ex mailer (with the directlabs.com or your own doctor's prescription). Nothing could be easier. Yet how many women do you think I've seen (who have had breast cancer) have had this test ordered by their family doctor, oncologist, gynecologist, or surgeon? And of course there are many other tests that should be done to prevent breast cancer initially. And if you have already had a cancer, these tests definitely should be done to prevent recurrence and metastases. One of the easiest ways to regulate the ratios to dissuade cancer is with adding more Brassica vegetables to the diet and 2 twice a day of each, **IndolPlex, Tocotrienols,** and **Calcium D-Glucarate** (you learned about this in the last chapter and there is more in *TW*).

Or look at the unknowledgeable recommendation of a **daily aspirin** that is mandated by Medicare overseers. It actually inhibits the enzyme UDP-glucuronyl transferase that you need to detoxify your unavoidable daily onslaught of phthalates, which then can go on to trigger every disease. In *The High Blood Pressure Hoax* and in *The Cholesterol Hoax* we went into the ridiculousness of this and then presented the actual doses of the nutrients that are far better at not only inhibiting unwanted clots, but also essential for strengthening your cardiac blood vessels and heart muscle at the same time, something aspirin is incapable of. Plus a daily aspirin can markedly increase your cataract, stroke, deafness, and other risks. But be sure to check 2013 *TW* on how **once you have a stent**, as an example, **this changes the rules. You need to adhere to medications until** you have proof of sufficient healing.

Or look at the amount of radiation women are exposed to for the diagnosis of osteoporosis (not to mention the prescription drugs like Fosamax which can rot out your jaw). Obviously their physicians are unaware of the **Bone Resorption** test which shows if the nutrient levels are sufficient to turn off osteoporosis now, or if folks are still silently continuing to lose bone. You don't need the radiation of a bone scan that takes 2 years to show osteoporosis. And even if you don't have osteoporosis this test shows if you are silently headed for it.

And yet the majority of folks are placed on biphosphonates like Fosamax® which not only can cause worse hip and other bone fractures, but rotting out of the jaw bones with loss of all the teeth. And its side effects don't stop there, for it can cause atrial fibrillation which is then treated with Coumadin (warfarin). This drags calcium out of the bones and dumps it into the coronary arteries and heart valves, thereby requiring surgery if you live that long. And it increases the risk of cancer of the esophagus, stomach and rectum (Sellmeyer, Migliorati, Howard, Green, Genuis). Do you see how too easily the unread public is continually duped?

Meanwhile, this easy noninvasive test also shows you (once you have chosen your program for healing osteoporosis) whether or not it is successful or needs "tweaking" with often neglected nutrients that are crucial for healing bone like **Vitamin K2, BioSil, Nutra**

Support Joint, Solar D Gems, Strontium, etc., and more (*TW*). This simple urine test done at home quickly shows you if you are still losing bone or if you are on the right track and have turned off bone loss now! You don't wait 2 years to find out. Clearly, to keep "nuking" folks with bone scans every year or two is ridiculous if you have a safer, quicker, less expensive, and far better measure of success.

Or if you want to delve into another newly emerged area of medicine which really stoops to the lowest level of knowledge, look at the **sleep apnea** crap. I've yet to see one person's records from a sleep center that included *any* nutrients that have to do with sleep. I think even a high school student could tell you to look at tryptophan and RBC magnesium. So I guess it shouldn't surprise me that they have not looked at any of the other chemistry that makes up the brain receptors of relaxation, much less the neurotransmitters like glycine, melatonin, etc. conducive for sleep. So far be it from them to ever even check levels of adrenal hormones like **DHEA**, important in relaxing the GABA membrane receptors (much less repairing them) in the brain as well as improving libido, memory, heart function, lipids, osteoporosis, and even diabetes. But how often do you see sleep docs do the **Adrenal Stress Panel** even though the adrenal gland is commonly attacked by plasticizers, heavy metals, nutrient deficiencies, and more? Just abnormal adrenal secretions can cause insomnia.

And when I review records of previous years, for non-patient reader phone consults, there is usually evidence that they were on their way to disease even on their conventional lab tests. But when I ask them what their doctors said about particular abnormalities on their blood tests (or x-rays), they say they were told the abnormalities were minimal and of no consequence. What he really meant was he didn't have the faintest idea of what minerals and vitamins and other cofactors are needed in the metabolic pathway to correct the "inconsequential" abnormalities before they reach more serious proportions.

For example, if there is a slight decrease in a liver enzyme LDH (lactic acid dehydrogenase) they usually don't know that that's a sign of zinc deficiency. They just tell folks that "We only worry about it if it is elevated, for then it can be a sign of liver abnormality, bone metastases, etc.". So when you develop diabetes later on from this ignored opportunity to correct an early zinc deficiency, they still are clueless that they missed the opportunity to prevent your diabetes. For through ignorant neglect eventually the "inconsequential lab abnormality" does become more serious. But you know what? This is not malpractice. Because currently the **definition of malpractice is that you are *not* doing what the rest of the herd is doing. If the majority are doing inferior drug-oriented medicine, you are blameless.**

And recall that zinc deficiency is very common, since everything from environmental pollutants like phthalates to common prescriptions like statin cholesterol-lowering and diabetes drugs can cause it. Yet who checks your RBC zinc, even when you have an obvious zinc-deficiency disease like diabetes?

As you are beginning to appreciate, no one book is sufficient to educate and protect you in this era of medicine. **Health education is an ongoing process**. For example, diabetics are known to have slow wound healing. As well, they often have hypertension and coronary artery disease. Yet as we discussed in *The High Blood Pressure Hoax* an inexpensive **Arginine Powder** can improve all of those (Witte). Now you can appreciate how not knowing this can make you a statistic after surgery as opposed to a success story. That's why **I never leave anyone out when I write a book**. Even if you don't have high blood pressure, the health of your blood vessels is paramount to the health of every organ, especially the pancreas. So regardless of the title you need to read every book, because I don't know any other way to protect and empower you, and at the same time so inexpensively. And another benefit is once you have the knowledge, it is yours forever.

Just look at the references below that I've selected from random out of thousands and then in back issues of the books and the *TW* newsletters and you will see how stagnant the practice of medicine is. In fact it's downright scary.

As I have said before, I think *people power* is the only thing that can turn medicine around, but then we need more people aware of the facts. At nearly 70 I don't need money or fame. I have had an exceedingly successful career for over 40 years in medicine, and am ecstatically happy to devote myself to God's greatest blessing, Luscious. I only keep this information coming because of you. If you want to encourage your friends to read the books and subscribe to the newsletters then I'll keep providing the information, but it is up to you. If not, I'm very happy improving my tennis and golf games and continuing to learn cocktail piano to produce those romantic tunes of the 30s and 40s....and pampering Luscious.

If you think your physician is salvageable and a potential Dynamo and you really like the guy/gal and trust him, start by giving him this book or an easier one like *Is Your Cardiologist Killing You?,* and maybe half a year subscription of *TW.* I use the newsletter of 25 years, *Total Wellness,* to keep folks abreast of the latest findings and updates since each book, and it is always referenced. Articles like how to reverse macular degeneration when the ophthalmologist says there is no cure, how one nutrient makes the brain 12 years younger in 3 months, how folks are totally healthy decades after they were given just days to live with wildly metastatic cancer, or how one mineral can make the abnormal prostate enzyme, PSA, revert to normal so the poor guy doesn't have to have a 12-point needle biopsy of his prostate are just a smattering of the articles already in *TW.* Meanwhile, a good sign of a hopeless Dinosaur doctor is one who doesn't have time to read 7-8 pages a month and a book of less than 200 pages that can save not only *your* life but *his.*

References:

• Wertenbruch T, et al, Serum **selenium levels in patients with remission** and a **relapse** of **Graves' disease**, *Med Chem* 3; 3:281-84, 2007

• Ruz M, et al, Single and multiple **selenium, zinc, iodine deficiencies affect** rats' **thyroid** metabolism and ultra structure, *J Nutr* 129; 1:174-80, 1999

• Montori VM, et al, **Fish oil supplementation in type II diabetes**: a quantitative systemic review, *Diabetes Care* 23; 9:1407-15, 2000

• Morris DW, et al, **Chromium supplementation improves insulin resistance in patients with type II diabetes mellitus**, *Diabetes Med* 19; 9:684-5, 2000

• Witte MD, et al, **L-arginine supplementation enhances diabetic wound healing**: involvement of the nitric oxide synthase and arginase pathways, *Metabolism* 51; 10:1269-73, 2002

• Moriyama K, et al, **Thyroid hormone is disrupted by bisphenol A** as an antagonist, *J Clin Endocrinol Metab* 87:5185-90, 2002

• Kitamura S, et al, Thyroid hormonal activity of the **flame retardant tetrabromobisphenol A** and tetrachlorobisphenol A, *Biochem Biophys Res Comm* 293:554-9, 2002

• Vandenberg LN, et al, **Bisphenol-A** and the great divide: a review of controversies in the field of **endocrine disruption**, *Endocr Rev* 30; 1:75-95, 2009

• Sellmeyer DE, et al, **Atypical fractures as a potential complication of long-term biphosphonates therapy**, *J Am Med Assoc* 304; 13:1480-4, 2010

• Migiorati CA, et al, **Biphosphonate-associated osteonecrosis of mandibular** and maxillary **bone**: an emerging oral complication of supportive cancer therapy, *Cancer*, 104; 1:83-93, 2005

• Howard PA, et al, Impact of **biphosphonates on the risk of atrial fibrillation**, *Am J Cardiovasc Drugs* 10; 6:359-67, 2010

• Green J, et al, Oral **biphosphonates and risk of cancer of esophagus, stomach, and colorectum**: case-control analysis within a UK primary care cohort, *Brit Med J*, 341 article ID C4444, 2010

• Genuis S, et al, Combination of Micronutrients for Bone (COMB) Study: bone density after micronutrients intervention, *J Environ Pub Health*, article ID 354151, 2012

Is Wellness Intentionally Stifled?

When we look at the statistics of a diabetic precursor like Syndrome X, which has been called "the epidemic of global proportions", it makes me wonder where the normal people are? For over 40% of the people over 40 years of age have Syndrome X, while 75% of diabetics have it. Plus 50% of folks with Syndrome X have high blood pressure and 50% go on to get peripheral neuropathy. Furthermore, Metabolic Syndrome or Syndrome X leads to not only diabetes, but obesity, NASH, high cholesterol, coronary artery disease, inflammation, kidney disease and cancers (Guan, Houston). Where are the healthy folks?

You have here at your fingertips a smattering of the overwhelming evidence that **disease is mainly caused by two things: deficiencies and toxicities**. And the proof of the pudding lies with the folks who have cured their "incurable" diseases by bringing the body back into sufficient balance so that it can heal itself. You have had a glimpse at the immutable evidence of God's awesome design of the intricacies of human molecular biochemistry, most of which is still a mystery to scientists. We have biochemical pathways to detoxify chemicals that were invented yesterday. We have foods with their nutrients that literally talk to and regulate and even repair genes. We have everything we need. But the money is in poisoning a malfunctioning part for immediate symptom stifling, rather than reversing or repairing and curing.

If you want one tiny more appalling fact to bring home the grisly nature of conventional 3-D medicine, consider these facts. You know how folks are brow-beaten into having a **colonoscopy** in hopes of finding an early colon cancer. Indeed, **this procedure has lowered the risk of dying from colon cancer 12-17%** (Parkin). But instead of this $500 (plus) procedure, pennies of vitamin D (for which there is documented epidemic deficiency in all walks of life) lowers colon cancer risk not double, not triple, not quadruple, but over five times more. **Vitamin D deficiency correction can lower the risk of colon cancer 80%** (Garland). Now which one will your colonoscopist choose for you? His $500 procedure or pennies of vitamin D coupled with learning more chemistry of the human body that he is licensed to treat? For as we have referenced in *TW*, even when a polyp is found, rarely do they assay the gut and body to see what needs correcting to keep the polyps from returning or turning cancerous. Sometimes it is as simple as more folinic acid (sublingual **Folixor**). Meanwhile, will he make his patient healthy enough to let God's chemistry keep

306

him from cancer, or use a technique over 5-times less effective but that helps him with his Mercedes payment? You decide.

References:

- Guan Y, Peroxisome proliferator-activated receptor family and its relationship to real complications of the metabolic syndrome, *J Am Soc Nephrol*, 15:2801-15, 2004

- Houston MC, et al, The metabolic syndrome, *JANA*, 8;2: 3-83, 2005

- Parkin DM, et al, Predicting the impact of the screening programme for colorectal cancer in the U.K., *J Med Screening*, 15;4:163-174, 2008

- Garland CF, et al, Serum 25-hydroxyvitamin D and colon cancer: eight-year prospective study, *Lancet* 2;8673:1176-8, 1989

- Genuis SJ, What's out there making us sick?, *J Environ Pub Health*, article ID 605137, 10 pg, 2012

Recent Cardiology Guidelines are a Joke.

One 53 year old surgeon literally died in the emergency room from a heart attack. With no pulse, breathing or blood pressure, they immediately did cardioversion (the dramatic paddles where you attempt to electrocute the heart back to life). After 5 unsuccessful attempts and all the modern medications, someone walked in and suggested IV magnesium. It supplied what the heart needed to start it beating again and he lived. And recall this is not unusual. Many folks I have consulted on were brought back from the dead with an injection of magnesium in the emergency room (*TW* 2011). But nowhere in their hospital records was there ever a measure of RBC magnesium, even though it was that minimally corrected deficiency that brought them back to life. Nor were they discharged with an order for an RBC magnesium test.

Clearly the **"medical experts" appear ignorant about healing via nutrients.** And why wouldn't they be when their own guidelines don't even mention such important things as magnesium? Instead they push drugs as though they were the only option. And it's interesting because there are thousands of papers showing that drugs are not the answer, while nutrients are. But then you only have to recall that **less than 11% of cardiologist's**

307

recommendations are based on science. The rest are based on pharmaceutical financial influence.

For example, in one study **giving calcium channel blockers** (like Norvasc, see *TW* 2010 for other names of these that rot the brain) had **no effect on total mortality** (Multi-Center Diltiazem Postinfarction Trial Research Group). Yet this class of drugs and others are still prescribed to this day even though **they actually increase the rate of heart attack** (Hine, Cardiac Arrhythmia Suppression Trial). And only you know why they make folks worse. They fail to repair the calcium channels and arrhythmia-causing deficiencies. They merely further poison the chemistry to temporarily attenuate the symptoms.

And why shouldn't *calcium channel blockers accelerate death*? After all, if you need a drug to block the membrane calcium pores, then hadn't you better find out why calcium is building up too fast inside heart cells and killing them? Sometimes the fix is as simple as magnesium or the membrane oil change that you learned about.

I know hearing about the intransigence of medicine is sometimes hard to believe, so I'll quote to you from the American College of Cardiology in association with the **American Heart Association's recent practice guidelines** written for physicians. I have to quote because you won't be able to believe it otherwise. "Allocation to metaprolol produced an average relative increase in cardiogenic shock of 30%" (page 301). "Metaprolol allocation was associated with significantly more persistent hypotension and more cases of bradycardia".

What are they saying? **Folks who were prescribed a beta blocker, like metaprolol (atenolol,** etc. other names in *The High Blood Pressure Hoax*) **have a 30% higher chance of heart death.** Yet the "expert" guidelines are that (and I again quote) "Oral beta blocker therapy should be administered promptly to those patients without contraindications". **So even though these "experts" realize folks die sooner who have the drugs (and no** corrections), they still recommend them. Why? Because their *only tools* are drugs and surgery. They are clueless about finding the causes and cures of heart disease, even though the solutions and scientific back-up are proven. Also the *PDR* repeatedly warns that **NSAIDs can counteract the effects of beta blockers yet aspirin is almost invariably prescribed with it.** Go figure.

I have yet to meet one cardiologist who has slugged his way through these ridiculous guidelines and I can't blame them. But how much easier and more productive it would be, and how many millions of lives could be saved if they would only read of the simpler causes and cures of heart disease, starting with *Is Your Cardiologist Killing You?* They can knock it off in 2 weeks at 10 minutes a day and change the draconian focus of medicine.

References:

- Multi-center Diltiazem Postinfarction Trial Research Group, The effect of diltiazem on mortality and re-infarction after myocardial infarction, *New Engl J Med* 319:385-92, 1988
- Antman EM, et al, 2007 focused update on the ACC/AHA 2004 **guidelines** for the management of patients with ST-elevation myocardial infarction. A report of the American College of Cardiology/American Heart Association Task Force on Practice Guidelines, *Circulation* 117:296-39, 2008
- Hine LK, et al, Meta-analysis of empirical long-term antiarrhythmic therapy after myocardial infarction, *J Amer Med Assoc* 262:3037-40, 1989
- Cardiac Arrhythmia Suppression Trial. Preliminary report: effectiveness of flecainide on mortality in a randomized trial of arrhythmia suppression after myocardial infarction, *New Engl J Med*, 321:406-12, 1989

Drugs Proven to be Useless in Disease and to Accelerate Death

Remember from Chapter I how **the current focus on drugs for diabetes is worthless? Drugs do not improve longevity, in fact they increase the death rate, sometimes doubling and tripling it.** No matter how aggressively docs lowered the sugar and glycosylated hemoglobin A1C, *drugs did not make diabetics live longer.* They merely made blood tests and some symptoms improve, and that was just temporary, until more drugs were added. In fact, **lowering the glycated hemoglobin for over three years actually increased the death rate 22%.** And that's not all.

309

Diabetes drugs increased retinopathy (the chance to go blind) and renal failure (the need for dialysis) 37%. And they increased swelling, weight gain, congestive heart failure, heart attack rates and cancers.

But does that stop U.S. doctors from trying to bludgeon every patient's Hgb A1C into a normal level with the drug? No way. Scientists **have proven that you can throw all the best drugs at a patient for diabetes, blood pressure and cholesterol, etc. and it makes no difference in death rate** compared with doing nothing. And in some cases medications increased the death rate, as they should since you have added a drug that depletes nutrients and ushers in a myriad of side effects and eventually new diseases. Did I remind you of this from the earlier chapters again on purpose? You bet your life I did! (Pardon the pun!)

There is no excuse, but mainstream medicine is somehow able to turn a blind eye to all this. Does it have anything to do with the fact from the *Wall Street Journal* that the average office visit is 7 minutes and the average time a patient gets to tell their symptoms is 18 seconds? You can't teach anything in that time. You can only write a "script" and bolt for the door. And further studies proved **diabetes medications did increase the number of strokes, vision loss problems, nerve damage, and hospitalizations**. And that is not all! They **increased dementia (severe memory and brain function loss) by 50%.** We are headed for a nation of idiots.

Euthanasia is Closer Than You Think

Did you know that in Britain under the National Health Service (which our government appears to want to emulate) that **one in 6 deaths come from legalized killing of old and sick folks? They are euthanized by an overdose of a drug** designed to kill them. Do you want some bureaucrat, physician or physician's assistant, who knows nothing about healing that you learned about here, deciding when you should be knocked off? I quote, "In Britain in

2007-2008 **16.5% of deaths came after 'terminal sedation'** ". I guess we don't have to worry about the planned rationing of health care. This is far more effective! If, like me, you thought all doctors know all the facts in this book, think again. **You need to be in control**, and *surreptitiously test perspective physicians by innocently asking some of the test questions you've learned about* here. Clearly, **the only way you can save yourself is with knowledge**. For example, I would suggest you put in your termination of life instructions that you want complete documented evidence that you have had a **Cardio/ION** done with an expert interpretation before you are ever "terminated".

• Darwell R, Government medicine versus the elderly, *Wall St J,* A21, Sept 15, 2009

FDA Condones Brain Deterioration and Blindness

Does it sound ridiculous? These are apparently acceptable side effects. But I'll let you be the judge. Hidden undiagnosed B12 deficiency is becoming a more serious problem. Why? Because medications like Metformin for diabetes, plus non-prescription Prilosec, Nexium and other acid inhibitors for heartburn, some common blood pressure medications, Dilantin for seizures, plus some antibiotics, birth control, hormone replacement, and other **medications can silently deplete B12**. At first, hidden B12 deficiency can cause bizarre numbness and tingling or pain sensations or neuropathies (all of which also are seriously painful side effects of diabetes). Later, **B12 deficiency causes the brain to literally deteriorate while it shrinks away from the skull**. Along with this loss of brain volume or size is also the onset of loss of intellect, memory and eventual emergence of depression, Alzheimer's or dementia. But it is chalked up to "normal" aging, especially since it can come on ever so slowly.

B12 is needed for making the covering (myelin sheath) around nerves, so it should always be checked in folks with diabetic neuropathy, as well as multiple sclerosis, etc.. Plus many other nutrients are involved. Furthermore, a low B12 elevates homocysteine which can then lead to early heart disease, strokes, Alzheimer's, cancers, and many other diseases, the very things you are taking diabetes medications to ostensibly prevent. Furthermore, a low B12 can be a major factor ushering in macular degeneration, the number one cause of blindness in people over 50, and a common problem accelerated in diabetics.

You can imagine how I nearly have a stroke every time I see someone's records from their ophthalmologist who never even checked so much as their B12, much less the fatty acids and the dozens of other factors that are completely curable that could have caused (and cured!) their macular degeneration. Yet he has the gall to tell them that the disease (macular degeneration, etc.) has no known cause and no known treatment, and that they will be blind in five years so they had better start preparing for it.

And even more sad is the fact that this **brain rot or shrinking away of the brain occurs at "normal" blood levels of B12.** As extensively referenced in *TW (Total Wellness,* our monthly referenced newsletter for over 24 years), government recommendations are decades behind current scientific facts. The result is decades of unnecessary diseases and ruined lives.

But the saddest part is that the acid inhibitors notoriously dramatically lower B12. Yet as soon as many of these medications lost their patents, the FDA decided they were magically safer and no longer in need of a prescription. So folks can buy **Prilosec, Pepcid, Tagamet, Zantac and other acid inhibitors** without a prescription. That means there's *nobody* protecting folks against the **silent brain destruction stemming from these medications stealthily lowering their B12 levels**. And the FDA does not even require a warning about developing B12 deficiency on the labels.

Your protection? I would definitely make sure you get 1000 mcg (1mg) of **Sublingual B12** every day, so that you by-pass any possible hidden gut problem that you don't yet know you have like *Helicobactor pylori* (called *H.pylori*) or *Candida*. These bugs can silently damage stomach cells so they no longer secrete the intrinsic factor which is necessary for absorption of oral B-12 (see *No More Heartburn* for their diagnoses and treatments). By using the sublingual form you by-pass the gut. I would use 1000 mcg (= 1 mg) of sublingual B12 daily. You don't want your brain to shrink or to go blind from such an easily preventable cause.

References:

*   Rogers SA, *No More Heartburn, Total Wellness*, prestigepublishing.com or 1-800-846-6687
*   Rochtchina E, et al, Elevated serum **homocysteine, low serum B12, folate**, and age-related **macular degeneration**: the Blue Mountains Eye Study, *Am J Ophthalmol*, 143 (2): 344-346, Feb. 2007
*   Vogiatzoglou A, et al, Vitamin **B12 status and rate of brain volume loss** in community-dwelling elderly, *Neurology*, 71:826-32, 2008
*   Pelton R, et al, *Drug-Induced Nutrient Depletion Handbook*, 1-800-837-5394, 1999
*   Goodwin JS, et al, Association between **nutritional status and cognitive functioning** in healthy elderly population, *J Am Med Assoc*, 249:2917-21, **1983**
*   Seshadri S, et al, Plasma **homocysteine as a risk factor for dementia and Alzheimer's** disease, *New Engl J Med*, 346:476-83, 2002

Are You Headed For an Amputation? Wait!

Painful diabetic neuropathy, loss of sensation, nearly gangrenous toes, non-healing ulcers, and glaucoma are some of the nastiest complications of diabetes. But don't despair. **You may be able to heal** them. If that sounds preposterous, it's only because there is so much more that you don't know about. So let's take a quantum leap. (Other aspects of glaucoma were dealt with in 2012 *Total Wellness*).

By now you know that everything in the body is not only chemical, but at a deeper level it's electrical. In fact every organ, every enzyme, every component of a cell has an electrical frequency of its own. In *Pain Free In 6 Weeks* I gave the evidence of how soldiers returning from battle who had non-union fractures were healed using the correct bone frequencies. Prior to this, these fractures were pinned and plated and casted, yet they would never knit together and heal. But then applying the correct frequency to the bone cells turned on the chemistry of healing. Likewise we know how to use this frequency for diabetic neuropathy, whether it's in the early stages with severe pain or the later stages with loss of sensation, as well as with areas of poor circulation, ulcers, poorly healed burns, erectile dysfunction, and even glaucoma. Let me give you a little background.

"And God said, 'Let there be light,' and there was light. God saw that the light was good" (*Gen* 1:3). But I didn't know that He had designed light so that it could be used for healing! I do know that giving you the science first is not the way to entice you to read on, but if you're like me, I needed a lot of scientific evidence before I could begin to believe the healing miracles that I saw. So let's start, backwards.

Light has a whole spectrum from short wavelengths all the way up to very long wavelengths. And having wavelengths, means that it also has energies or frequencies. God has programmed receptors for light in living organisms. Plants use light for photosynthesis to grow and move. Animals have receptors for light in the visual part of the brain, the eye, plus photo-receptors are in the skin for making the hormone vitamin D. But more exciting regarding His phenomenally unfathomable molecular biochemistry of the body is that inside cells we also have enzymes that respond to light and specific frequencies, like NAD and cytochrome C oxidase.

Physicists have learned that they could harness the energies of light through laser technology. High frequencies of lasers are more precise than a surgeon's knife and can cauterize at the same time to stop bleeding. Low frequency levels of lasers have been used to heal, but they are not without side effects and the machines are very expensive and require training.

This is where the LED (light emitting diode) comes into play. Compared to laser, it is safer, cheaper, easier to use, there is no risk of eye damage (in fact it is used to heal eyes), it penetrates a broader surface area at once, it is gentler, without side effects, and has greater healing energy. If you are a skeptic like me, who has seen hundreds of useless devices and supplements, you're probably saying about now, "Yeah, yeah, yeah, everything sounds too good to be true. Where's some proof that will bowl me over?"

LED light protects the toxic eye. Proof? Methanol, also known as wood alcohol, is notorious for causing blindness as many prohibition era medical case histories have confirmed. It does so by changing into formaldehyde, which is highly toxic to the optic nerve in the retina (back) of the eye. After testing their vision, researchers at the Medical College of Wisconsin injected methanol into rats. One group of rats was left alone while the other group was treated with the LED only three times in the next two days. The untreated rats lost so much vision that they could hardly recognize light. In those that had only three treatments of LED, their vision was markedly better, 72% of normal. There's nothing in medicine that can protect like that.

And you guessed it. When the researchers did a microscopic examination of the retinas, inside the cells of the untreated animals *the mitochondria* (which you are now knowledgeable in) were swollen and abnormally disrupted. But for the LED-treated animals, their retinal cells' mitochondria looked normal under the microscope. The LED in only three treatments saved the eye cells from permanent damage from the notoriously toxic chemical. There is no drug in medicine that can do that (and without side effects)!

Further studies by the same researchers showed that they could give one of the most potent toxins in the world and reverse its damage inside cells. Tetrodotoxin causes death by poisoning the enzyme, *cytochrome oxidase*, again inside cellular *mitochondria* where energy is made. **Once the enzyme cytochrome oxidase is poisoned, the mitochondria are powerless to make the energy** needed to sustain life. But **the LED reversed the damage to cytochrome oxidase.** This enzyme is actually turned on by light in the far-red (visible) to near-infrared spectra as it strongly

315

absorbs this stimulating energy. *This energy transfusion* in turn increases electron transfer *in the mitochondria*, leading to *increased energy synthesis for healing.* And you can have one of these devices in your home, because this LED red light with the specific frequency for the enzyme has been used for well over a decade. It is called the **Lumen** (lumenphoton.com).

LED can turn on other beneficial body chemistries, for cytochrome oxidase is just one of several enzymes that can be turned on by light. This small hand-held LED unit, called the **Lumen**, has been used to accelerate wound healing after surgery, after a heart attack, in broken bones, non-union fractures, in diabetic mice, in burns, skin ulcers, resistant infections including teeth root infections, plus **regenerate nerves**, and stop pain. It has been used to destroy tumors, accelerate the healing of skin, muscle, nerve, tendon, cartilage, bone, dental and periodontal tissues.

So why am I so excited about this particular one? Because it empowers you and I more than ever to heal. In addition, it is FDA approved, and is the most efficacious, cost-effective and safest device I have seen. My husband and I play tennis two hours a day often 3-6 days a week so we've had lots of opportunity to use it on ourselves and friends. On the other end of the spectrum, folks have rescued themselves from needless surgeries. Clearly, I can't imagine a home without one.

For example, one time during the aftermath of a hurricane I absentmindedly grabbed onto a frying pan handle that had been inside a 450° grill for 25 minutes. As a former emergency room physician I had visions of skin grafts, tendon repairs and permanent tendon damage. I immediately alternated the **Lumen**, cycling with ice. Within 4 hours my screamingly painful burned hand was painless and looked totally normal. The white blanched palm and fingers were pink. This is in stark contrast to a scar I still have from a quick touch of my wrist on an oven rack when I didn't use the **Lumen**. And this was not anywhere near the intensity of the burn I had used the Lumen to heal.

As we age, our chances of developing hidden infection in the tiny teeth roots increases exponentially. Having root canals, implants, extracted teeth which leave cavitations or cracks in teeth all increase the chance of hidden infection. Therefore it makes a great deal of sense to wrap the Lumen pad around your mouth twice a day while you're reading or watching TV. This can strengthen the immune function of the area, **tighten the tiny ligaments that hold the teeth** in, and ward off infection (and don't forget to use your enzymes for biofilms, see *TW* 2011). Many of us have used the Lumen to avoid extraction. *If this machine did nothing else, it would be important for everyone to have one just for this indication alone, since none of us wants to lose any teeth as we age.*

The **Lumen** (1-828-863-4834) has a fascinating track record with pain relief after surgery or accidents, arthritis, accelerating the healing of sports injuries, healing of recalcitrant chronic problems like low back pain and neck arthritis, herpes and regenerating nerves damaged by accidents or surgery. **If you have diabetic ulcers or are contemplating amputation** I would check this out first. And do your Cardio/ION with expert interpretation.

However, remember, **because it works on the mitochondria it does not work in people's mitochondria if they are deficient in things like copper or zinc for example, or are poisoned by fatty acid and phosphatidylcholine deficiencies** (this all clearly shows on the **Cardio/ION**). Everyone has pain at one time or another: hips, knees, shoulders, backs and more get tendonitis, fasciitis, bursitis, arthritis, burns, sprains, strains, ruptures, breaks, non-union or failure to heal fractures, localized chronic infections, falls, surgeries, and auto accidents, and more. I can't imagine a home without a **Lumen**.

Would I recommend using the Lumen for cancer? I can't, merely because (1) I haven't had the opportunity to check it for this, (2) have seen no huge studies, and (3) that is not its FDA indication. Having said that, if I had a cancer and had done the Cardio/ION, corrected nutrient deficiencies, identified and gotten rid of major toxins that caused the cancer, and was on a macrobiotic strict phase diet (start with *You Are What You Ate*, then proceed to *The Cure Is In The Kitchen*), the little scientist that lives inside me would be very tempted to evaluate it. In fact I can't think of a medical reason not to use it, whereas a lot of evidence supports its use.

For starters, the **Lumen revs up cytochrome C oxidase,** a crucial detoxification enzyme in mitochondria that is needed by all cancer patients. But remember key is to have repaired the nutrient deficiencies that caused the cancer in the first place, and next to get rid of the toxicities that caused the cancer, and also eventually make it metastasize and make it chemotherapy-resistant. For remember, **if your mitochondria are poisoned** (proven by over a dozen indicators on the Cardio/ION), **they can't make cytochrome C, necessary in turn for turning on the p53 gene that makes cancer cells commit suicide**!

This is one more piece of evidence also demonstrating that **if an oncologist isn't starting with your Cardio/ION, how in the world does he help you cure your cancer ?** (unless of course, that isn't the goal). Unfortunately most don't even know what role cytochrome C plays in healing cancer. In fact I've never met one who even knows the most rudimentary facts that I've referenced in *TW* that show why the carrot juicing in *Wellness Against All Odds* is so crucial. Yet Harvard researchers showed decades ago that **beta-carotene makes the p53 mutated cancer gene revert back to its normal function of killing cancer** cells (2009 *TW*). And so do tocotrienols, silymarin. and more that you have learned about here. Meanwhile, without making you a chemist, **revving up cytochrome C is important for making cancer cells commit suicide** (called *apoptosis*), one of several major mechanisms involved in cancer cure. Again, I frankly can't imagine a home without a **Lumen**.

318

References:

• Eells JT, Henry MM, Whelan HT (Medical College Wisc.), Therapeutic photobiomodulation for methanol-induced retinal toxicity, *Proc Natl Acad Sci,* 100;6:3439-3444, Mar 18, 2003

• Karu T, Molecular mechanism of the therapueutic effect of low-intensity laser radiation, *Lasers in Life Science,* 2:53-74, 1988

• Hug DH, Photoactivation of enzymes, *Photochem Photobiol Rev* 6:87-138, 1981

• Smith KC (Stanford Univ.), The photobiological basis of low level laser radiation therapy, *Laser Therap,* 3;1, Jan-Mar 1991

• Shamir MH, et al, Double-blind randomized study evaluating regeneration of the rat transected sciatic nerve after surgery and post-operative low-power laser treatment, *J Recon Microsurg,* 17: 133-37, 2001

• Moore KC, Hira N, Broome IJ, Cruikshank JA, The effect of infra-red diode laser irradiation on the duration and severity of post-operative pain: a double blind trial, *Laser Therapy,* 4:145-49, 1992

• Rochkind S, et al, Effects of laser: irradiation on the spinal cord for the regeneration of crushed peripheral nerve in rats. *Lasers Surg Med,* 28:216-19, 2001

• Nakaji S, Shiroto C, Liu Q, et al, Retrospective study of adjunctive diode laser therapy for pain attenuation in 662 patients: detailed analysis, by questionnaire, *Phytomed Laser Surg,* 23;1:60-65, 2005

• Bonnet S, et al, A **mitochondria-K+ channel axis is suppressed in cancer and its normalization promotes apoptosis and inhibits cancer** growth, *Cancer Cell* 11:37-51, Jan 2007

• Platoshyn O, et al, **Cytochrome c activates K+ channels before inducing apoptosis,** *Am J Physiol,* 283:C1298-1305, 2002

• Green DR, et al, **Mitochondria and apoptosis,** *Science* 281:1309-12, 1998

• Hanahan D, et al, The hallmarks of cancer, *Cell,* 100:57-70, Jan 7, 2000

• Wang Z, Roles o f **K+ channels in regulating tumour cell proliferation and apoptosis,** *Pflugers Arch-Eur J Physiol,* 448:274-86, 2004

• Depreter M, et al, *J Endocrinol* 175:779-92, 2002

• Robertson JD, et al, Caspace-2 acts upstream of **mitochondria to promote cytochrome c release** during etoposide-induced **apoptosis,** *J Biol Chem* 277:29803-9, 2002

• Li F, et al, Cell-specific **induction of apoptosis by** microinjection of **cytochrome c,** Bcl-xl has activity independent of cytochrome c release, *J Biol Chem,* 272:30299-305, 1997

Heal Diabetic Stasis Ulcers Without Antibiotics

One of the common nasty side effects of diabetes is stasis ulcers. They begin with damaged blood vessels which finally break down, ooze and get infected. They can become so severe that underlying bone becomes infected and combined with progressively more compromised circulation, this can lead to amputation. Therefore, you want to prevent leg ulcers, and once they have started, learn how to nip them in the bud. And if you can, you would also like to avoid antibiotics so you don't then get overgrowth of Candida in the gut leading to auto-immune arthritis or MS or colitis, or thyroiditis, fibromyalgia, etc.

First step is to make sure you have enough **Arginine Powder** and **Magnesium** on board to heal the vessel. You want to do everything you can to heal the blood vessels that supply diabetic stasis ulcers, beginning with not only rudimentary arginine and magnesium that you learned about here, but if you need, you can take it too much higher levels in the book about vascular health, *The High Blood Pressure Hoax.* Meanwhile healing the vessels could be something as simple as 1-2 **NSC-24 Beta Glucan Circulatory Formula** twice a day. As well, be sure your Cardio/ION is expertly interpreted. The **Lumen** that you just learned about is also indispensable.

But, **how to avoid antibiotics**? Silver has been used to prevent infection in severe ulcers and even total body burns. The standard form used for decades in hospitals, sulfadiazine, is not without problem, however. It can accumulate in the skin and organs causing silver toxicity (argyria), create auto-immune disease, anemias, blistering (bullous) rashes, fatal kidney disease, grayish skin color, etc. And folks can develop resistance to it.

Wouldn't it be great if there were a form of silver that didn't do any of that and yet could kill the worst bacteria like methicillin-resistant *Staphylococcus aureus* and fungi like *Candida albicans*? That would be too perfect to imagine because usually a bacteria requires an antibiotic, while fungi require an anti-fungal. Meanwhile antibiotics act like fertilizer for fungi like Candida, and make them grow even more wildly than they already do in the system of a diabetic. But **Argentyn 23 Professional First Aid Gel** takes care of both categories of bugs and without the side effects (Brandt). Plus it helps relieve pain and itching and facilitates healing all the while it is fighting potent bacteria and fungi in a non-toxic homeopathic manner. In fact it not only accelerates healing but improves the strength of the tissues (Jain, Liu). Apply it 3-4 times a day as needed.

References (more in *TW*):

• Brandt O, et al, Nanoscalic silver possess broad-spectrum antimicrobial activities and exhibits **fewer toxicological side effects than silver sulfadiazine**, *Nanomed Nanotechnol Biol Med,* 8:478-88, 2012

• Kwan KH, et al, **Modulation of collagen alignment by silver** nanoparticles results in better mechanical properties **in wound healing**, *Nanomed Nanotechnol Biol Med,* 1; 7:457-504, 2011

• Jain J, et al, **Silver nanoparticles** in therapeutics: development of an **antimicrobial** gel formulation for topical use. *Mol Pharmacol* 6; 138-401, 2009

• Liu X, et al, Silver nanoparticles mediated differential responses in keratinocytes and fibroblasts during the skin who wound healing, *ChemMedChem* 5; 468-75, 2010

Diabetes Leads to Destruction Only if You Let It

Clearly no matter who you are or what disease you have or don't have, you want to control your sugars. **A fasting glucose over 85 mg/dL gives a 40% increased risk of death** from cardiovascular disease (Bjornholt). And higher sugars lead to an increased risk of cancers (Noto). And in fact there's a 38% increase in deaths just from digestive tract cancers in folks with a higher glucose from merely metabolic syndrome and not even having diabetes (Matthews). On the flipside, once you get diabetes you have to consider whether it's really an early pancreatic cancer (Pannala, Chari, Gapstur). And yet *zinc can cause cultured pancreatic cancer cells to die* while not affecting normal insulin producing cells (Jayaraman). So this little mineral (that you have already learned is often deficient) **zinc is important for not only** *normal* **function of the pancreas, but for** *making pancreatic cancer cells die.* So where are the diabetologists (and oncologists) who should be measuring and regulating the best dose for you? Don't you see how your first question should always be, *"And what is your plan doctor for helping me find the cause and cure of my disease?"*. The answer will usually save you enormous time and money by helping you exit the wrong office as soon as possible.

And you have learned that having diabetes not only gives you risk for all of the things we've talked about, but you have a **70% greater risk of developing Alzheimer's** as you get older (Rosick). You've learned enough here to begin to make the right choices.

References:

* Bjornholt JV, et al, Fasting blood **glucose: an underestimated risk factor for cardiovascular death.** Results from a 22 year follow-up of healthy non-diabetic men, *Diabetes Care* 22; 1:45-9, 1999

* Noto H, et al, Substantially **increased risk of cancer in patients with diabetes mellitus,** *J Diab Complic* 24; 5:345-53, 2010

* Matthews CE, et al, **Metabolic syndrome and risk of death from cancers** of the digestive system, *Metabol* 59; 8:1231-9, 2010

* Pannala R, et al, **New-onset diabetes: a potential clue to the early diagnosis of pancreatic cancer.** *Lancet Oncol* 10; 1:88-95, 2009

* Chari, ST, et al, **Pancreatic cancer-associated diabetes mellitus**: prevalence and temporal association with diagnosis of cancer, *Gastroenterol* 134; 1:95-101, 2008

* Gapstur SM, et al, **Abnormal glucose metabolism in pancreatic cancer mortality,** *J AM Med Assoc,* 283; 19:2552-8, 2000

* Jayaraman AK, et al, Increased level of exogenous **zinc induces cytotoxicity** and up-regulates expression of the ZnT-1 zinc transporter gene **in pancreatic cancer cells**, *J Nutr Biochem* 22:79-88, 2011

* Rosick ER, **The deadly connection between diabetes and Alzheimer's**, *Life Extension* 33-41, Dec. 2006, Fort Lauderdale Florida, 800 678-8989, www.lef.org

Are You Worth It?

Some folks do not focus on their health because they actually don't feel they are worth it. So if you're guilty of this, don't forget the important books I told you about in Chapter 5, namely Dr. Gil Gockley, PhD's *Inner Journey: Finding Happiness Within* and Dr. Art Mathias, PhD's *In His Own Image*, and *Biblical Foundations Of Freedom.* They are excellent for your self-esteem, as well as showing how a remorseful, guilty, jealous, angry or unforgiving thought poisons your body chemistry.

As William P. Young said in *The Shack* (www.theshackbook.com), "Forgiveness is not about forgetting,... it is about letting go of another person's throat". You don't have to love them or even

322

incorporate them into your life, and they certainly don't have to be your next best friend. On the other hand let God deal with it and don't let this emotion (which can be as damaging as any mycotoxin, chemical or nutrient deficiency) steal from your life.

Clearly mental and physical aspects of the body have been ignored. Combating mental stress, hostility, anger, unforgiveness, plus incorporating exercise, stretching and strengthening are crucial. Just remember that a mere bad emotion can make platelets abnormally clot (more in *TW)* leading to a heart attack or stroke.

Likewise, if you can't take a few moments each day to do some body work, whether its is exercise, stretching, trigger points, myo-fascial release, cranial-sacral, stretching, strengthening, inversions, or any combinations of the above, how much more time will you spend in doctors' offices? We'll be addressing more of this in *TW* since body work is a very neglected aspect of healing, but way beyond the focus of this tome.

References:

• Mathias A, *In His Own Image,* followed by *Biblical Foundations Of Freedom,* 1-907-563-9033, www.akwellspring.com

• Benson H, Systemic hypertension and the relaxation response, *New Engl J Med,* 296:1152-6, 1977 (also see his book **The Relaxation Response**)

• Haft JI, et al, Intravascular **platelet aggregation in the heart induced by stress,** *Circulation* 47:353-8, 1973

• Chaput LA, et al, **Hostility predicts** recurrent events among postmenopausal women with **coronary heart disease,** *Am J Epidemiol,* 156:1092-99, 2002

• Williams JT, et al, **Effects of an angry temperament on coronary heart disease risk**: the Atherosclerosis Risk in Communities Study, *Am J Epidemiol,* 154:230-5, 2001

• Pischke CR, et al (includes Ornish), Long term effects of lifestyle changes on well-being and cardiac variables among coronary heart disease patients, *Health Psychology* 27; 5:584-92, 2008

• Schiffer F, et al, Evidence for emotionally induced coronary arterial spasm in patients with angina pectoris, *Brit Heart J* 44:62-6, 1980

• Ornish D, Mind/heart interactions: for better and for worse, *Health Values* 2:266-9, 1978

• Ornish D, et al, Effects of stress management training and dietary changes in treating ischemic heart disease, *J Am Med Assoc,* 249; 1:54-9, 1983

• Nerem RM, et al, Social environment as a factor in diet-induced atherosclerosis, *Sci* 208:1475-6, 1980

Exercise/Stretching

Mattes A, Active Isolated Stretching, 1-941-922-3232
Mattes A, Active Isolated Strengthening, 1-941-922-3232

• Daubenmier JJ, et al (including Ornish), The contribution of **changes in diet, exercise, and stress management to changes in coronary risk** in women and men in the Multi-site Cardiac Lifestyle Intervention Program, *Ann Behav Med* 33; 1:57-68, 2007

• Froelcher V, et al, A randomized trial of exercise training in patients with coronary artery disease, *J Am Med Assoc* 252:1291-7, 1984

• Ehsani AA, et al, Effects of 12 months intense exercise training on ischemic ST-segment depression in patients with coronary artery disease, *Circulation* 64:1116-24, 1981

• Schuler G, et al, Perfusion **and regression of coronary artery disease in patients on a regimen of intensive physical exercise and low fat diet,** *J Am Coll Cardiol* 19; 1:34-42, 1992

• Blumenthal JA, et al, **Effects of exercise and stress management training on markers of cardiovascular risk** in patients with ischemic heart disease: a randomized controlled trial, *J Am Med Assoc,* 293:1626-34, 2005

• Ernst EEW, et al, Intermittent claudication, exercise and blood rheology, *Circul* 76:110-4, 1987

• Most AS, et al, Effect of a reduction in blood viscosity on maximal myocardial oxygen delivery distal to a moderate coronary stenosis, *Circulation* 74:1085-92, 1986

• Nolewajka AJ, et al, Exercise and human collateralization: an angiographic and scintographic assessment, *Circulation* 60:114-21, 1979

• Slattery ML, et al, Leisure time physical activity and coronary heart disease death, *Circulation* 79:304-11, 1989

• Verani MS, et al, Effects of exercise training on left ventricular performance and myocardial perfusion in patients with coronary artery disease, *Am J Cardiol* 47:797-803, 1981

• Koertge J, et al (including Ornish), Improvement in medical risk factors and quality of life in women and men with coronary artery disease in the Multicenter Lifestyle Demonstration Project, *Am J Cardiol* 91:1316-22, 2003

• Schuler G, et al, Low-fat diet and regular, supervised physical exercise in patients with symptomatic coronary artery disease: reduction of stress-induced myocardial ischemia, *Circulation* 77:172-81, 1988

A Planet Gone Awry

Diabetes has tripled in the United States in the last three decades. To quote the *Wall Street Journal*, according to the study (*Lancet*), the U.S. had 24.7 million diabetics in 2008, nearly triple the level of three decades ago." (Naik). Yet researchers reporting on this in the *Lancet* are literally clueless about the causes. They **blame it on the diet but never mention phthalates**. They **blame**

it on obesity but again don't look at any proven causes like **phthalates**. As well, they **blame it on lack of physical activity. But who can exercise when their mitochondria are poisoned and not repaired?** The sad thing is they never mentioned anything about the dwindling levels of nutrients and the rising levels of toxicities. These are the proven causes and you have seen only a smattering of the evidence.

And true to form other articles keep emerging showing how they hope an old tuberculosis vaccine (BCG), which is also used for bladder cancers, might hold promise (Winslow).   While when other government funded studies have already proven that giving insulin did not delay getting diabetes, they're now looking at drugs whose side effects include creating cancers (Wang)! And then of course the pharmaceutical folks are still pushing **diabetes drugs like Actos®, even though there's already an increased risk of getting bladder cancer,** as there should be since drugs do not fix what's broken (Dooren). Just look at all the money and lives that could be saved if docs would merely read and learn how to cure, and if insurance companies covered nutrient assays and nutrients as well as detoxification. Only *people power* can change this.

As just 2 miniscule examples, vitamin D3 is now a recognized under-appreciated epidemic in the United States.   And **just correcting the vitamin D3 levels has healed the insulin receptors in the pancreas** in experimental animals (Kumar). But I've never heard of one diabetologist who even checks vitamin D levels much less recognizes they should be far above the antiquated cut-off used by most commercial labs, as you've seen the evidence for. And you've seen how the ratio of omega-3 oils has changed 60-fold from 3:1 to 1:20 (or other sources say 4:1 to 1:15) over the decades, while simple DHA (omega-3, as part of cod liver oil) is a potent anti-diabetic agent (Yamamoto). Now you see why I've taken the time from my life and from Luscious to bring you this information on how to heal diabetes (and in fact any other thing that you have), because I don't know of any other place that you're going to get this package.

References:

- Wang SS, Trying to prevent type I diabetes, *Wall St J,* D1, D4, June 7, 2011

- Dooren JC, **FDA says diabetes drug might raise cancer risk**, B9, *Wall St J,* June 16, 2011

- Winslow R, Drug offers hope in diabetes study, *Wall St J,* A2, June 25, 2011

- Naik G, **Diabetes cases double to 347 million**, *Wall St J,* A3, June 27, 2011

- Kumar PT, et al, **Vitamin D3 restores** altered cholinergic and **insulin receptor** expression in the cerebral cortex and muscarinic M3 receptor expression **in pancreatic islets** of streptozotocin-induced diabetic rats, *J Nutr Biochem*, 22:418-25, 2011

- Yamamoto K., et al, Identification of putated metabolites of **docosahexaenoic acid as potent PPAR** gamma agonists and **antidiabetic agents**, *Bioorg Med Chem Lett* 15:517-22, 2005

Why Is There So Much More Diabetes ?

As the song goes, "B-B-B-Baby, you ain't seen nothing yet!". Forty-eight years ago in medical school diabetes was not a common disease. Now it's an epidemic out of control with more than 1 in 12 Americans affected. And not only is it an epidemic out of control, but in some areas as many as 1 in 8 children has it, which is unheard of in the history of this planet. If that were not scary enough, millions of folks have either **NASH (non-alcoholic steatohepatitis, the newest liver disease) or metabolic syndrome (Syndrome X) which are proven precursors to diabetes**. And of course the epidemics of obesity, high blood pressure, high cholesterol, and high triglycerides contribute to this avalanche of U.S. folks into the sickest nation in the history of the world. Yet we have the most expensive medical system complete with unparalleled high tech medical resources.

And most do not know that diabetes can begin even in the womb. Many **environmental triggers program** the child, adolescent and adult **for diabetes, starting in the uterus**. Long before the child is even born, genetic changes driven by poor diet, nutrient deficiencies, plastic pollution and a host of other environmental chemicals have already turned on the genetics for diabetes. Yet the

FDA, while busy torturing nutrient companies, doesn't even have a cut-off for a permissible level of phthalates in foods, even though they are a major part of packaging and permeate our diets so profusely that they are the #1 pollutant in the human body. And along with hundreds of other unavoidable environmental pollutants the phthalates are environmental endocrine disruptors, which also can trigger diabetes by yet another route.

However Medicare does not even allow the comprehensive nutrient assay needed to reverse diabetes. In fact they are the only government medical institution which does not bargain for the lowest drug prices. As one example they pay $2000 for an injection that other insurances pay $50 for (*TW* 2011). And the FDA condones labeling on foods that say they are "heart healthy" when they contain trans fatty acids hidden in vegetable oil, soybean oil, or GMO canola, or contain high fructose corn syrup or Olestra, as examples. And as the *Journal of the American Medical Association* **has repeatedly shown us, the "authoritative expert" practice guidelines that dictate the practice of medicine are over 87% controlled by physicians who are under the influence of the drug industry.** No wonder you've been brainwashed to think that the word "cure" should be equated with quackery.

As you have learned here we know how to cure diabetes, whether it's in the young or the old. We know what nutrients are important and how to assay them in the pregnant female and even before she gets pregnant. We know how to repair the mitochondria and the peroxisomes and get rid of the phthalates and other pollutants. Will we see this done routinely in your lifetime? Not a chance! But luckily for you, you have the tools with which to do this now, and many already have. We can never go back to a less polluted society, but *with the gifts from millions of researchers who have each added their own pieces to the puzzle, we have been able to reverse and actually cure diabetes.* I invite you to do the same.

327

References:

- Sundaresan S, et al, A mouse model of nonalcoholic steatohepatitis, *J Nutr Biochem*, 22:979-84, 2011

- Theys N, et al, Maternal malnutrition programs pancreatic islet mitochondrial dysfunction in the adult offspring, *J Nutr Biochem* 985-94, 2011

- Reusens B, et al, **The intrauterine metabolic environment modulates the gene expression** patterns in fetal rat islets: prevention by maternal taurine supplementation, *Diabetologia* 51:836-45, 2008

- Wallace DC, **A mitochondrial paradigm of metabolic and degenerative diseases, aging, and cancer: a dawn for evolutionary medicine**, *Annu Rev Genet* 39:359-407, 2005

- Patane G, et al, Role of ATP production and uncoupling protein-2 in the **insulin secretory defect induced by chronic exposure to** high glucose or free fatty acids and effects of **peroxisome** proliferator-activated receptor-gamma **inhibition**, *Diabetes* 51:2749-56, 2002

- Simmons RA, **Developmental origins of diabetes: the role of oxidative stress**, *Free Rad Biol Med* 40:917-22, 2006

- Remacle C, et al, <u>**Intrauterine programming of the endocrine pancreas**</u>, *Diabetes Obes Metab*, 9 (supple 2): 196-209, 2007

- Maechler P, et al, Novel <u>**regulation of insulin secretion: the role of mitochondria**</u>, *Curr Opin Investig Drugs*, 4:1166-72, 2003

- Schinner S, et al, **Inhibition of human** insulin **gene** transcription **by peroxisome** proliferator-activated receptor gamma and thiazolidinedione oral **antidiabetic drugs**, *Brit J Pharmacol* 157:736-45, 2009

- Leloup C, et al, **Mitochondrial** reactive oxygen species **are** obligatory **signals for** glucose-induced **insulin** secretion, *Diabetes* 58:673-81, 2009

- Theys N, et al, Early low protein diets aggravates unbalance between antioxidant enzymes leading to islet dysfunction, *PloS ONE*, 4:e6110, 2009

- Chen JQ, et al, **Regulation of mitochondrial** respiratory chain biogenesis **by estrogens/estrogen receptors** and physiological, pathological and pharmacological implications, *Biochim Biophys Acta*, 10:1540-70, 2009

How to Recognize the Dangerous Draconian Dinosaur Diabetes Doctor

In closing I'm thinking about a professional Olympic athlete with whom I recently consulted on the phone. He has devoted his life to eating well and being healthy. And now at 52 has serious heart disease and innocently asks, "How can I be sick when I've devoted my life to being healthy?". The answer is simple. **The work of living in this world depletes nutrients and raises toxins to unprecedented levels. To make matters worse, assay and repair**

328

of these is not part of conventional medicine. But for a cure there's no substitute for these for reversing the dual cause.

I just can't let you go without another example of how important it is for you to be able to protect yourself regardless of what diseases you get as you go through life. Even the most obtuse dinosaurs realize that at the very base of every disease is inflammation. **And this inflammation sets up the cascade of destruction that we call chronic disease. It can only be stopped by repairing the nutrient deficiencies and getting rid of the toxicities that caused it all.** The dinosaurs have heard that fish oil is important so they recommend it. But such a casual recommendation smacks of ignorance. That's why it rarely works for anyone.

Why? Because the dinosaur has not (1) assayed and balanced the amount of omega-3 versus omega-6 and repaired the ratio, (2) has not checked the indican, elastase, Candida overgrowth, etc. and other manifestations of pancreatic insufficiency to see if enzymes are needed to promote absorption of the fats, nor has he (3) prescribed the **PC Powder** which is the innards of the electrical membranes and (4) supplemented the **ALC Powder** that is damaged by the ubiquitously unavoidable phthalates, but is absolutely necessary to carry the fats into the cell and especially into the mitochondria. And he has failed to (5) assay the damage done by phthalates, heavy metals, pesticides, PFOA, PBDEs, VOHs and other xenobiotics that are the basis of disease in this century. Nor has he (6) assayed the other nutrients needed to protect that fish oil in the cell membrane such as the **tocotrienols** and tocopherols. And when he does check a magnesium level, for example, he uses the wrong assay. Or when he checks nutrients like vitamin D he uses the antiquated commercial labs cut-off.

And then the guys who check the genetics without checking all of the above are really dinosaurs pretending to be dynamos or you might say Dynamo wanna-be's. For anyone who really knows about genes knows that **foods and nutrients not only talk to**

genes, but control them. That is an enormously phenomenal part of God's orchestration of human molecular biochemistry.

So this is a very rudimentary example, but one that is applicable to just about everyone as we unavoidably develop these deficiencies and toxicities. For clearly God-given nutrients have the power to rescue us. Somebody up there knew we were going to poison ourselves in this era and provided an answer. Recall, I'm no smarter than any other doctor, and I am one solo country practitioner, not affiliated with the enormous financial benefits of a medical school/university complex. Yet by just looking for the evidence of how **God has designed the body to heal**, I was able to collate all of this as the sole researcher, clinician, writer, and editor. Surely the physician concerned about his patient can go one step further and read all this now that the groundwork has been done for him. Meanwhile, **a simple test to identify a dinosaur** is to coyly ask if he will be measuring your EPA and DHA. Only a dynamo would enthusiastically say, "Of course! I wouldn't have it any other way". Any other response is a dinosaur.

Further surreptitious tests would be to inquire what nutrient must be corrected before the fatty acids can get into the mitochondria (carnitine), and what nutrient holds the fatty acid layers together in the membrane sandwich (phosphatidyl choline), and what nutrient is lowered by crucial mitochondrial lipoic acid (biotin), and what test shows its deficiency (beta hydroxyl iso-valerate). If he gets all 4 right off the bat, he's a keeper, a definite **Dynamo Doc.**

If you feel overwhelmed at this point (as you should since you are on the hugest learning curve of your life), **let me leave you with something incredibly easy yet powerful. If you do nothing else today**, start your **Lemon-Flavored Cod Liver Oil, PC Powder**, eight forms of vitamin E, Magnesium, and **ALC Powder** and see what happens with a *three-month oil change* for your cellular, nuclear, endoplasmic reticular, and mitochondrial membranes.

References:

• Watkins BA, et al, **Dietary PUFAs and flavonoids as deterrents for environmental pollutants**, *J Nutr Biochem*, 18:196-205, 2007

• Wang L, et al, **Changing ratios of omega-6 to omega-3 fatty acids can** differentially modulate polychlorinated biphenyl **toxicity** and endothelial cells, *Chemico-Biolog Interact* 172:27-38, 2008

• Rahimi R, et al, A review on the mechanisms involved in **hypoglycemia induced by organophosphorus pesticides**, *Pesticide Biochem Physiol* 88:115-21, 2007

• Hennig B, et al, **Using nutrition for intervention and prevention against environmental chemical toxicity and associated diseases**, *Environ Health Persp* 115:493-5, 2007

• Hennig B, et al, **Modification of environmental toxicity by nutrients,** Implications in atherosclerosis, *Cardiovasc Toxicol* 5:153-60, 2005

The Great Divide is Ever Widening

In summary, you have learned that the level of the number one pollutant in the human body is over 1000 times higher than the other over 80,000 pollutants, while previous studies have grossly underestimated the amounts (Grob, Vandenberg). And **there are 2000 new chemicals introduced each year, but the EPA does not routinely assess the safety or risks associated with these new chemicals** (Vandenberg). Not only are **low concentrations very toxic** as they silently accumulate, but they never occur alone. In reality **our daily exposures are the result of mixtures of hundreds** of other toxic chemicals (Muncke). And **there's no way to avoid them** since they are in personal care products that we all use daily (Preau, Schecter), foods, medicines, household construction materials, appliances, baby bottles, mattresses and bedding, clothing, furnishings, in the air from industrial and auto pollutants, and even in un-packaged fresh foods (Schecter). And they are used as fragrances, flame retardants as well **as pesticides disguised as package linings so that they can even be used secretly in <u>organic</u> foods** (Grob, Schecter, Preau).

Once in the human body, **pollutant damage begins even in the unborn fetus, where he has been programmed for diseases like not only diabetes**, but cancers of the prostate and breast that won't emerge until adult life. And no wonder bisphenol A, a common

331

accompanying cousin to phthalates is also a carcinogen since it contains two benzene rings, known for starters to cause of leukemia (Vandenberg). But these ubiquitous unavoidable chemicals bind thyroid receptors, adrenal, testicles, ovaries, and in fact any gland. Since the pancreas is the gland we're most concerned with here, it is no surprise that **even low doses of plasticizers create diabetes** as well as all of its precursors like insulin resistance, high blood pressure, high cholesterol, obesity, high triglycerides, non-alcoholic steatohepatitis (NASH or fatty liver disease), cancers, coronary artery disease, and more, since they poison the body's cellular mechanisms in dozens of ways (Vandenberg, Lang, Feige, Alonso-Magdalena, Newbold).

Clearly regardless of what diseases you have, and especially anything related to diabetes, screenings for assay of **Phthalates, Heavy Metals, Porphyrins, Volatile Solvents, Pesticides** as well as a **Cardio/ION** can be paramount. Anything less when stumped is pure dinosaur medicine. And if you can only afford one test, it would be the latter because we all have these toxins in us with the potential to create diabetes (Lee, Vasiliu). *So it merely boils down to repairing the deficiencies and getting rid of the toxins* (Majkova). For remember **these unavoidable chemicals that are found everywhere** <u>create diabetes and its related problems at levels far below what the EPA says are safe</u> (Ropero).

Unfortunately every time I pick up a book or a medical paper regarding any of the aspects of diabetes, there is not one mention of phthalates. They are dinosaurs. They are ignorant of the last 3 decades of proof of the fundamental underlying causes of disease in the 21st century. And in fact this goes for every disease from cancer to heart to hormonal, arthritic, neurologic, MCS, or whatever you have. **The label of a disease is inconsequential**. It is meaningless. Our everyday pollutants have the ability to create every dysfunction in the human body. Fortunately you know how to prove it and correct it, and (as with most of us) make your bodies healthier than they've ever been before.

332

References:

- Alonso-Magdalena P, et al, The estrogenic effect of **bisphenol A disrupts pancreatic** beta-cell function in vivo and **induces insulin resistance**, *Environ Health Persp* 114; 1:106-12, 2006

- Lee DH, et al, A strong dose response relation between serum concentrations of persistent organic pollutants and diabetes: results from the National Health and Examination Survey 1999-2002, *Diabetes Care* 29; 7:1638-44, 2006

- Ropero AV, et al, **Bisphenol-A disruption of the endocrine pancreas** and blood glucose homeostasis, *Int J Androl* 31; 2:194-200, 2008

- Newbold RR, et al, Effects of endocrine disruptors on obesity, *Int J Androl*, 31; 2:201-8, 2008

- Vom Saal FS, et al, An extensive new literature concerning **low-dose effects of bisphenol A** shows the need for new risk assessment, *Environ Health Persp* 113; 8:926-33, 2005

- Lang IA, et al, **Association of urinary bisphenol A concentration with medical disorders and laboratory abnormalities in adults,** *J Am Med Assoc,* 300; 11:1303-10, **2008**

- Preau JL, et al, Variability over one week in the urinary concentrations of metabolites of diethyl phthalate and di (2-ethylhexyl) phthalate among eight adults: an observational study, *Environ Health Persp*, 118; 12:1748-54, 2010

- Grob K, et al, **Food contamination** with organic materials in perspective: **packaging materials** as **the largest and least controlled source?** A view focusing on the European situation, *Crit Rev Food Sci Nutr* 46:529-35, 2006

- Muncke J, Exposure to **endocrine disrupting compounds via the food chain**: is **packaging** a relevant source? *Sci Total Environ* 407:4549-59, 2009

- Feige JN, et al, The pollutant diet ethylhexyl **phthalate regulates** hepatic energy metabolism by species-specific **PPAR** a-dependent mechanisms, *Environ Health Persp* 118; 2:234-41, 2010

- Vandenberg LN, et al, Bisphenol-A and the great divide: a review of controversies in the field of endocrine disruption, *Endocr Rev* 30; 1:75-95, 2009

- Schecter A., et al., Bisphenol a (BPA) in US food, *Environ Sci Technol* 44:9425-30, 2010

- Majkova Z, et al, Omega-3 fatty acid oxidation products prevent vascular endothelial cell activation by coplanar and polychlorinated biphenyls, *Toxicol Appl Pharmacol*, 251; 41-9, 2011

- Wang L, et al, <u>**Changing ratios of omega-6 to omega-3**</u> fatty acids can **differentially** modulate polychlorinated biphenyl **toxicity** in endothelial cells, *Chem Biol Interact* 172:27-38, 2008

Your Role Has Just Quadrupled in Importance

If you think things are going to get better and that with all of this scientific back-up the world of medicine couldn't possibly ignore the overwhelming evidence that you've just learned, think again. Let me give you just some highlight quotes from recent *Wall Street Journal* articles and you'll see that **you must take control for yourself.**

As one example, Lantus is a top-selling form of artificial insulin (glargine) in the United States which made over $4.9 billion in 2011. So you would think it's a pretty good drug especially since it has to be injected every day. But let me quote to you from the *Wall Street Journal*: "A large study looked at the use of Lantus by people in early stages of diabetes or with blood sugar problems and found **the product** <u>**failed**</u> **to cut the risk of heart attacks** and strokes compared with standard treatments." (Dooren). So who needs it? Even more interesting was that the article bragged that it didn't cause cancer. But they only did the study for 3 years which hardly gives cancer a chance to get started, since it takes about 10 years on average.

And then another article showed how **46% of the users of Lantus had hypoglycemia** that could cause fainting, seizures or even a heart attack (Loftus). But the title of the article was that it did beat out its oral form competitor (by 0.6%)! It wasn't even 1% better at reducing the hemoglobin A1C than its competition, that could be taken as a once a day pill. Now which would you choose.... a daily shot or pill? And of course they knew nothing of the alternative non-toxic cures that you have learned about here!

Meanwhile, Lantus' daily long-acting injection was supposed to be a step up from drugs like Byetta that had to be injected twice a day. Three companies have since merged so that this older diabetes drug, Byetta, given twice daily will be replaced by **Bydureon**, which is a once a week injection (Loftus). This can raise havoc with side effects, even though it is the same ingredient, but with a sustained action. By now you have got to be wondering what the awful trade-off is that manufacturers and prescribers think you should make. For one, the *PDR* warns that it **can cause thyroid cancer**, as well as fatal rotting of the pancreas (fatal necrotizing pancreatitis), you can develop antibodies to the pancreas, or kill your kidneys (renal failure) necessitating dialysis (that you are trying to avoid by taking a drug).

So let's look at newer oral diabetes drugs like Jentadueta. It adds the old and cheap metformin to the new linaglyptin. Although its dangers include lactic acidosis (which is fatal in 50% of cases), they never mention thiamine (vitamin B1) which is a crucial first step in curing it (*MPR*). Lactic acidosis begins silently with flu-like achiness and muscle soreness progressing to trouble breathing, arrhythmia and trouble staying awake. How much more sense it makes to fix what is broken (as you have learned here), instead of adding new and increasingly potent chemicals to an already poisoned and deficient body.

Then another *WSJ* article was bemoaning the fact that there has been a **23% jump in type I diabetes among American youth**. Sadly one of the specialists was quoted as saying "We don't know yet what is triggering diabetes or why it is increasing" (Linebaugh). I guess they've been under a rock for the last three decades so they have never heard of phthalates, trans-fatty acids, PFOA's (stain and water resistant products), PBDEs (flame retardants), heavy metals, etc. Then they got even more stupid and discussed a study that found no improvement in diabetes when they gave large doses of vitamin D supplements. I guess they were also under the rock again when they were supposed to learn that D is not a solo act in the body. You can't treat it as though it's a drug. It must work in harmony with other nutrients like the fatty acids, tocotrienols, vitamin K2, minerals, etc.

And if you think the government will sooner or later hire enough people smart enough to rectify all this, remember that **the Medicare prescription drug plan does not even allow Medicare to even negotiate for the lowest price**. Do you know of any other institution in the entire world that has that ridiculous restriction? I don't. And I think you'll find it even more interesting when you **read this quote from the *Wall Street Journal*: "The pharmaceutical industry wrote into the prescription drug plan that Medicare could <u>not</u> negotiate with drug companies"**. I'll continue to quote, "And you know what? The chairman of the committee who pushed the law through (Tauzin) went to work for the pharmaceutical industry shortly after that, making $2 million a year" (op-ed). My opinion? Truly we are on our own indefinitely.

And it just gets worse. A *Wall Street Journal* article explained how "drugstore chains (like CVS and Walgreens) are **training pharmacists** to specialize in conditions like diabetes". "At some drug stores, **the pharmacist** meets privately with patients to review medications." "He **checks if statins and blood pressure drugs are prescribed, as recommended, for diabetes patients.**" "If the patient agrees he calls the physician to suggest prescribing these drugs if they are missing." This is **because "widely accepted guidelines suggest that statins and blood pressure medications should be prescribed, in addition to diabetes medications, for diabetes patients."** The fox guarding the hen house!

After all that you have just read and learned about the practice guidelines (and how repairing nutrient deficiencies and toxicities actually cures diseases) are you as speechless about this as I am? If he wanted to do something useful, he should at least tell each person on a statin to take CoQ10, selenium, etc. Instead, **pharmacies are training their employees to police physicians who are not using the drug-oriented practice guidelines, that are proven to neither prolong life nor cure.**

References:

• Dooren JC, et al, Leading insulin doesn't heightened cancer risk, studies find, *Wall Street Journal*, B2 June 12, 2012

• Linbaugh K, Type I diabetes on rise among youth, *Wall St J*, A5, June 11, 2012

• Loftus P, Sanofi insulin treatment gets boost. Company-funded clinical trial finds Lantus is more effective than rival drug, *Wall St J* B2, June 11, 2012

• op-ed, ObamaCare's secret history. **How a Pfizer CEO and big Pharma colluded with the White House at the public's expense,** *Wall St J* A12, June 12, 2012 and Emails reveal **how the White House bought big Pharma,** *Wall St J*, A13, June 12, 2012

• Landro L, **The pharmacist is in and nudging you to take your pills,** *Wall Street J*, D1-2, June 26, 2012

• *MPR* (Monthly Prescribing Reference), p 140-5, July 2012 ((www.eMPR.com, 1-800-436-9269)

And the Beat Goes On

I'll have to stop reading the world's medical news if I'm ever going to close this *first volume* on healing diabetes. The evidence just gets heavier every day. Glaxo just pled "guilty to criminal charges of illegally marketing drugs and withholding safety data from U.S. regulators, and to pay **$3 billion** to the government in what the Justice Department called **the largest health-care fraud settlement in U.S. history**." (Whalen). And of course this settlement includes a diabetes drug that you've already learned about here that has the ability to more than double your heart attack risk. In fact, the Justice Department said **"Glaxo failed to report certain safety data to the FDA about Avandia, formerly one of the top-selling diabetes treatments in the world. The missing data included two studies that examined the cardiovascular safety of Avandia". Avandia now merely carries a blackbox warning about heart risk.** The FDA put tight curbs on its use in 2010, while European regulators ordered it withdrawn from the market." (Whalen). And the power of the pharmaceutical industry is multiplying like a cancer.

And there's no level at which they feel shame. You all recall the most abused narcotic on the market in the U.S. is OxyContin. A *WSJ* headline for the summary of Business & Finance section reads, "Purdue Pharma hopes to extend patent protection for OxyContin by testing the painkiller's safety for children." They don't even pretend to cover their intentions. In order to extend the patent life of this narcotic pain reliever, the makers are targeting the only market left, children ages 6-16 (Martin). There's no level to which they will not stoop. As one physician stated, clinics that take money from the pharmaceutical company to put children with chronic pain on long-term addicting OxyContin are "unethical", to say the least. And they are not alone. The Eli Lilly blockbuster anti-depressant Cymbalta had six more months added to its exclusivity for testing it on children. Unfortunately for them the tests results were inconclusive. Since they couldn't prove the drug worked, they are not going to seek regulatory approval to market the drug to children. However that doesn't stop the FDA from giving the company their 6-month extension on the patent, even after it viewed this negative study (Loftus). Go figure.

And they don't know the half of it. For just how many of these children with cancer or depression had benefit of a **Cardio/ION, Undercarboxylated Osteocalcin, GI Effects, Adrenal Stress Panel, Phthalates, Volatile Solvents, Porphyrins** and **Heavy Metal Provocation Assays** to find the causes, much less the nutrients, hormones and other corrections needed to rally against their cancers or depression (*TW*)?

And lest you still think there is anything magnanimous about chronic medications without first looking for the correctable causes and cures, remember that most medications are stolen from Nature, from antibiotics which come from bacteria and fungi to protect themselves, down to the cholesterol-lowering statins derived from food fermentation products. And when researchers hit bottom and don't know where else to go, they steal from the human body. For example, one of the latest prostate cancer drugs is actually made from the patient's own God-given cancer-fighting substances. His blood is drawn and cultured in the lab to concentrate these cytokines then given back to the owner, for a charge of around $98,000 (*TW*). And then life is extended often 5 months at best. Wouldn't it be better to make the body healthy enough to concentrate and boost its *own* cytokines that God designed in him? Besides, he has a much better fighting chance when he does that because he makes *every* cell healthier, not just certain ones.

I feel like the mother wren reticent to push her fledgling babies out of the nest for the first time. As I'm trying to let you go and close this book, the *Wall Street Journal* comes out with a huge article "New strategies for treating diabetes". The "experts" of course bemoan the fact that there are **over 24 million Americans with diabetes and this will double in the next decade.** They talk about such ridiculous things as letting folks get away with a little higher

338

laboratory level of sugar, and they mentioned dangerous bariatric surgery as an option. This is while they bemoan the side effects of weight gain, bone loss, serious heart problems and cancers from the diabetes drugs. But the best is yet to come.

Then they are honest enough to even say, "Although available drugs all improve blood-sugar levels, **there is a lack of data to show whether they actually prevent or delay development of diabetes' long-term consequences.**" In essence *there is no evidence that the best drugs help.* Then they go on to explain the new updated (dinosaur) guidelines, which only you can appreciate. For if patients fail to control their blood sugars (which was just shown not to be the determining factor of longevity) with Metformin, diet and exercise, **the new guidelines call for a second diabetes drug** like Januvia, Actos, Victoza or Lantos which you've also learned about.

This of course is all in spite of the fact that there are "hardly any trials comparing these drugs against each other on long-term benefits". And they further admit that typically many diabetics progress through 3-4 treatment tiers (drugs) before adding insulin. And in spite of all of this they state that "such a graduated **treatment strategy does little to change the disease progress** and means that patients' own insulin producing beta cells remain continuously exposed to high blood sugar." (Winslow). No kidding. There is not one mention of finding cause and cure. I had to put all these quotes in because with all the evidence that you have seen here, only you folks can appreciate what a ridiculous waste of time and money and precious lives this represents. And only you know how to reverse and cure all of this. The ball is in your court.

References:

* Whalen J, et al, Glaxo sets guilty plea, $3billion settlement, *WS,J* B1-2, July 3, 2012

* Loftus P, Bristol puts focus on diabetes treatment, *WSJ,* B7, July 3, 2012

* Martin TW, **OxyContin trial planned for kids**, *WSJ,* B3, July 3, 2012

- Loftus P, **Cymbalta maker gets extension for drug**, *Wall Street J*, D5, July 10, 2012
- Winslow R., New strategies for treating diabetes, *WSJ*, D1, D4, July 10, 2012

What's Ahead?

Because heart disease is the number one cause of death and diabetics are even at more risk for early heart attacks, 2013 *TW* focuses (not exclusively, but as one example) on what to do after you have had your first heart attack and stent. Why? Because having a hunk of chicken wire mesh (which is a literal clot magnet in your coronary arteries) changes all the rules of medicine. For starters the stunned patient exits the hospital with a basketful of drugs that include beta blockers like metaprolol that poison adrenaline receptors in the heart, ACE inhibitors to lower blood pressure that work by poisoning kidney enzymes, and statins to lower cholesterol which deplete selenium, vitamin E, zinc, fatty acid chemistry, carnitine, and much more, while they usher in sudden amnesia and insidiously create Alzheimer's.

The **stents themselves put out chemotherapy** which merely extends the restenosis time by about six months and slows down healing of the infarcted area so much that practice guidelines dictate using **Plavix one month for bare metal stents, but 12 months for drug-eluting stents**. Meanwhile the drug stents also elute phthalates which resemble "crazy glue" (methyl acrylate), toxic fluorinated copolymers which resemble Teflon, plus metals and more. And while these folks are on clopidogrel (Plavix) in attempts to reduce clotting, by poisoning platelets you also poison infection control. Is this why many of these folks end up in the hospital again shortly afterwards with sepsis?

To make matters worse, **Lipitor and other statins actually lower the effectiveness of Plavix**. And up to **45% of folks are resistant to it**. It doesn't stop clots in them because their detox systems have not been repaired. Plus omeprazole (**Nexium**, etc.) not only also lowers the effectiveness of Plavix, but **increases the chance of getting pneumonia in the hospital 30%**. And it **lowers B12** which can mimic depression, Alzheimer's, or bizarre nerve conditions. It just doesn't stop once you start down the drug path. Meanwhile, nutrients like arginine, ALC, glycine, taurine, CoQ10, D-ribose, the eight forms of vitamin E, ascorbate, fatty acids, and other nutrients (*TW* 2012-13) have a huge role in regulating and repairing not only the platelets, but the lining of the coronary arteries and the damaged heart muscle itself.

Meanwhile, folks can present to their doctors complaining of something as simple as fatigue and/or shortness of breath. But when a cardiology workup does not reveal any problem they are left with the suggestion of psychiatric help. When, in fact, the person who needs the help is the physician who failed to look at the BNP (B-type natriuretic peptide) and molecular biochemistry of cardiac tissues starting with such simple things as thiamine, cod liver oil, phosphatidylcholine, the eight forms of E, etc. And of course when folks have shortness of breath and fatigue one of the main causes is that the oxygen carried in the hemoglobin of the red blood cells has had its chemistry severely damaged by environmental chemicals as well as prescription drugs. But how many dinosaurs even know to start with the most rudimentary test to diagnose this, the **Porphyrins**? They think porphyria is the old-fashioned extremely rare disease that we learned about in medical school. They are clueless about the proven causes and cures of diseases in the last decade.

TW will go into more of all this in 2013-2014. And as usual we will also go into all the other diseases and answer many readers' (snail-mailed in, please, not e-mailed) questions. So stay tuned.

References:

• Ferroni P, et al, Platelet function in health and disease: from molecular mechanisms, redox considerations to novel therapeutic opportunities, *Antioxidants & Redox Signaling*, 2012

• Liu Y, et al, **Mixed tocopherols inhibit platelet aggregation in humans**: potential mechanisms, *Am J Clin Nutr* 77:700-706, 2003

• May JM, How does ascorbic acid prevents endothelial dysfunction?, *Free Rad Biol Med* 28:1421-9, 2000

- Pignatelli P, et al, **Vitamin C inhibits platelet expression** of CD40 ligand, *Free Rad Biol Med* 38:1662-6, 2005

- Radomski M, et al, A **L-arginine**/nitric oxide pathway present **in human platelet regulates aggregation**, *Proc Natl Acad Sci US*A 87:5193-7, 1990

- Zymek P, et al, The role of platelet derived growth factor signaling in healing myocardial infarcts, *J Am Coll Cardiol* 48:2315-23, 2006

- Kerrigan SW, et al, **Platelet-bacterial interactions**, *Cell Molec Life Sci* 513-23, 2010

The Seven Top Reasons For Failure to Get Well

Do you ever wonder why you never got well, why you couldn't heal your diabetes? I'll give you the seven top reasons. If you take the last 100 people who thought they had done everything that medicine has to offer to heal their diabetes or any other serious disease, the following are the **seven top reasons for failure**. The good news is that by addressing aspects of this total load of causes, they have learned to heal the impossible....because the body was miraculously designed to do so.

(1) Number one is failure to do a **diet**. You have seen there are numerous diet choices that have enabled folks to heal the impossible, from macrobiotic (which has healed end-stage cancers given 48 hours to live) to the Ornish/Esselstyn-type markedly reduced fat diet (which has healed end-stage heart disease resistant to anything else medicine has to offer), as well as live/raw foods, yeast-free, whole foods and others. Equally important is what foods to avoid.

(2) Next most common reason for failure is to ignore the identification and correction of **nutrient deficiencies** that invariably accrue in this era in the human body. **Nutritionists**, dietitians, and other health professionals **are literally "working blindly" if they are not measuring precisely what you need.** Plus if they don't do organic acids (part of the Cardio/ION) they will never know if you need twice as much of certain nutrients as the average person. Another common mistake is some physicians will order minerals one month, some vitamins next month, some hormones the next month, etc. The best way to see what the total

342

problem is and what needs correcting first is when you have **the maximum amount of total information all at once.** What good is the mechanic who just checks your spark plugs when your car won't run because it has no spark plugs, but also no fuel, two flat tires and no carburetor? And **some practitioners are even scarier and more dangerous because they start right out detoxifying people without ever knowing the status of their detoxification chemistry,** much less mitochondria, cell membranes, etc. They make folks worse. Clearly the best test to adequately accomplish all of this is the 13-page assay of the **Cardio/ION.**

(3) Failure to check the health of the **gut** since it houses over half the immune system and over half the detoxification system for the whole body. Sometimes it can be as simple as three each of **Para-Gard** and **Phytosan** 2-3 times a day for a few weeks to kill the bad bugs followed by a bottle of **ABX Support** to restore the good probiotics (*TW*).

(4) Failure to check **hormone** deficiencies as well as their membrane receptor capabilities, remembering that most toxins are environmental endocrine disruptors, damaging not only the hormones but the membrane docking sites. It's difficult to assimilate nutrients no matter how much they are needed if the basic glandular support chemistry of the thyroid, adrenal, etc. need a temporary boost.

(5) Failure to identify and get rid of the **toxic** load that is poisoning fundamental body chemistry. Sometimes it's as simple as repairing an identified deficiency so that folks can get off a prescription medication which is silently poisoning multiple pathways. Clearly **detoxification is a lifelong process in this era**, since we are the most unprecedentedly poisoned populace in the history of the planet. Also most people are not aware of the toxicities hidden not only in their daily diets and water, but the very air in their homes, vehicles and offices. As a simple example, if you have become silently sensitive to EMF but have on your nightstand a clock radio, you may never clear your insomnia. Or if you have become

sensitive to formaldehyde/pesticides/flame retardants but are sleeping on a new mattress or an old one loaded with mites, your asthma or body aches or sinusitis may never clear. Remember many environmental toxins are able to create new allergies almost overnight (*The E.I. Syndrome* has more).

(6) A neglected aspect is **bodywork**. Getting the toxins out of the muscles, tendons, fascia and other tissues may involve anything from increased exercise to learning trigger point therapy, myofascial release, yoga with proper stretching, strengthening, self-adjusting chiropractic techniques, learning activation technique (2012-13 *TW*), etc. As well, scar tissue can interrupt electrical flow in meridians and needs to be detoxified (*TW* 2003).

(7) Taking more personal **responsibility** in reading and continually growing in knowledge about the workings of the body. Remember you would not take your brand-new car to a mechanic who refused to read the new manual on how it works and how to repair its malfunctions. Another aspect of personal responsibility is to re-evaluate your whole emotional investment in your health, and to realize that if you don't think you are worth the effort, who else will?

So there you have the total load and **the 7 most common reasons why many people will never get well.**

Dinosaurs Blame Genes and Age, While Ignoring Cure

If you want another absolute sign of a dinosaur doc, consider the poor guy who blames your genetics. As you've learned, **nutrients talk to genes and regulate them**, making the difference of whether or not genes are expressed (Genuis, 2006A). Or worse yet is the guy who likes to blame everything on the fact that you're just plain getting older. Then how does he explain the fact that not only do the animals in the wild have human diseases, but **children now get the diseases of old age** (Perrin, Genuis 2006B). We can no

344

longer blame age! He is so close-minded and under-trained it's pathetic. But such is the history of medical science:

Over 300 years ago Dr. Lind proved that food could be a cure for mysterious deaths on British Royal Navy ships at sea. His findings were mocked and disregarded, while decades of death passed before his simple idea was accepted. *A mere lemon was the cure.* Likewise, when one out of five women died in childbirth, Semmelweis *merely suggested that medical folks wash their hands* after doing autopsies before delivering babies. But true to the ignoble field of medicine, rather than thank him for this simple life-saving approach, his medical colleagues, true-to-form, scorned him with contempt. To this day doctors are too lazy to wash their hands so they have a little alcohol powder device at the door of every hospital room thinking that this will kill germs. So why is there more methacillin-resistant *Staphylococcus aureus* infection in hospitals now than ever before in history? Plus aerosolized powders add to patient's load to detox. The history of science is full of this disgustingly egocentric and jealous denial of reality and unscientific approach to medicine (Genuis 2011). And the beat goes on.

Some doctors will argue that it's too difficult to learn this chemistry, yet how difficult is a heart transplant that necessitates a life of cancer-provoking chemotherapy so that your body does not reject the new heart? Or how hard is it to live with an amputation for the rest of your life? It's ironic that we physicians spend thousands of dollars to go to a medical meeting for a week to learn about drugs. Yet for less than $500 a physician could get the last 10 years of *TW* and books and bring himself into the 21st century of medicine. And all the work including references has been done for him. It's all laid out. It couldn't be any simpler.

Meanwhile, most of the greatest societies of history have disappeared. Yet whether it be the Babylonians, the Greeks, the Roman Empire, or the British Empire, on their way out they had a

345

few things in common. They became gluttonous, obese, and denied responsibility for the health. We are following the same formula.

Over four decades ago the most respected journals showed that the I.Q. of children were severely damaged by environmental toxins with environmental lead as an example. Yet we still have the proof that the government's authoritative cut-off for a "safe" level of lead is dangerously high. What do they do about it? It stays ignored while they're busy attacking nutrient companies that produce a safe and valuable detoxification chemical that the FDA itself approved over 50 years ago. We know now that babies are born already toxic from the heavy metals, plasticizers, fire retardants, and more that they have received from their mothers while still in the uterus. The time in their lives when their brains are most vulnerable and must grow the most rapidly to supply them for the rest of their lives is seriously compromised. And worse, these brain toxins can spawn juvenile delinquents and a life of crime. We know the fatty acids and minerals that are compromised by environmental toxins but that are so crucial for infant and toddler brain development. Yet the average physician does not check mothers or children for these.

We know how disease happens, we know how to prevent it, we know how to fix it when it happens, yet we don't. Just ask your average pediatrician how he plans to check your child for lead and get it out as well as the other unavoidable bio-accumulated brain-damaging pollutants like phthalates, PBDE fire retardants, Teflon-type stain resistant PFOAs, etc. If he doesn't even know what you're talking about he has never read even *DOD*. And all of this **early toxicity programs the innocent child for adult cancers, brain deterioration, allergies** and a host of other diseases including the dreaded *diabetes*.

References:

• Genuis S, What's out there making us sick?, *J Environ Publ Health* (article ID 605137, 10 pages) 2012

• Perrin JM, et al, The increase of childhood chronic conditions in the United States, *J Am Med Assoc* 297; 24:2755-9, 2007

• Genuis S, et al, Time for an oil check: the role of essential omega-3 fatty acids and maternal and pediatric health, *J Perinatology* 26; 6:359-65, 2006A

• Genuis S, Nowhere to hide: chemical toxicants and the unborn child, *Reprod Toxicol* 28; 1:115-6, 2009

• Genuis S, The chemical erosion of human health: adverse **environmental exposure and in-utero pollution -- determinants of congenital disorders and chronic disease**, *J Perinat Med 34*; 3:185-95, 2006 B

• Genuis S, Health issues and the environment -- an emerging paradigm for providers of obstetrical and gynecological health care, *Human Reprod* 21; 9:2201-8, 2006

• Genuis S, Sensitivity-related illness: the escalating pandemic of allergy, food intolerance and chemical sensitivity, *Sci Total Environ* 408; 24:6047-61, 2010

• Genuis S, et al., **Celiac disease presenting as autism**, *J Child Neurol* 25; 1:114-9, 2010

• Lanphear BP, et al, **Low-level** environmental **lead** exposure and **children's intellectual** function: an international pooled analysis, *Environm Health Persp* 113:894-99, 2005

• Genuis S, et al, Blood, Urine, and Sweat (BUS) Study: monitoring and elimination of bioaccumulated toxic elements, *Arch Environ Contam Toxicol*, (publ. online Nov. 6, 2010, DOI 10.1007/S00244-010-9611-5) 2010

• Canfield RL, et al, **Intellectual impairment in children with blood lead concentrations below 10 mcg/dl,** *New Engl J Med* 348; 16:1517-26, **2003**

• Counter SA, et al, Mercury exposure in children: a review, *Toxicol Appl Pharmacol* 198; 2:209-30, 2004

• Grandjean P, et al, Developmental neurotoxicity of industrial chemicals, *Lancet* 368; 9553:2167-78, 2006

• Nevin R, How **lead exposure relates to** temporal **changes in IQ, violent crime, and unwed pregnancy**, *Environ Res* 83; 1:1-22, 2000

• Nevin R, Understanding international **crime** trends: the legacy of **preschool lead** exposure, *Environ Res* 104; 3:315-36, 2007

• Schnaas L, et al, **Reduced intellectual** development in children with **prenatal lead** exposure, *Environ Health Persp 114*:791-7, 2006

• Schwartz BS, et al, Past **adult lead** exposure is associated with longitudinal **decline in cognitive** function, *Neurol* 55:1144-50, 2000

• Needleman HL, et al, Bone **lead levels and delinquent behavior**, *J Am Med Assoc* 275; 5:363-9, 1996

• Needleman HL, et al, **Deficits in** psychological and **classroom performance of children with** elevated **dentin lead** levels, *New Engl J Med* 300:689-95, 1979

• Holick MF, **Vitamin D: importance in the prevention of** cancers, **type I diabetes**, heart disease, and osteoporosis, *Am J Clin Nutr*, 79; 3:362-71, **2004**

Last Chance For a Mulligan

In golf, we have a Mulligan, a free shot or re-try with no penalty. That's what this book is. It is a last chance opportunity to heal yourself. You have the tools. Now you need to *re-read and organize and do the work*. This is your life's mulligan.

You have seen the evidence. **We possess the ability to heal not only diabetes, but the vast majority of ailments that are still touted as having no known cause, and no known cure.** Why doesn't medicine do it? Because there is no money in it. A well person does not buy thousands of dollars of drugs each year. And the practice of medicine is basically controlled by the pharmaceutical industry, one of the most powerful groups in the world. Instead we practice medicine in the Neanderthal era, by bludgeoning every symptom with the latest drug. Patients are in and out of the office in a flash (the *Wall Street Journal* tells us the average patient visit is seven minutes, and the time the patient gets to explain his symptoms is 20 seconds). But on the flipside, dinosaur patients don't have to clutter their minds with information about how to heal. And when drugs fail, we stent, replace, burn or cut out and throw away the non-responding part.

You can empower yourself to learn how to use food, nutrients, and detoxification to restore God's chemistry. For we are warned that we "are destroyed from lack of knowledge" (*Hos* 4). And since **"you yourselves are God's temple"** (*I Cor* 3), why would you be like those whose "God is their stomach" (*Phi* 3) and fill that temple with disease-producing trans fats, Teflon, plastics, flame retardants, heavy metals, and junk food? For **"If anyone destroys God's temple, God will destroy him; for God's temple is sacred, and you are that temple."** (*I Cor* 3). Fortunately, we are "fearfully and wonderfully made" (*Ps* 139).

The unsuspecting and contentedly ignorant patient can continue to remain unencumbered by knowledge, and content with **the farce that the absence of symptoms means the problem has been solved**. Clearly "the wisdom of this world is foolishness in God's sight" (*I Cor* 3). As one example, **all cancer drugs eventually cause cancer**. I have witnessed folks who have exhausted all that medicine has to offer and were given literal days to live with wildly metastatic cancer. Then they chose real healing and many of them are alive decades later (2006 *TW*). "Has not God made foolish the wisdom of this world?"(*I Cor* 1).

In fact "God chose the weak things of the world to shame the strong."(*I Cor* 1). I've witnessed this not only in myself in curing over 20 dead-end diagnoses, but in many of you with far worse diseases. When we were down and out and thought there were no more options for us, then we learned how to heal. Many of us, myself included, had to be literally brought to our knees in order for God to get our attention. Yet, because of this, you and I have at our fingertips more knowledge about how to heal (and totally referenced from the best journals) than any hundred highly specialized physicians.

And don't be suckered in by catchall terms such as "holistic", "integrative", "functional", "alternative", "environmental" or "comprehensive" medicine. I've been to all of those courses and I've taught in them. I've seen some of the worst medical records come from practitioners "certified" with these designations. How do you know if you have a Dynamo versus a Dinosaur? **Go right ahead and test him with any of the things you have learned here. It can be done so surreptitiously** he won't even know he has been tested.

Life is a big **C**: a **challenge**, a **choice**, to **change** and learn how to take **charge** of your health. So there you have it. Are you staying with your Dinosaur doctor until he becomes extinct in another few decades? Some folks are too old or too sick to wait that long. They don't have that much time. Or are you off to find, educate and become a partner with your Dynamo doctor? In a nutshell, **dinosaur docs do drugs; while dynamo docs focus on cause and cure**. Dinosaur docs don't take the time to learn how God designed the body to heal.

And I know from consulting with many of you readers that there is often a forced choice. "My way or the highway" has been proclaimed by many physicians. They have told you that they do drug medicine, and if you don't like it you should go elsewhere. So even though you may be temporarily stranded, you have learned enough here (and **surely you will have to re-read this book several times**) to get yourself better in spite of them, or until you find your Dynamo. Clearly you have sufficient tools to learn to heal yourself. Sure, it's tough to be a pioneer, "For wide is the gate and broad is the road that leads to destruction and many enter through it. But **small is the gate and narrow the road that leads to life, and only a few find it.**" (*Mat* 7).

Is it not ironic "that the ancient serpent (snake) called the devil, or Satan, who leads the whole world astray" (*Rev* 12) is the symbol of drug-driven medicine's pagan caduceus? Clearly you cannot rely on someone else to cleanse your temple; you have to do it yourself. And when you chose a doctor as a partner, sure, you want one who goes by the book. But which book?

References:

• Strobel L, *The Case for the Creator*, Zondervan, Grand Rapids MI, 2004

• Clifford R, *Leading Lawyers' Case for the Resurrection*, Canadian Institute for Law, Theology & Public Policy, Inc., Edmonton, Alberta, Canada, 1996

• Strobel L, *The Case for Christ, A Journalist's Personal Investigation for the Evidence for Jesus,* Zondervan, Grand Rapids MI, 1998

• Strobel L, *The Case for the Real Jesus*, Student Edition, Zondervan, Grand Rapids MI, 2008

In closing, remember from the Bible how Eve was duped by the serpent into disobeying God's commands? The serpent gave bad advice.

"Now the serpent was more crafty than any of the wild animals the Lord God had made. He said to the woman, "Did God really say,' You must not eat from any tree in the garden'?" (Genesis 3: 1).

Later that day, "the Lord God said to the woman,' What is this you have done?'"

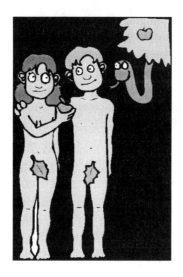

"The woman Said, The serpent deceived me, and I ate."
(Genesis 3: 13)

"The serpent deceived me"

Is it a coincidence that the caduceus symbol for organized, drug-driven pharmaceutically-focused organized medicine is a winged staff with two serpents entwined? For I humbly submit to you to consider that the serpent is *still* deceiving us.

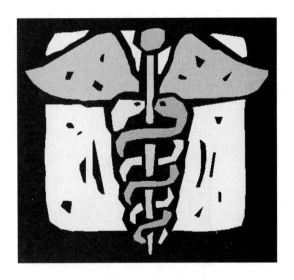

The serpent is still deceiving us.

Books and Services
By Sherry A. Rogers, M.D.

Is Your Cardiologist Killing You?

Medicine has had a free ride by drugging every symptom for long enough. The evidence is clear that drugs merely work by poisoning a pathway that makes the symptoms subside. However, in doing so you have missed a golden opportunity to actually cure the problem. So eventually the problem worsens and requires more medications.

As well, all drugs use up or deplete nutrients from the body in the work of detoxifying them. So by a second mechanism drugs also create new symptoms and diseases that seem unrelated and are often unsuspected as being caused by medications.

The exciting part is that we now know so much molecular biochemistry of the body, and how it is orchestrated to harmonize with foods and nutrients that we have enormous **power to actually cure conditions** that are currently relegated only to drug therapies. This book focuses on cardiology problems from high blood pressure, cholesterol, arrhythmias, cardiomyopathy, angina, and congestive heart failure to the first steps of what to do after a heart attack, stents, bypass, or to reverse coronary calcifications. (*TW* 2012-2013 goes even further).

It contrasts the current practice guidelines and pharmaceutical focus, as well as cardioversion and ablation, with the overwhelming evidence on how to actually cure much of this and not need drugs, devices or destruction at all. Furthermore, it details (with thorough references) the serious and often life-threatening drawbacks of the pharmaceutical approach.

353

The Cholesterol Hoax

Cholesterol is not the biggest cause of heart disease nor is it predictive of heart disease. In fact, over half the folks who die of a heart attack never had high cholesterol. But they did have other warnings that could have saved their lives, had they been checked. And the cure for these is spelled out here via safe non-prescription nutrients.

Cholesterol is merely the messenger, the smoke detector, alerting you to a curable problem. Why shoot the messenger with a drug when you can find the cause and cure once and for all?

Statin drugs prescribed for high cholesterol poison cholesterol synthesis, which then leads to Alzheimer's, impotence, tooth loss, depression, sudden heart attack, fibromyalgia, chronic fatigue, polyneuropathy, tendon ruptures, insulin resistance, amnesia, suicide, heart failure and cancers. Plus statins produce deficiencies of vitamin E, folic acid, and CoQ10, ushering in more diseases and shortening life. Fortunately, there are many non-prescription, cheaper, safer, and more effective agents to control cholesterol damage.

Juicy steaks, cheeses, and wine are not forbidden, but one bite of a more common food ingredient (recommended by dieticians) sends thousands of damaging molecules to every one of your body's trillions of cells and creates high cholesterol. As well, Teflon, plasticizers, PCBs, lead, arsenic, mercury and other unavoidable toxins that we all harbor can trigger coronary artery disease, with or without high cholesterol, as can hidden infections that stem from the teeth, the gut, or former "colds".

Since half the folks who have a heart attack never make it to the hospital in time, you will also learn here how to thwart death with your own home emergency box, plus crucial steps for those who have already survived one. Furthermore, complete with over 700 scientific references for evidence, you will learn more about the prevention and reversal of heart disease than most physicians know, because you need to. For no one can heal you, but you can learn how to heal yourself. Yes, **having high cholesterol is one of the luckiest things that ever happened** to you, because it led you to this book, which can save your life, regardless of who you are. Clearly, **even if you never had high cholesterol** you need this book to show you how to thwart the number one cause of death, cardiovascular disease.

The High Blood Pressure Hoax

Blood pressure drugs guarantee you will get worse, for they actually deplete the nutrients that cause high blood pressure, making sure you will need even more medications as your pressure goes higher and you also develop new symptoms. High blood pressure is not a deficiency of blood pressure-lowering drugs, which also shrink the brain and raise your risk of heart attack, senility, cancer and blindness. But there are dozens of ways you can permanently cure your blood pressure without drugs.

And since healthy blood vessels determine the longevity of every organ in the entire body, **you need this book even if you don't have high blood pressure, for vascular health is key to total body health and longevity.** First of all the health of every single cell of your body depends on the health of your blood vessels that supply them. For example, if you don't want to get Alzheimer's, then you need a healthy brain, but it is only as healthy as its blood supply. Likewise, if you don't want cancer (or you are trying to heal it), it starts (and spreads) in areas of poor circulation. Furthermore, obvious conditions like impotency or erectile dysfunction plus painful neuropathies and vasculites scream for blood vessel health to be restored.

The High Blood Pressure Hoax will show you that for every ailment, even one as simple as high blood pressure, there are multiple causes and multiple cures. You have a lot to choose from. In fact I would suggest you read the entire book before you chose your program. For by understanding how the various causes work, you (who know your body and medical history better than anyone else) have the optimum opportunity for choosing the best solution for you.

This is the ultimate plan for vascular health, but it doesn't stop there. **This book is also the sequel to the classic,** *Detoxify or Die*, because it takes off from where *DOD* left off, bringing you to even more powerful levels of detoxification. For **it is unprecedented in showing you how to detoxify heavy metals with non-prescription items that are safer, easier, and more efficacious than IV chelation.** Dr. Rogers can't wait to empower you! So let's get started.

Detoxify or Die

If you don't own this book, you're missing out on the most surefire and thoroughly documented way to begin to "heal the impossible" and reverse aging, regardless of how "stuck" you might feel. Environmental toxins are ubiquitous, impossible to escape. For example, the phthalates from plastic wrap of foods to Styrofoam trays and cups, plastic bottles for water, soda, juices and infant formula leach into our foods. Once inside our bodies they can create any disease and indefinitely stall the chemistry of healing. EPA studies show this pollutant is in every person and is thousands of times more plentiful than the hundreds of other environmental toxins that insidiously stockpile in the body, taking sometimes decades to produce disease seemingly overnight. Luckily there are a multitude of ways to boost your body's ability to detoxify them, starting with the *Detox Cocktail* that you can make at home every day.

Our lifetime accumulation of pesticides, volatile organic hydrocarbons, heavy metals and more contribute to every disease and symptom. The most exciting part is the proof that **getting rid of environmental toxins reverses diseases for which medicine claims there is no known cause and no known cure!** Contrast this with medicine's solution that consists of a lifetime sentencing to costly medications with a laundry list of side effects. Once you peel away the underlying causes, the body is able to heal itself and disease melts away, as scientific studies in leading medical journals from the Mayo Clinic, for example, clearly prove. **Detoxification is equally crucial for the addicted individual trying to get free from alcohol or addiction to prescription or street drugs.** This is the most thorough program for medical detoxification, including detoxification for folks with infertility and parents-to-be, showing you how to do it safely at home, avoiding the pitfalls. The Resources chapter is complete with where to find everything in this book, 1-800 numbers, addresses, web sites and more, plus over 700 complete scientific references. If you buy only one book this year, make it the classic, ***Detoxify or Die.***

Pain Free in 6 Weeks

All pain has a cause, and once you know the cause, you have the cure. We don't all just look different; we have different chemistries and different underlying causes for our pain.

Old injuries, old age, autoimmune disease, chronic degeneration and even cancer are not the *reasons* for pain. They are mere *labels and excuses* for not finding the true cause and getting rid of it. In fact, the very medications prescribed for pain actually cause deterioration of bone and cartilage, guaranteeing that hip and knee replacements will be needed in the future. And total cure from pain need not be difficult, for the solution may be as simple as eliminating an unidentified newly emerged food antigen, correcting a nutrient deficiency, healing the gut, or killing an unidentified stealth infection.

For others it has required getting rid of a lifetime's accumulation of everyday toxic chemicals. U.S. EPA studies of chemicals stored in the fat of humans showed that 100% of people harbor environmental chemicals that trigger mysterious back pain, hip pain, arthritis, osteoporosis, painful burning skin, migraines, prostatitis, fibromyalgia, sciatica, degenerating back discs, cystitis, neuropathies, tic doloreau, and even end-stage cancer. When folks get symptoms, they are told that they are a normal consequence of aging, and that there is no known cause or cure. This is totally wrong, as the over 500 scientific references prove. And it is written by a medical doctor who had rheumatoid arthritis, osteoporosis, broke her back 6 times, blew out a shoulder, knee, elbow, and more and healed with no drugs or surgery. The exciting part is that the majority of folks have total power over their pain. Sometimes it is as simple (as it is for 3 out of 4 folks) as eliminating one botanical category of food that overnight becomes an allergen attacking joints. Are you ready to reverse years of pain and become truly **pain free**?

357

No More Heartburn

The chance of healing any condition in the body is slim to none until the gut is healthy first. Heartburn, indigestion, irritable bowel, spastic colon, colitis, gall bladder disease, gas and bloating are far from benign, for they are all signs of an ailing gastro-intestinal tract. And disease and death began in the gut.

Learn how the many prescription and over-the-counter drugs guarantee that you will not only have worse gut symptoms eventually, but that you can pile on new symptoms, seemingly unrelated to the gut, within the next few years like arthritis, heart problems or cancer.

Come learn how to find the many hidden causes of symptoms like food allergies, Candida overgrowth, Helicobacter pylori, leaky gut, nutrient deficiencies, toxic environment and thoughts, and more. Then learn how to use non-prescription remedies to heal, not merely mask every symptom from mouth to rectum.

Since the gut houses over half the immune system and over half the detoxification system, a silently ailing gut holds back healing for any condition indefinitely. This book is also full of new non-prescription Candida and other yeast fighters and protocols, since this is a common unsuspected cause of many diseases.

Learn how **heartburn masked with drugs is a fast road to a heart attack or cancer**, chronic fatigue, chronic pain or fibromyalgia. Explicit, clear directions are given for every gut symptom, their causes and cures. For an unhealthy gut is a primary reason for many folks to be stuck at a standstill, unable to heal any further. **If your healing is stalled, chances are you need to start healing the gut first.** You need to heal from the inside out, for **the road to health is paved with good intestines.** (Over 350 references)

Depression Cured at Last!

Just when you think all has been accomplished, along comes one of the most important books of all. Unique in many ways, (1) it is written for the layperson and the physician, and is appropriate as a medical school textbook. In fact, it should be required reading for all physicians regardless of specialty. (2) It shows that it borders on malpractice to treat depression as a Prozac deficiency, to drug cardiology patients, or any other medical/psychiatric problems without first ruling out proven causes.

With over 700 pages and 1,000 complete references, it covers the **environmental, nutritional** and **metabolic** causes of all disease, using depression as an example. It covers leaky gut syndrome, intestinal dysbiosis, hormone deficiencies, hidden sensitivities to foods, molds, and chemicals, dysfunctional detoxification, heavy metal and pesticide poisonings, toxic xenobiotic accumulations, and much, much more.

It is the best blueprint for figuring out what is wrong and how to fix it once and for all. If no one knows what is wrong with you, you need this book. If they know, but say there is no cure, you need this book. If they say you need medications to control your symptoms indefinitely, you need this book. **Using depression as an example, it is the protocol for the environmental medicine work-up for all disease: how to systematically find the causes** that conventional medicine ignores.

It is inconceivable that there is anyone who would not benefit from this book, as it surely leaves drug-oriented medicine in the dust of the 21st century. And it does so by using the only disease that by definition sports a lack of hope. We chose this disease, depression, as a prototype; to be sure to drive home the message that **just when you least expect it, there is always hope. Every symptom has a cause and a cure**. Come learn how to find the causes of yours.

Chemical Sensitivity

This 48-page booklet is the most concise referenced booklet on chemical sensitivity. It is for the person wanting to learn about it, but who is leery of tackling a big book. It is ideal for teaching your physician or convincing your insurance company, as it is fully referenced. And it is a good reference for the veteran who wants a quick concise review.

Most people have difficulty envisioning **chemical sensitivity as a potential cause of everyday maladies.** But the fact is that a lack of knowledge of the mechanisms of chemical sensitivity can be the solo reason that holds many back from ever healing completely. **Some will never get truly well, simply because they do not comprehend the tremendous role chemical sensitivity plays.** For failure to address the role that chemical sensitivity plays in every disease has been pivotal in failure to get well. The principles of environmental controls are of especially vital importance for cancer victims.

If you are not completely well, you need to read this booklet. If you have been sentenced to a lifetime of drugs, whether it is for high blood pressure, high cholesterol, angina, arrhythmia, asthma, eczema, sinusitis, colitis, learning disabilities, chronic pain or cancer, you need this booklet. **It matters not what your label is. What matters is whether chemical sensitivity is a factor that no one has explored that is keeping you from getting well.** Most probably it is, and this is an inexpensive way to start you on the path toward drug-free wellness. Then give one to your physician and friends who need to learn about pervasive everyday chemicals and their underappreciated power to cause any disease.

Wellness Against All Odds

This revolutionary book **should be the "first read" for every cancer patient**. It contains the ultimate healing plan that people have successfully used to beat cancer when they were given 2 weeks, some even 2 days to live by esteemed medical centers. These people had exhausted all that medicine has to offer, including surgery, chemotherapy, radiation and bone marrow transplants. Some had even been macrobiotic failures. And one of the most unbelievable things is that the plan costs practically nothing to implement and most of it can be done at home with non-prescription items, even by folks new to the idea taking control of their health.

Of course, in keeping with the other works and going far beyond, this contains the mechanisms of how these principles heal and is complete with the scientific references for physicians. In fact, this program has been proven to more than quadruple cancer survival in the most hopeless forms of cancer (Gonzales, *Nutrition & Cancer*, 33(2): 117-124, 1999). Did you know, for example, that Harvard physicians have shown how vitamins actually cure some cancers, and over 50 papers in the best medical journals prove it? Likewise, did you know that there are non-prescription enzymes that dissolve cancer, arteriosclerotic plaque, and auto-antibodies like lupus and rheumatoid? Did you know that there is a simple inexpensive, but highly effective *way to detoxify the body at home to stop the toxic side effects of chemotherapy within minutes*? Did you know that this procedure *can also reduce chemical sensitivity reactions (from accidental chemical exposures)* from 4 days to 20 minutes? Did you know that there are many hidden causes for "undiagnosable" symptoms that are never looked for? Clearly it is easier and quicker to prescribe a pill than find (and fix) the cause.

The fact is that **when you get the body healthy enough, it can heal anything. You do not have to die from labelitis.** It no longer matters what your label is, from chronic Candida, fatigue, MS, or chronic pain to chemical sensitivity, an undiagnosable condition, or the worst cancer with only days to survive. If you have been told there is nothing more that can be done for you, you have the option of kicking death in the teeth and healing the impossible. Are you game? And **if you can give only one book to a friend with cancer,** start here, then progress to *The Macro Trilogy*.

361

You Are What You Ate

This book is indispensable as the primer and introduction to the macrobiotic diet. The macrobiotic diet is the specialized diet with which many have healed the impossible, including end-stage metastatic cancers. This is after medicine had given up on them and they had been given only months or weeks to live. Yes, they have rallied after surgery, chemotherapy and radiation had failed. Life was seemingly, hopelessly over, yet they kicked death in the teeth.

Understandably, this diet has also enabled many chemically sensitive universal reactors, and highly allergic and even "undiagnosable people" to heal. It has also enabled those to heal who had "wastebasket" diagnostic labels such as chronic fatigue, fibromyalgia, MS (multiple sclerosis), rheumatoid arthritis, depression, chronic infections, colitis, asthma, migraines, lupus, chronic Candidiasis, sarcoidosis, neuropathies, diabetes, high cholesterol, cardiac disease and much more.

Although there are many books on macrobiotics, this is one that takes the special needs of the allergic person and those with multiple food and chemical sensitivities as well as chronic Candidiasis into account. It provides details and case histories that the person new to macrobiotics needs before he embarks on the strict healing phase, as meticulously described in the sequel, *The Cure is in the Kitchen*.

Even people who have done the macrobiotic diet for a while, will find reasons why they have failed and tips to improve their success. When a diet such as this has allowed many to heal their cancers, any other medical condition "should be a piece of cake". It is book #1 in *The Macro Trilogy*.

The Cure is in the Kitchen

This is the next book you should read *after* **You Are What You Ate** to fully understand how to successfully implement the healing macrobiotic diet. It is the first book to ever spell out in detail what all those people ate day to day who cleared their incurable diseases like MS, rheumatoid arthritis, fibromyalgia, lupus, chronic fatigue, colitis, asthma, migraines, depression, hypertension, heart disease, angina, undiagnosable symptoms, and relentless chemical, food, Candida, and electromagnetic sensitivities, as well as terminal cancers.

Dr. Rogers flew to Boston each month to work side by side with Mr. Michio Kushi, as he counseled people at the end of their medical ropes. As their remarkable case histories will show you, nothing is hopeless. Many of these people had failed to improve with surgery, chemotherapy and radiation. Instead their metastases continued to spread. It was only when they were sent home to die within a few weeks that they turned to the diet.

Medical studies confirm that this diet has more than tripled the survival from cancers. And many are documented cures. And the beauty of this diet is that you use God-given whole foods to coax the body into the healing mode. It does not rely on prescription drugs, but allows the individual to heal himself at home.

If you cannot afford a $500 consultation, and you choose not to accept your death sentence or medication sentence, why not learn first hand what these people did and how you, too, may improve your health and heal the impossible. It is book #2 in *The Macro Trilogy*.

La Cura Se Encuentra En La Cocina
(The Cure is in the Kitchen in Spanish)

Este libro explora la relación entre dieta, medio ambiente, salud, y enfermedad y explica como la dieta macrobiótica, basada en cereales integrales, porotos y sus productos y otros alimentos naturales integrales puede prevenir enfermedades y restablecer la salud.

Nos explica cómo una dieta muy artificial contribuye a una variedad de problemas de salud y cómo ciertos aspectos de la vida moderna también nos pueden debilitar.

Un programa macrobiótico consiste de dos fases; pasar gradualmente a una dieta macrobótica o ponerse en una fase curativa estricta de carácter temporario. El objectivo de la fase curativa de esta dieta es aclarar una condición en particular. Es necesariamente, muy estricta e individualizada, y por eso razón, la persona debe consultar un doctor entrenado en la macrobiótica.

Otros libros escritos por Dra. Rogers que tienen que ver con prevenir enfermedades y restablecer la salud son **Cansancio o Intoxicación?, Eres lo que Has Comido,** y **El Síndrome de E.A.**

Macro Mellow

This book is designed for 4 types of people: (1) For the person who doesn't know a thing about macrobiotics, but just plain wants to cook and eat better to feel better, in spite of the 21st century. (2) It solves the high cholesterol and triglycerides problem without drugs, and is the preferred diet for heart disease patients. In fact, it is the only proven diet to dissolve cholesterol deposits from arterial walls (described in the *Journal of the American Medical Association*, Ornish, 1996). (3) It is the perfect transition diet for those not ready for macro, but needing to get out of the chronic illness rut. (4) It spells out how to feed the rest of the family members who hate macro, while another family member must eat stricter in order to clear "incurable" symptoms.

It shows how to convert the "grains, greens, and beans", strict macro food, into delicious "American-looking" food that the kids will eat. This helps save the cook from making double meals while one person heals. The delicious low-fat whole food meals designed by Shirley Gallinger, a veteran nurse who has worked with Dr. Rogers for over two decades, uses macro ingredients without the rest of the family even knowing. It is the first book to dovetail creative meal planning, menus, recipes and even gardening so the cook isn't driven crazy.

Most likely your kitchen contains a plethora of cookbooks. But you owe it to yourself and your family to learn how to incorporate healing whole foods, low in fat and high in phytonutrients into their diets. **Who you have planning and cooking your meals has been proven to be as important, if not more important, than who you have chosen for your doctor.** Medical research has proven time after time the power of whole food diets to heal where high tech medicines and surgery have failed. It is book #3 in *The Macro Trilogy*.

Tired or Toxic?

This is the first book that describes the mechanism, diagnosis and treatment of chemical sensitivity, in 400 pages complete with scientific references. It is written for the layman and physician alike and explains the many vitamin, mineral, essential fatty acid and amino acid analyses and treatments that help people detoxify everyday chemicals more efficiently and hence **get rid of baffling symptoms**, including chronic pain.

It is the first book written for laymen and physicians to describe xenobiotic detoxification, the process that allows all healing to occur.   You have heard of the cardiovascular system, you have heard of the respiratory system, the gastrointestinal system, and the immune system. But **most have never heard of the chemical detoxification system, which is the main determinant of whether we have chemical sensitivity, cancer, and in fact, every disease.**

This program shows you how to diagnose and treat many resistant everyday symptoms and use molecular medicine techniques. It also gives the biochemical mechanisms in easily understood form, of how Candida creates such a diversity of symptoms and how the macrobiotic diet heals "incurable" end stage metastatic cancers. It can be a great book for the physician you are trying to win over, as it shows how chemical sensitivity masquerades as common symptoms. It then explores the many causes and cures of chemical sensitivity, chronic Candidiasis, brain fog or toxic encephalopathy, and other "impossible to heal" medical labels.

Cansancio o Intoxicacion?
(Tired or Toxic? In Spanish)

El lego informado reconoce que a medida que el mundo se vuelve más tecnológico, el hombre pierde proporcionalmente más control sobre su vida. Este libro le permitirá recuperar el control de su salud, ofreciéndole mayor capacidad para formar equipo con su medico para diagnosticar y tratar su condición.

Esta información es vitalmente importante ahora ya que a todos toca con cualquier síntoma tal como la sensibilidad química, alto colesterol, fatiga crónica, complejo relacionado a Cándida, depresion, Alzheimer, hipertensión, diabetes, enfermedad cardíaca, osteoporosis y más.

Dra. Rogers se encuentra en la avanazada de la educación pública sobre los efectos del medio ambiente en el individuo.

Otros libros escritos por Dra. Rogers que tienen que ver con prevenir enfermedades y restablecer la salud son **Eres lo que Has Comido, El Síndrome de E.A.,** y **La Cura Se Encuentra En La Cocina:** La Fase Curativa Estricta de la Dieta Macrobiotica.

The E.I. Syndrome, Revised

This 635-page book is necessary for people with and without **environmental illness**, since it is the basis of all illness. It explains chemical, food, mold allergies, and Candida sensitivities, nutritional deficiencies, testing methods and how to do the various environmental controls and diagnostic diet in order to get well.

Many docs buy this by the hundreds and make them mandatory reading for patients, as it contains many pearls about getting well that are not found anywhere else. In this way it increases the fun of practicing medicine, because patients are on a higher educational level and office time is more productive for more sophisticated levels of wellness. It covers hundreds of facts that make the difference between E.I. victims versus E.I. conquerors. It **helps patients become active partners in their care and thereby get better results**, while avoiding doctor burnout. It covers the gamut of the diagnosis and treatment of environmentally induced symptoms, which masquerade as any disease.

Because the physician author was a severe universal reactor who has recovered, this book contains mountains of clues to wellness. As a result, many have written that they healed themselves of resistant illnesses of all types by reading this book. This is in spite of the fact that no consulted physicians were able to diagnose or effectively treat them. **If you are not sure what causes your symptoms**, this, Dr. Rogers' very first book, is still a necessary classic and is a great start.

Many veteran sufferers have written that they had read many books on aspects of allergy, chronic Candidiasis and chemical sensitivity and thought that they knew it all. Yet (they wrote that) what they learned in *The E.I. Syndrome, Revised* enabled them to reach that first pinnacle of wellness.

Scientific Basis for Selected Environmental Medicine Techniques

Contains the scientific evidence and references for the techniques of environmental medicine. It is designed with the patient in mind who is being denied medical payments by insurance companies that refuse to acknowledge environmental medicine.

With this guide a patient may choose to represent himself in small claims court and quote from the book justifying special allergy treatments. For example, the *Journal of the American Medical Association* states that "titration provides a useful and effective measure of patient sensitivity". Or he may need to prove to his HMO that a **U.S. Government agency stated, "an exposure history should be taken for every patient".** Failure to do so can lead to an inappropriate diagnosis and treatment.

It has sections showing medical references of how finding hidden vitamin deficiencies have, for example, enabled people to heal carpal tunnel syndrome without surgery, or heal life threatening steroid-resistant vasculitis, or stop seizures, or migraines, or learning disabilities.

This book is designed for patients who have chosen to *learn how to begin to find the causes of their illnesses, rather than merely mask their symptoms with drugs for the rest of their lives.* It is also for those who have been unfairly denied insurance coverage, or denied appropriate diagnosis by an HMO that is more concerned about profit than finding the cause of their patients' symptoms. And it is the ideal book with which to educate your PTA, attorney, insurance company, or physicians who still doubt your sanity or want to drug your child for ADD.

In this era, HMO's tell people what diseases they can have, how long they can have them, and what treatments they can have. And all diseases seem to be deficiencies of drugs, for that is how they are all treated. It is as though arthritis were an Advil deficiency. This book arms you with the ammunition to defend your right to find the causes, get rid of symptoms and drugs, and get reimbursed for it by your insurance company.

Total Wellness Newsletter

Did you miss these articles?

Did you miss the article on how to prepare for surgery? Or the one on what to do when you get home from the hospital and feel worse than ever? Or better yet, the one on, as an example, how to clean out the gall bladder rather than having it removed? Did you miss the enzymes that are needed to stop cancer metastases, or the vitamins that make cancer cells commit suicide, or the amino acid that can turn off schizophrenia or another one that stops alcohol cravings? Did you miss what minerals are needed to rejuvenate the thyroid and its receptors to turn off exhaustion, weight gain, constipation, and hair loss? Did you miss the over-the-counter (non-prescription) every day medications that are silently causing the epidemics of congestive heart failure, joint replacements, intestinal hemorrhage, Alzheimer's, and high blood pressure?

Did you properly prepare your family to be able to survive the emergency room? Did you miss the crucial nutrients that stop chemotherapy from killing the heart and other organs? Did you miss the mineral that can reverse brain fog, obesity, diabetes, chemical sensitivity or sulfite sensitivity? Did you miss the non-antibiotic treatments for H. pylori which mimics heartburn as well as coronary heart disease? Did you miss the articles on a fatty acid that increases brain cells matter and builds new synapses, actually making you smarter? Or what about the article on how one common mineral deficiency can make the prostate's PSA go back to normal or how one amino acid and mineral can correct erectile dysfunction (without provoking a heart attack like the prescription can)? Did you miss how to find the cause and cure of "undiagnosable" bizarre neurological symptoms with fabricated names? Or did you miss the **simple nutrient that can make the brain 12 years younger in 3 months**? Or how about the non-medical way folks have cured years of arthritis within weeks?

You can either empower yourself every month with new information that doesn't exist elsewhere in this form, or be unwell. **The body was designed to heal.** Only drug-oriented medicine ignores healing and prefers to label diseases as "chronic", or "having no known cause and no known cure". It is a lie. Every malady has a cause, and you can make yourself smart enough to find the cure. Your choices are clear. Either pile on symptoms and medications, or continually learn how to eliminate each disease as you reach maximum wellness.

In its nearly 25th year, this tightly referenced monthly 8-page newsletter is available in hard copy for only $54/year or $39.95/year for the electronic version. At 80¢ a week you actually cannot afford to be without it.

370

Non-Patient Phone Consultation
With Dr. Sherry A. Rogers

Many people are stuck. They have an undiagnosable condition, or they have a label but have been unable to get well. Or they have a "dead-end" label that means nothing more can be done. These people could benefit from a non-patient consultation with Dr. Rogers to explore what diagnostic and treatment options may exist that they or their health care providers are not aware of. For this reason we offer prepaid, scheduled phone consultations with the doctor. Call her office, 315-488-2856 for more information. It is a good idea to read at least three of her latest books and a couple of years of the *TW* newsletter in order to help you ask more informed questions that will save you time an money and take the consult to higher levels.

Many schedule for interpretation by Dr. Rogers of their Cardio/ION that she collates with all their other laboratory data. The molecular biochemistry of healing plus reversal of the damage created by environmental pollutants have evolved into a new medical specialty. Healing hinges on the knowledge which goes far beyond mere checking of what lies outside the "normal range" or using computer generated suggestions. Maximum benefit is achieved by having as much information about you (past, present and future) as possible all at once, not piece-meal. This includes all exams, labs, x-rays, and other procedures, environmental, dental, surgical, obstetrical, major illness, traumas, psychological, a recent photo, etc. In other words, your total package.

Make sure to include your recent medical reports from the last few years, as this promotes more precise tailoring of biochemical parameters to your individual case (and make copies for yourself as the ones you send are non-returnable).

371

PRESTIGE PUBLISHING
1-800-846-6687
www.prestigepublishing.com

Price List

Books

How To Cure Diabetes	$23.95
Is Your Cardiologist Killing You?	$19.95
The Cholesterol Hoax	$23.95
The High Blood Pressure Hoax	$19.95
Detoxify or Die	$22.95
Pain-Free In 6 Weeks	$19.95
No More Heartburn	$15.00
Depression Cured At Last!	$24.95
Chemical Sensitivity (booklet)	$ 3.95
Wellness Against All Odds	$17.95
You Are What You Ate	$12.95
The Cure Is In The Kitchen	$14.95
Macro Mellow	$12.95
Tired or Toxic?	$18.95
The E.I. Syndrome Revised	$17.95
The Scientific Basis for Environmental Medicine Techniques	$17.95

Spanish Translations

Cansancio o Intoxicacion? (Tired Or Toxic?)	$30.00
La Cura Se Encuentra En La Cocina	
(The Cure Is In the Kitchen) .	$30.00

Total Wellness Newsletter

Monthly referenced newsletter on current wellness and healing information

Current 1 year subscription (12 issues, 8 pages, referenced)	$54.00
Current 1 year subscription (via e-mail)	$39.95
Back issues/1 year (12 issues)	$36.00
Individual back issues	$ 4.00

Radio Shows

Here are a few examples of where you can often hear Dr. Rogers live and call in with your questions. Also these shows often are available on tape, CD, or archived on the net for months after a show. And you can contact them to ask for future shows and request specific topics with Dr. Rogers.

www.hwwshow.com
www.thepowerhour.com
www.healthiswealthlive.com
www.frankieboyer.com
www.ksevradio.com or www.hotzehwc.com
www.radiomartie.com

To have Dr. Rogers speak at your local hospital, church or organization, contact: orders@prestigepublishing.com

For a list of the
Scientific Papers Published by Sherry A. Rogers, M.D. and International Scientific Presentations by Sherry A. Rogers, M.D., see ICKY. (*Is Your Cardiologist Killing You?*)

Summary of Product Sources

Appendix

Sources of products mentioned in each chapter (Remember that companies get sold, owners retire or die, inventories are dropped, base ingredients become unavailable, and some companies do not sell (small quantities) to the public, etc. When you cannot find something, begin with needs.com):

Chapter 1

carlsonlabs.com call 1-800-323-4141
Acetyl-L-Carnitine, Cod Liver Oil, Arginine Powder, Niacin-Time (B3), P5P, Chelated Magnesium (glycinate), B6, E-Gems Elite, Tocotrienols, Vitamin K2, B6, Biotin, B1 (Thiamine), Super DHA, B12 Sublingual, Solar D Gems,

intensivenutrition.com 1-800-333-7414
R-Lipoic, Magnesium (as ascorbate chelate), Folixor (folic/folinic acid sublingual), ALC Powder, Glycine Powder

happybodies.com 1-800-happybodies
PC (Phosphatidyl Choline) Powder, HB-Mag

allergyresearchgroup.com 1-800-545-9960
Natural Gamma E (to replace Gamma E Gems that are no longer available).

Chapter 2

DOC (Diagnostic Outpatient Center) 1-727-896-0000 or 1-800- 890-4452
Ultrafast heart scan Orlando or St. Petersburg/Tampa

carlsonlabs.com 1-800-323-4141
Chelated Selenium, Chelated Vanadium, Chelated Zinc, Chelated Chromium, Chelated Manganese, Chelated Copper, Cod Liver Oil, D-Ribose Powder, Arginine Powder, Niacin-Time (B3), E Gems Elite, Tocotrienols, Solar D Gems, Vitamin K2, B6, B1 (Thiamine), Biotin, Super DHA, P5P, Chelated Magnesium, Acetyl L-Carnitine (ALC), B Compleet-100, D-Ribose Powder

intensivenutrition.com 1-800-333-7414
Q-ODT (CoQ10 sublingual), R-lipoic Acid, Mag C (magnesium ascorbate), Chelated Chromium, ALC Powder, Glycine Powder, Vitamin C Powder

Metametrix.com 1-800-226-4640
Cardio/ION

wakunaga.com 1-800-429-2998
Kyolic Liquid

happybodies.com 1-800-happybodies
PC Powder (phosphatidylcholine), HB-Mag

allergyresearchgroup.com 1-800-545-9960
Natural Gamma E (since Gamma E Gems is no longer available).

Chapter 3

Wakunaga.com 1-800-421-2998
Kyo-Chrome

intensivenutrition.com 1-800-333-7414
R-Lipoic Acid, Stress Guard (BCAA, branched chain amino acids), QODT (sublingual oral dissolving tablet of CoQ10), Lutein, Folixor (folic/folinic acid), Chelated Chromium, ALC Powder, Glycine Powder, Vitamin C Powder

Natural Calm: use NEEDS.com, 1-800-634-1380 or happybodies.com 1-800-happybodies (**Happy Bodies Mag**)

happybodies.com 1-800-happybodies
HP-PC (Happy Bodies Phosphatidyl Choline Powder)
Happy Bodies Mag

metametrix.com 1-800-226-4640 Cardio/ION, Phthalates, Pesticides, Volatile Solvents, Adrenal Stress Panel

allergyresearchgroup.com 1-800-545-9960
Natural Gamma E (since Gamma E Gems is no longer made)

carlsonlabs.com 1-800-323-4141
Chelated Chromium, Chelated Vanadium, Chelated Selenium, Solar D Gems, Super DHA, Super D Omega-3, Vitamin K2, Acetyl L-Carnitine, ACES with Zinc, Chelated Magnesium, E Gems Elite, Tocotrienols, Cod Liver Oil, Chelated Manganese, Moly B, Chelated Zinc, B6, P5P, D-Ribose Powder, (sublingual) B12, Arginine Powder, Super 2 Daily, Lutein with Kale, Chelated Copper

needs.com 1-800-634-1380
NOW Pure Magnesium Citrate 650mg/tsp.

Chapter 4

Naturallifestylemarket.com 1-800-752-2775
Cinnamon, all sorts of organic foods and cooking supplies
Natural Lifestyle is the most complete place I know of to fill all your culinary needs, including foods and tools, regardless of diet type and where you live.

Doctorsdata.com 1-800-323-2784
Comprehensive Stool with Purged Parasites X3

Integrativeinc.com 1-800-931-1709, use NEEDS1-800-634-1380 or needs.com
ParaGard, Grapefruit Seed Extract, Recancostat

Wakunaga.com 1-800-421-2998
Kyolic Liquid

Protherainc.com 1-888-488-2488
ABX Support (triple probiotic)

Argentyn23.com 1-888-328-8840
Argentyn 23 (homeopathic silver), Sovereign Silver

Jarrow.com 1-800-726-0886
Zinc Balance

Carlsonlabs.com 1-800-323-4141
Digestive Aid #34, NAC (N-Acetyle Cysteine)

Metametrix.com 1-800-221-4640
GI Effects (genetic stool test), Cardio/ION

indigotea.com 1-866-248-3516
Sencha organic green tea

hightechhealth.com 1-800-794-5355
Far infrared sauna, alkaline water machine

happybodies.com 1-800-427-7926
Detox Cocktail, HB-Mag, PC Powder

intensivenutrition.com 1-800-333-7414
R-Lipoic Acid, Vitamin C Powder, Q-ODT, Folixor, DHEA, ALC Powder

BOOKS:

Love, Sanae. My healing journey, by Sanae Suzuki (www.LoveEricInc.com or 1-310-450-6383)

376

Chapter 5

intensivenutrition.com 1-800-333-7414
Silboron, SeaSel, Q-ODT, R-Lipoic Acid, Folixor, Germanium 132, Lutein, Vitamin C Powder, DHEA, Chelated Chromium, ALC Powder, Glycine Powder, Vitamin C Powder, Hemp seed oil

happybodies.com 1-800-HAPPY Bodies (also carries other items)
Phosphatidyl Choline Powder, BioSil, Happy Bodies Mag, Detox Cocktail

jarrow.com 1-800-726-0886
Zinc Balance, Glucose Optimizer

druckerlabs.com 1-888-881-2345
IntraMin

integrativeinc.com 1-800-931-1709, use NEEDS.com, 1-800-634-1380
Super Milk Thistle X (silymarin)

doctorsdata.com 1-800-323-2784
Comprehensive Stool Study with Purged Parasites X3, RBC Minerals and Toxic Elements

hightechhealth.com 1-800-794-5355
far infrared sauna, alkaline spring water machine

metametrix.com 1-800-221-4640
GI Effects, Cardio/ION, Adrenal Stress Panel

carlsonlabs.com 1-800-323-4141
Cod Liver Oil Lemon-Flavored, GLA, E-Gems Elite, Gamma E-Gems, Tocotrienols, Solar D Gems 4000, Vitamin K2, Lutein with Kale, Moly B, Chelated Vanadium, Chelated Chromium, ACES with Zinc, Acetyl L-Carnitine Powder, Arginine Powder, Chelated Manganese, Nutrient Support Joint, D-Ribose Powder, B Complete-100, Niacin Time, P-5-P, Vitamin B1 (Thiamine), Lutein with Kale, Digestive Aid #34, PS-100, Glycine Powder

allergyresearchgroup.com 1-800-545-9960
Natural Gamma E (since Gamma E Gems is no longer made)

Magnesium Chloride Solution 200 mg/cc (Rx written by your doctor as follows:
Disp. 18 oz
Sig. ½ tsp b.i.d., ref 20),

then call the Windham Pharmacy (Windham, NY) to get it properly filled (518-734-3033). If you cannot get a prescription, at least use 1-2 heaping teaspoons (spread into 2-4 doses) daily of Natural Calm (NEEDS.com, 1-800-634-1380) or Happy bodies Mag (happybodies.com or 1-800-happybodies).

Nystatin Pure Powder, Paddock (for Rx use the NDC # 00574040405)

optimox.com use needs.com   1-800-634-1380
Iodoral

Captomer (DMSA), thorne.com   use needs.com, 1-800-634-1380

Detoxamin Suppository (now Rx through compounding pharmacy as 750mg EDTA in glycerin suppository)

Excellent yoga/trigger point/cranial sacral/massage therapist, Linda Lee (healthdoesmatter@comcast.net, 941-365-72270).

Books:

Rescued By My Dentist. New Solutions To a Health Crisis, Dr. Douglas L. Cook, DDS

Biblical Foundations Of Freedom, Dr. Art Mathias, Ph.D., akwellspring.com, or 1-907-563-9033

Inner Journey: Finding Happiness Within (1-585-872-0688 or ww.gockley.com/gockleyinstitute@gockley.com, or 1-877-buy-book or www.buybooksontheweb.com

Active Isolated Stretching: The Mattes Method and *Active Isolated Strengthening: The Mattes Method,* by Aaron Mattes, both available from 1-941-922-3232 or 1-941-922-1939, or 2932 Lexington St., Sarasota, FL 34231-6118 or fax one-941-927-6121 or www.stretchingUSA.com

Love, Sanae. My healing journey, by Sanae Suzuki (www.LoveEricInc.com or 1-310-450-6383)

Chapter 6

hightechhealth.com 1-800-794-5355
far infrared sauna

lumenphoton.com 1-828-863-4834
Lumen

intensivenutrition.com 1-800-333-7414
R-Lipoic Acid, DHEA 25 mg, ALC Powder, Chromium, Vitamin C Powder, Glycine Powder

econugenics.com 1-800-308-5518
Pectasol Chelation Complex

integrativeinc.com 1-800-931-1709, use NEEDS.com, 1-800-634-1380
Super Milk Thistle X (silymarin), IndolPlex, Calcium D-Glucarate

happybodies.com 1-800-HAPPY Bodies (also carries other items)
Happy Bodies Mag, Detox Cocktail

Nnaturallifestylemarket.com 1-800-752-2775
cellophane bags

metametrix.com 1-800-221-4640
ION Panel, Cardio/ION, Adrenal Stress Panel, Porphyrins, Volatile Solvents (VOHs), Pesticides, Phthalates

carlsonlabs.com 1-800-323-4141
Cod Liver Oil Lemon-Flavored, Acetyl L-Carnitine Powder, Arginine Powder, Chelated Zinc, Chelated Magnesium, Scooter Rabitt Chewables, Super DHA, Tocotrienols

Captomer (DMSA) use needs.com, 1-800-634-1380

Detoxamin Suppository (now Rx through compounding pharmacy, see above)

elfoust.com 1-800-elfoust
Auto and home air purifiers

directlabs.com (to order your own lab tests)

anylabtestnow.com (to get your blood drawn)

Chapter 7

argentyn23.com 1-888-328-8840
Argentyn 23 Professional First Aid Gel

lumenphoton.com 1-828-863-4834
Lumen

intensivenutrition.com 1-800-333-7414
DHEA 25 mg, alc Powder, Vitamin C Powder, Glycine Powder

integrativeinc.com 1-800-931-1709, use NEEDS.com, 1-800-634-1380
ParaGard, Phytosan, IndolPlex, Calcium D-Glucarate

happybodies.com 1-800-HAPPY Bodies (also carries other items)
PC Powder (Phosphatidyl Choline), Detox Cocktail, BioSil, HB-Mag

metametrix.com 1-800-221-4640
Estronex, Bone Resorption, Phthalates, Heavy metal Provocation, GI Effects
(Gastrointestinal), Cardio/ION, Adrenal Stress Panel, Porphyrins, Volatile
Solvents, Pesticides, Undercarboxylated Osteacalcin [NOTE: at this writing
MetaMetrix has been bought by Genova Labs]

carlsonlabs.com 1-800-323-4141
Cod Liver Oil Lemon-Flavored, Acetyl L-Carnitine Powder, Arginine Powder,
Chelated Zinc, K2, Nutra Support Joint, Solar D Gems 4000 mg, B12
Sublingual, Scooter Rabbit Chewables, B2 (Riboflavin), Tocotrienols

protherainc.com or 1-888-488-2488
ABX Support

hightechhealth.com 1-800-794-5355
far infrared sauna

nsc24.com or 1-888-541-3997
NSC-24 Beta Glucan Circulatory Formula

use **needs.com or 1-800-634-1380**
for strontium, NOW Magnesium Citrate Powder

Books:

Biblical Foundations Of Freedom, Dr. Art Mathias, Ph.D., akwellspring.com, or
1-907-563-9033

Inner Journey: Finding Happiness Within (1-585-872-0688 or
ww.gockley.com/gockleyinstitute@gockley.com, or 1-877-buy-book or
www.buybooksontheweb.com

stretchingUSA.com 1-941-922-3232
Active Isolated Stretching: *The Mattes Method*

INDEX

As you can see, an index is ludicrous when you are learning to heal the whole body. It would entail listing every medical condition mentioned, every nutrient, every toxin, every drug, every chemical pathway and concept. Then add all the pages on which you find each of these and you would have doubled the volume of this book. Therefore you are much better served by making notes that pertain to your own joyful discoveries.

NOTES to self: